Crohn's & Colitis
Diet Guide
SECOND EDITION

Dr. A. Hillary Steinhart, MD, MSc, FRCP(C)
Division Head, Gastroenterology, Mount Sinai Hospital
& Julie Cepo, BSc, BASc, RD

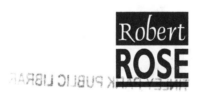

Robert
ROSE

For complete cataloging information, see page 336.

Disclaimer
This book is a general guide only and should never be a substitute for the skill, knowledge and experience of a
qualified medical professional dealing with the facts, circumstances and symptoms of a particular case. The
nutritional, medical and health information presented in this book is based on the research, training and
professional experience of the authors, and is true and complete to the best of their knowledge. However, this
book is intended only as an informative guide for those wishing to know more about health, nutrition and
medicine; it is not intended to replace or countermand the advice given by the reader's personal physician.
Because each person and situation is unique, the author and the publisher urge the reader to check with a
qualified health-care professional before using any procedure where there is a question as to its appropriateness.
A physician should be consulted before beginning any exercise program. The authors and the publisher are not
responsible for any adverse effects or consequences resulting from the use of the information in this book. It is
the responsibility of the reader to consult a physician or other qualified health-care professional regarding his or
her personal care.

This book contains references to products that may not be available everywhere. The intent of the
information provided is to be helpful; however, there is no guarantee of results associated with the information
provided. Use of brand names is for educational purposes only and does not imply endorsement. The recipes in
this book have been carefully tested by our kitchen and our tasters. To the best of our knowledge, they are safe
and nutritious for ordinary use and users. For those people with food or other allergies, or who have special
food requirements or health issues, please read the suggested contents of each recipe carefully and determine
whether or not they may create a problem for you. All recipes are used at the risk of the consumer.

We cannot be responsible for any hazards, loss or damage that may occur as a result of any recipe use. For
those with special needs, allergies, requirements or health problems, in the event of any doubt, please contact
your medical adviser prior to the use of any recipe.

Design and Production: Joseph Gisini/PageWave Graphics Inc.
Editors: Bob Hilderley, Senior Editor, Health; and Sue Sumeraj, Recipes
Proofreader: Sheila Wawanash
Indexer: Gillian Watts
Illustrations: Kveta
Cover Photography: Colin Erricson

Cover photograph: Crunchy Citrus Chicken (page 211)

The publisher gratefully acknowledges the financial support of our publishing
program by the Government of Canada through the Canada Book Fund.

Published by Robert Rose Inc.
120 Eglinton Avenue East, Suite 800, Toronto, Ontario, Canada M4P 1E2
Tel: (416) 322-6552 Fax: (416) 322-6936
www.robertrose.ca

Printed and bound in Canada

1 2 3 4 5 6 7 8 9 MI 22 21 20 19 18 17 16 15 14

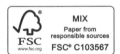

Contents

Acknowledgments

We would like to thank Mount Sinai Hospital and Robert Rose Inc. for the opportunity to develop this diet guide. A special thank you to Bob Dees, Bob Hilderley, Sue Sumeraj and the staff at Robert Rose Inc. for their expertise and professionalism. We also wish to thank Aura Bessin for completing chosen nutritional analyses and Roula Tzianetas, who volunteered her time to validate selected nutrition information.

From Hillary:
This book is intended to help all people suffering with IBD, but I would like to dedicate it, in particular, to those individuals with IBD whom I have had the privilege of being able to help during my years of practice at Mount Sinai Hospital. They have been a source of inspiration.

I would especially like to thank my family — Tracey, Zachary, Candace and Courtney — without whose support and patience I could not have seen this through to completion.

From Julie:
I dedicate this edition to Luke Joshua and Anthony Jakob with love.

Thank you to my husband, family, friends and colleagues for their support. I am humbled and inspired by the courage and strength of individuals living with IBD. I hope this book improves their relationship with food.

Introduction

Diet is a topic of high priority not only for people living with Crohn's disease and ulcerative colitis, but also for their families and friends. Perhaps you have been diagnosed with one of these inflammatory bowel diseases (IBD) and are wondering if your current diet is appropriate. Maybe your spouse or child has been diagnosed and you are unsure whether the foods you usually buy at the grocery store can still be part of your family's diet. Or maybe you've been living with IBD for a long time but are still afraid to try new foods.

Although individual food products or food types have not been proven to cause, propagate or cure Crohn's disease and ulcerative colitis, many patients, families, dietitians and physicians believe that diet has an impact on managing the painful and discomfiting symptoms of these conditions. Patients have found that certain foods or food types seem to relieve their symptoms and other types seem to aggravate their symptoms, particularly when their illness is flaring. In response to these food experiences, one of the most common requests we receive from IBD patients and their families is for a "Crohn's diet" or a "colitis diet." Unfortunately, just as there is no one cause of IBD and no one medical or surgical therapy for IBD, there is no one diet that will always improve symptoms or prevent a flare-up in all patients.

However, there is no question that dietary therapy can help manage IBD symptoms in most cases. How diet can do so is the subject of this book. We provide general guidelines regarding specific foods that might cause you problems in specific situations if you have IBD, and present recipes that will allow you to maintain proper nutritional balance within these constraints, while enjoying good taste.

Managing your own diet can provide a sense of control when you're living with an unpredictable and uncontrollable chronic disease, such as Crohn's disease and ulcerative colitis. Understanding how your food choices help contribute to your health is an extremely powerful motivation for modifying and improving your diet. To promote this understanding, we describe the normal functioning of the digestive system and the problems that may arise if you have IBD. We trust that we have provided reliable answers to most of your questions about your diet and your condition — and that you will enjoy preparing the recipes and eating a wider range of foods.

If you need further information, consult your family doctor or gastrointestinal specialist, who may refer you to a registered dietitian (RD) for specific dietary advice on managing your symptoms. Registered dietitians are nutrition experts in food science who have completed a university education, as well as a nationally accredited internship program. The title "Registered Dietitian" is protected in Canada under the Regulated Health Professionals Act, whereas the title "nutritionist" has no minimum qualifications in Canada. Similar restrictions on the use of the title "Registered Dietitian" apply in the United States.

This means that a dietitian is accountable to the public for providing reliable and safe information. Dietitians are professionals qualified to consult, assess and evaluate nutritional status and to provide advice for preventing and treating disease. Dietitians work in health care, industry, research and government. Look for these initials behind the professional's name: RD, RDN, P.Dt., Dt.P. or R.Dt.

For more medical information on IBD, consult Dr. Steinhart's authoritative book *Crohn's & Colitis: Understanding and Managing IBD*, Second Edition, published by Robert Rose Inc., which includes a list of patient resource books, medical texts and journal articles on IBD.

Part 1

Crohn's and Colitis Basics

What Is Inflammatory Bowel Disease?

Inflammatory bowel disease (IBD) is not a single disease. The term describes, in a general way, any condition that results in excessive or uncontrolled inflammation of the gastrointestinal tract, including infections of the intestine, but it refers primarily to two similar disorders: ulcerative colitis and Crohn's disease.

Excessive Inflammation

Inflammation is a natural defensive reaction in the body that occurs in response to any sort of injury, whether the injury is a life-threatening infection or something as small as a paper cut.

In a healthy person, there is normally a certain amount of inflammation present in the intestines in the form of defensive white blood cells. The amount of inflammation is closely regulated so that there is just enough immune response to protect against potentially harmful bacteria, viruses, parasites and foreign proteins, but not enough to cause pain or loss of function.

As with most things in life, too much of a good thing can be bad, and the amount of inflammation in the intestinal lining is no exception. If there is too much inflammation, or if it is not properly controlled, it can cause swelling and damage to the tissues of the gastrointestinal (GI) tract, also called the digestive system or gut. This damage can lead to problems with the normal functioning of the GI tract, functions that include absorbing nutrients and fluids, retaining and expelling stool at appropriate times and warding off infections.

When the damage is particularly severe, the internal lining of the GI tract can slough off, leading to further inflammation, which can, in turn, lead to abdominal pain, diarrhea, blood in the stools and weight loss. Children with excessive inflammation may fail to thrive or grow properly.

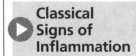

Classical Signs of Inflammation

- Pain
- Swelling
- Redness
- Loss of normal function

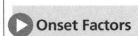

Onset Factors

Excessive or uncontrolled inflammation is central to the onset of ulcerative colitis and Crohn's disease.

Q **Does what I eat affect the amount of inflammation in my gut?**

A In someone *without* inflammatory bowel disease, the type of food eaten is not known to increase or decrease the amount of inflammation normally present in the GI tract. However, if you have Crohn's disease involving the small intestine, the elimination of one or more specific foods or food types could result in reduced inflammation. In addition, it has been shown that, for children with Crohn's disease in the small intestine, placing them on a diet consisting of only a liquid nutritional formula (known as a defined formula diet) can result in reduced inflammation and reduced symptoms. Unfortunately, this direct relationship to diet does not appear to apply in Crohn's disease involving the large intestine, nor to ulcerative colitis.

Kinds of IBD

Excessive inflammation in the gut can lead to ulcerative colitis or Crohn's disease. These inflammatory bowel diseases should not be confused with irritable bowel syndrome (IBS), which is not caused by excessive inflammation in the gastrointestinal tract.

Ulcerative Colitis

Ulcerative colitis was first fully described in the late 19th century and is sometimes called ulcerative proctitis, ulcerative proctosigmoiditis or ulcerative pancolitis. These names relate primarily to the extent of the inflammation in the colon rather than to any fundamental differences in the presumed causes of ulcerative colitis. In the first half of the 20th century, the treatment of ulcerative colitis was surgical and, unfortunately, many patients died of complications of the disease or the surgery. Since the 1940s, there has been a consistent improvement in the surgical and medical management of ulcerative colitis. Death due to complications of the disease or its treatment is now exceedingly rare.

Inflammation Site

In ulcerative colitis, the inflammation is limited to the colon, or large intestine, which includes the rectum. The rest of the gastrointestinal tract is not involved. The rectum is always diseased or inflamed, but the extent of the inflammation within the colon varies from person to person. It may also vary within an individual over the course of the illness.

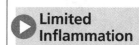
Limited Inflammation

The fact that the inflammation in ulcerative colitis is limited to the colon determines, to a large degree, the strategies used to manage the disease, including dietary therapy. Diet modifications can be especially effective at reducing symptoms in these cases.

When the inflammation extends upwards above the rectum, it usually does so in a continuous fashion. In about half of the people with ulcerative colitis, the entire colon is inflamed. In some cases, only the rectum, the lowest portion of the colon, is inflamed. This particular type of ulcerative colitis is often called proctitis or ulcerative proctitis and is probably a form of the same disorder.

Typical Symptoms

The inflammation in the inner lining of the colon typically results in blood and mucus in the stools, abdominal cramps, diarrhea, frequent trips to the toilet and an urgent need to move the bowels that often can't be delayed. Because of these symptoms, patients with ulcerative colitis often feel they have to stay close to a bathroom when their disease is active. Chronic inflammation of the intestinal lining, found in some cases of ulcerative colitis, can result in an increased risk of cancer of the colon and rectum.

Prognosis

Because the inflammation in ulcerative colitis is generally limited to the innermost lining of the colon and rectum, when the inflammation is controlled the bowel is able to heal and, in many cases, return to normal or to near normal without leaving much scarring.

Crohn's Disease

Crohn's disease probably dates back to the early 19th century, based on descriptions of similar ailments in the medical literature of that era. In 1932, Drs. Crohn, Ginzburg and Oppenheimer at Mount Sinai Hospital in New York first described the condition as a specific disease entity. The form of the disease they described focused on inflammation of the ileum, the lower part of the small intestine. They called the condition regional ileitis, with "ileitis" indicating inflammation of the ileum. Several years after Dr. Crohn and colleagues described the condition, it was given the name "Crohn's disease." In the early 1950s, doctors recognized that Crohn's disease did not necessarily affect just the ileum; other parts of the gastrointestinal tract, such as the colon, could be affected.

Inflammation Sites

In Crohn's disease, inflammation can occur in any part of the gastrointestinal tract but is seen most often in the ileum and the colon. Crohn's disease can also affect the esophagus, stomach and upper parts of the small intestine (duodenum and jejunum). The areas of the intestine affected by Crohn's disease

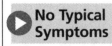
No Typical Symptoms

Because of the variation from person to person with respect to the locations within the intestinal tract affected by Crohn's disease, there is no typical patient or typical symptom.

may not be adjacent to one another. These cases are called skip lesions because the inflammation appears to skip over areas of normal bowel.

Unlike ulcerative colitis, where the inflammation is usually limited to the innermost lining of the gut, in Crohn's disease the inflammation has a tendency to penetrate from the inner lining, where inflammation and ulcers first occur, through the deeper layers of bowel to the outer surface. This results in a defect or hole in the bowel wall, which can lead to localized infections (abscesses) in the abdominal cavity or communications (fistulas) from the bowel to other organs, the abdominal wall or even the skin.

Treatment Variations

The wide variation in the sites affected by Crohn's disease can lead to important differences in how individual patients experience Crohn's disease and how they receive treatment, including the use of medications, surgery and dietary therapy.

Indeterminate Colitis

In a small proportion of individuals with inflammatory bowel disease that involves the colon, it is impossible, based upon the features, to differentiate between ulcerative colitis and Crohn's disease. In these instances, physicians usually classify the person as having indeterminate colitis. To some extent, the differentiation is not critical, since these people clearly have a form of IBD and since many of the treatments for the two conditions are the same. Differentiation becomes much more important if surgery is contemplated as a means of treatment, because the surgical approaches in ulcerative colitis and Crohn's disease can be quite different.

 Q What is the difference between IBD and IBS?

A Inflammatory bowel disease (IBD) and irritable bowel syndrome (IBS) are often confused because their names are so alike. IBS is a poorly understood condition of the gastrointestinal tract. Although IBS is characterized by chronic abdominal discomfort or pain and an alteration in the normal bowel habit, it is quite different from Crohn's disease and ulcerative colitis. In IBS, there is no clear or consistent evidence that inflammation plays a role in causing the symptoms. Inflammation is the defining characteristic of IBD, and treatment against inflammation will help control the disease and reduce its symptoms. In IBS, treatment is usually aimed at modifying the motility of the gastrointestinal tract or the transmission of the pain impulses from the intestine to the brain.

Incidence of IBD

The onset of inflammatory bowel disease may be influenced by age, gender and geography.

Age Factors

Crohn's disease and ulcerative colitis most commonly begin in young people. Although it is unusual to see these disorders in children under the age of 5, there is an increase in the occurrence of IBD up until the age of 20, with maximum incidence in the age group between 20 and 40. First onset of disease is less common among people in their 50s and 60s and quite rare in the elderly. When symptoms first occur in someone over 50, the attending doctor will usually consider other causes more likely than IBD.

 Gender Factors

IBD appears to occur in males and females at roughly the same rate, although some studies have suggested that there may be slightly higher incidence in females. If such a difference exists, it is likely to be minor and of no real significance.

Q Do the ethnic foods I eat affect my risk of getting IBD?

A Although they are thought to be more prevalent in developed countries, Crohn's disease and ulcerative colitis have been observed in every ethnic group that has been specifically studied. The incidence of IBD has generally been higher in North America and Northern European countries and lower in countries at more southerly latitudes. This has been described as a "north-south gradient." IBD is also much less common in Asia, though this may be changing. In Japan, for example, Crohn's disease was almost unheard of in the middle of the 20th century, but there appears to have been a steady increase in the incidence since then. The incidence in the Jewish population is among the highest of any ethnic or racial group. These variations provide clues to the possible contributing factors or causes and have led to a number of interesting theories, including those about the role of ethnic foods in the onset and control of IBD.

Onset of IBD

Inflammatory bowel disease usually first develops in one of three patterns: gradual onset, sudden onset, or relapsing or remitting onset.

Gradual Onset

Most often, Crohn's disease and ulcerative colitis develop very gradually, so that it takes many weeks, months or in some cases years before patients recognize the symptoms and mention them to their doctor for diagnosis.

Sudden Onset

Infrequently, though certainly not rarely, IBD develops abruptly. Symptoms may come on so suddenly that the disease seems to develop virtually overnight, with the patient going from a state of good health to a serious and severe illness without any obvious warning. Important medical management decisions, including the choice of medications and the possibility of undergoing surgery, may be required.

Relapsing or Remitting Onset

IBD may also develop in a relapsing or remitting course. Patients can present with mild episodes, or flares, that occur for days, weeks or even months at a time. During these flares, symptoms get noticeably worse, but then they seem to go away spontaneously (also called "going into remission") and the person returns to a state of normal health with no symptoms for many weeks, months or years before another episode, or flare, occurs.

Because the flares often subside on their own, patients sometimes do not go to the doctor for investigation or treatment until an episode is more severe, lasts longer than usual or is of more concern in some way.

IBD Anatomy

Inflammatory bowel disease tends to occur in specific sections of the gastrointestinal tract, which extends from the mouth to the anus.

Functions of the Gastrointestinal Tract

The gut has two vital functions critical to keeping us alive: nutrient absorption and immune protection. It allows nutrients to enter our body while keeping out harmful substances.

Nutrient Absorption

The primary job of the gut is to take in and absorb nutrients. These nutrients provide the building blocks and fuel that are needed to maintain all other bodily functions. The gut absorbs water, minerals and vitamins from the food and drinks that are ingested.

Immune Protection

At the same time that it allows or promotes absorption of nutrients, the gastrointestinal tract must also provide a barrier to prevent bacteria, viruses and parasites that may cause disease from entering the body through the gut.

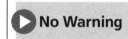

No Warning

Crohn's disease and ulcerative colitis typically develop in people who were previously in good health and who had no prior bowel symptoms or digestive problems.

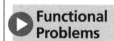

Functional Problems

The normal functioning of the gastrointestinal tract may go awry in inflammatory bowel disease, resulting in problems with nutrient absorption.

Principal Parts of the Gastrointestinal Tract

The gastrointestinal tract is a tubular structure that extends from the mouth all the way down to the anus. It has seven major components: the mouth, esophagus, stomach, small intestine, large intestine and anus.

Mouth

The mouth, teeth and tongue are involved in the ingestion of food. The teeth grind food into small particles that are more easily digested by the enzymes farther down in the intestine. The tongue assists with the chewing and swallowing of food.

Esophagus

The esophagus (or gullet) is a tube that transports food, once it is swallowed, from the mouth to the stomach. A valve at the bottom of the esophagus prevents food and stomach acid from coming back up into the esophagus, where it can cause heartburn or damage to the inner lining of the esophagus. When you vomit, this valve opens to allow acid and food to come out; when you burp, it opens to allow gas to come out.

Stomach

This saclike structure receives and holds food that has recently been eaten and slowly pushes it down into the small intestine, where most nutrient absorption occurs. The stomach lining secretes an enzyme, called pepsin, that helps with the breakdown of proteins in food. The stomach also secretes acid from its lining that helps protect against infections and assists in absorbing nutrients.

Small Intestine

The small intestine (or small bowel) is a tubular structure approximately 15 feet (5 m) long. It is divided into three segments; from top to bottom, these are the duodenum, the jejunum and the ileum. It is in the small intestine that most of the nutrients in food are absorbed into the body.

Large Intestine

The large intestine, also known as the colon, is about 3 to 4 feet (1 m) in length. Although shorter than the small intestine, it is called the large intestine because its width, or diameter, is greater than that of the small intestine. The large intestine's primary function is to absorb fluid (water) and minerals, such as sodium and potassium, from the intestinal contents into the tissues and the bloodstream. By absorbing fluid, the colon

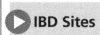

IBD Sites

The esophagus, stomach and especially the small intestine, large intestine and anus may all be affected by inflammatory bowel disease.

Principal Parts of the Gastrointestinal Tract

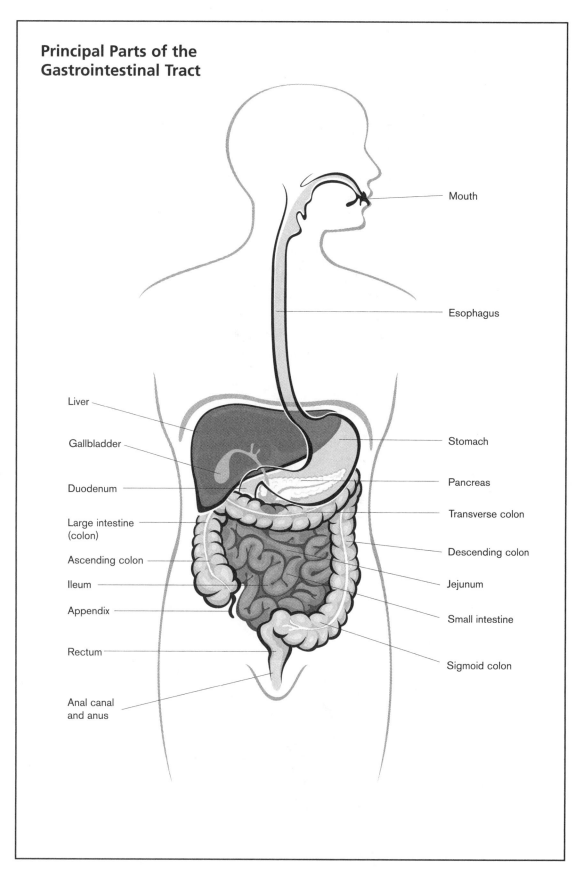

Mouth

Esophagus

Liver

Gallbladder

Duodenum

Large intestine (colon)

Ascending colon

Ileum

Appendix

Rectum

Anal canal and anus

Stomach

Pancreas

Transverse colon

Descending colon

Jejunum

Small intestine

Sigmoid colon

Small Intestine

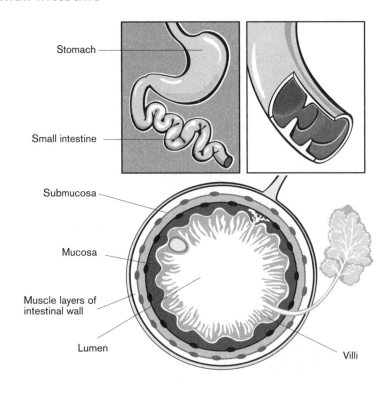

- Stomach
- Small intestine
- Submucosa
- Mucosa
- Muscle layers of intestinal wall
- Lumen
- Villi

Large Intestine

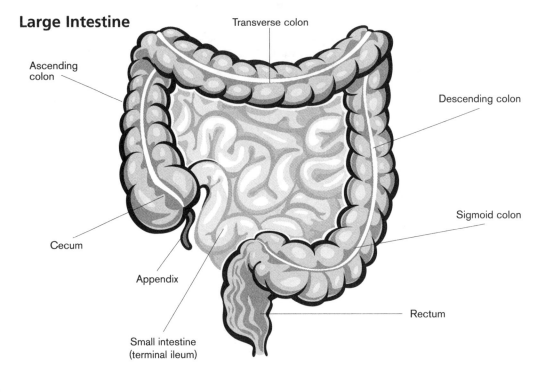

- Transverse colon
- Ascending colon
- Descending colon
- Cecum
- Sigmoid colon
- Appendix
- Rectum
- Small intestine (terminal ileum)

causes stool to be solid rather than liquid and helps the body prevent fluid loss and dehydration. It is divided into several sections: the cecum, ascending colon, transverse colon, descending colon, sigmoid colon and rectum.

Q How does IBD affect the gut's ability to absorb nutrients?

A The absorption of nutrients is dependent upon the presence of a highly specialized inner intestinal lining (or mucosa). The mucosal lining is made up of cells whose main reason for being is to absorb nutrients from the inside (or lumen) of the intestine and pass them through into the body, where they are available as building blocks or fuel for other body functions. The surface of the mucosa is folded into many tiny finger-like projections, called villi, which effectively increase the surface area and, therefore, the number of cells available for absorption of nutrients.

The surface of these cells contains enzymes that help break down food into smaller components so it can be absorbed more easily. When the intestine is inflamed, as is the case in inflammatory bowel disease, the villi may be reduced in number or size, or may be wiped out altogether so that the inner lining of the intestine appears flat. The loss of normal villi results in a reduced ability to absorb nutrients. When the inflammation is severe, the mucosal lining may be completely gone, leaving the underlying tissue exposed to the inside of the intestine.

IBD ULCERS

An area that has lost its mucosal lining is called an ulcer. When people talk about ulcers, they are usually referring to duodenal or gastric (stomach) ulcers. When ulcers occur in Crohn's disease and ulcerative colitis, they are typically seen in the last part of the small intestine (the ileum) and large intestine. They are much less common in the stomach and the first part of the small intestine (the duodenum).

Rectum

The rectum is the last part of the large intestine. The wall of the rectum can stretch, up to a certain point, to keep stool inside until there is an appropriate time to evacuate. When the rectum is inflamed or diseased in some other way, its ability to hold stool is reduced, and you may feel the need to go to the bathroom frequently and urgently. In some instances, this can result in associated loss of bowel function control, otherwise known as fecal incontinence. The need for frequent bathroom visits can be one of the most troubling symptoms of inflammatory bowel disease.

Anus

The anus (or anal canal) is the passageway that stool follows when it leaves the body. The primary role of the anus is to keep the stool in the rectum. In other words, it helps prevent fecal incontinence. Within the anal canal, two muscular sphincters (or valves) help prevent stool from coming out involuntarily.

Related Parts of the Gastrointestinal Tract

Other parts of the gastrointestinal tract are involved to a greater or lesser extent in digestion and nutrient absorption. These organs, which are typically connected to the tubular part of the gastrointestinal tract by small channels (or ducts), include the gallbladder, pancreas and liver. The gallbladder and pancreas are not usually affected by inflammatory bowel disease, but the liver may be affected in a small proportion of patients. Rarely, this can lead to liver damage and complications of liver disease.

IBD Complications

There are several serious complications that can occur as a result of inflammatory bowel disease. Some of the complications are similar in Crohn's disease and ulcerative colitis, while others are unique to one form of IBD or the other. Generally, the complications can be divided into two categories: 1) those that are a direct result of the inflammation or ulceration in the intestine; and 2) those that are not directly related to the intestinal inflammation and occur in areas of the body outside the gastrointestinal tract.

Intestinal Complications

In Crohn's disease, there are three main types of complications related to the intestinal inflammation and ulceration: strictures, abscesses and fistulas. If these complications are not properly managed, they can lead to further tissue damage, uncontrolled infection and possibly death. While these complications are often seen in Crohn's disease, they are very rare in ulcerative colitis. Chronic inflammation of the colon, from either Crohn's disease or ulcerative colitis, also appears to increase the risk of cancer of the colon and rectum.

Crohn's Disease Complications:
Strictures, Abscesses and Fistulas

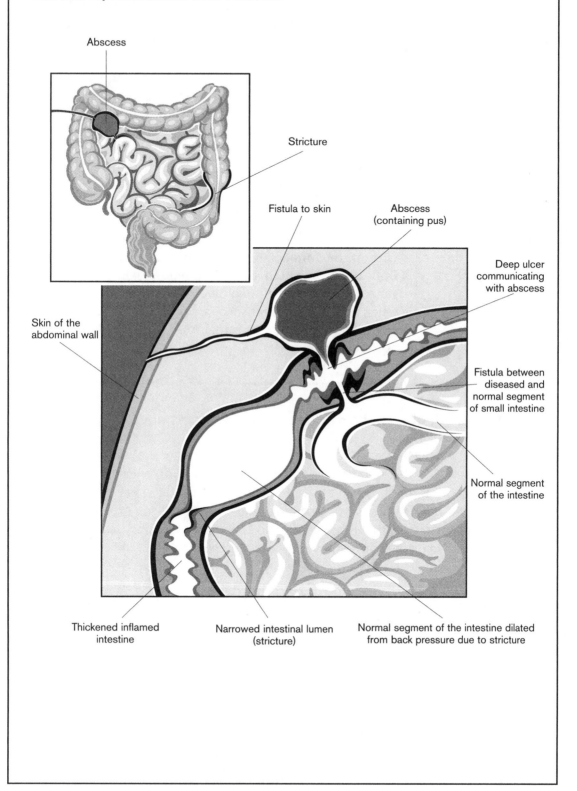

Abscess

Stricture

Fistula to skin

Abscess
(containing pus)

Deep ulcer
communicating
with abscess

Skin of the
abdominal wall

Fistula between
diseased and
normal segment
of small intestine

Normal segment
of the intestine

Thickened inflamed
intestine

Narrowed intestinal lumen
(stricture)

Normal segment of the intestine dilated
from back pressure due to stricture

Strictures

Strictures are segments of the intestine in which the normally large internal opening becomes narrowed. This can be due to swelling in the tissues of the intestinal wall as a result of active inflammation, similar to the swelling you get when you experience an injury, such as a broken bone. More often, the stricture is caused by scarring of the intestinal tissues following repeated or ongoing episodes of inflammation and healing.

Strictures are not necessarily a problem unless they cause a bowel obstruction, or blockage, when food or other material becomes caught in the stricture, preventing anything else from passing through. This produces pressure in the intestine "upstream" from the stricture, causing sharp, often crampy pain, a distended abdomen and nausea and vomiting.

Medications are not very effective at relieving obstructions, particularly when the narrowing is due to scarring. Fortunately, most obstructions caused by Crohn's disease strictures settle without the immediate need for surgery, but repeated obstructions usually mean that surgery is required. In that instance, the surgery can be scheduled electively, so that it is performed when you are well nourished, are otherwise in good health and are not taking medications that might affect healing and recovery after surgery.

Immediate Medical Attention

If symptoms of bowel obstruction are accompanied by fever or frequent vomiting, or if by 6 to 8 hours the symptoms are not starting to clear, as evidenced by reduced pain, decreased abdominal distension and resumption of normal bowel motions and passing gas, seek immediate medical attention.

Q **Are bowel obstructions related to the food I eat?**

A Not everyone with a stricture develops intestinal obstruction. Warning signs that a stricture may be worsening or leading to an obstruction include frequent or recurrent pain in the center of the abdomen after eating, along with a feeling of distension or bloating of the abdomen. If you experience a bowel obstruction that is not severe and know the symptoms, you can sometimes manage it on your own by avoiding solid food and drinking only fluids for several hours or even a few days.

If you have a stricture, avoid foods that aren't easily digested and, as a result, may get lodged in the narrowed part of the intestine.

Foods to Avoid with Strictures
- Popcorn
- Nuts
- Seeds
- Corn
- Raw vegetables (particularly stringy ones like celery)
- Skins of fruits

Not all of these symptoms are necessarily present when a bowel obstruction has occurred, particularly if it is partial or incomplete.
- Crampy severe pain, usually in the center of the abdomen
- Distension or bloating of the abdomen
- Reduced number of bowel motions
- No passing of gas
- Nausea and vomiting

Abscesses

When a deep ulcer penetrates through all the layers of the intestine, the contents of the intestine, primarily bacteria and fecal material, can leak into the abdominal cavity and tissues around the intestine. When a lot of this material leaks out suddenly, it can produce a serious and occasionally fatal infection called peritonitis.

In Crohn's disease, this leakage normally occurs very gradually, and the tissues around the intestine have a chance to react, forming a barrier against free leakage of the bacteria into the abdominal cavity. As a result, the bacteria accumulate in a localized area that is effectively walled off. The bacteria grow in the center of this walled-off region, causing a localized infection known as an abscess. An abscess typically contains pus in its center.

Fistulas

Fistulas are abnormal channels, or tracts, joining one part of the intestine to another part of the intestine or to another organ. When an area of the intestine becomes inflamed and ulcerated, the ulcer can penetrate through the full thickness of the intestine wall into an adjacent tissue. This is promoted by the fact that inflamed intestine tends to be "sticky" on its outer surface and will attach to adjacent segments of intestine, to surrounding organs or to the undersurface of the abdominal wall.

When a fistula goes from the intestine to the skin of the abdominal wall, intestinal fluid or stool comes out through the opening of the fistula on the skin. In addition to being unsightly, the intestinal fluid makes it difficult to keep the area clean and can be irritating to the surrounding skin. Fistulas can also pass from the intestines to adjacent organs, such as the bladder, which, in turn, leads to recurrent urinary infections.

Serious Bacterial Infection

When an abscess is not properly treated, it can grow in size. Eventually, the bacteria can spread into the bloodstream and throughout the body, or the abscess can burst into adjacent organs and tissues or into the abdominal cavity, causing the pus to spread throughout the abdomen. Any of these situations can be extremely serious or life-threatening.

Q **Can fistulas lead to nutritional problems?**

A When a fistula forms between two segments of intestine, there may be no obvious bad consequences, but it is possible that ingested food could bypass large segments of the intestine, which could cause decreased absorption of nutrients, leading to weight loss and malnutrition.

IBD Complications Outside the Intestine

- Joint symptoms (pain, stiffness, swelling)
- Sacroiliitis (inflammation of the lower spine or sacroiliac joints)
- Skin lesions
- Eye inflammation
- Liver disease (primary sclerosing cholangitis)

Bone Density Tests

Most IBD patients, particularly those with Crohn's disease or those treated with steroid medications, should have their bone density measured. If it is lower than normal, it should be checked periodically (every 1 to 2 years). Bone density is measured using a safe and easy test called a DEXA (dual energy x-ray absorptiometry), which does not require injections.

Perianal Fistulas

The most common type of fistula occurs in the area around the anus and can eventually open onto the skin in the area outside the anus. These fistulas, also called perianal fistulas or perineal fistulas, can be extremely distressing and, for some individuals, dominate all other manifestations of their Crohn's disease.

People with perianal fistulas can have ongoing episodes of pain around the area of the anus, along with swelling and drainage of mucus, pus, blood and stool. In women, the inflammation and fistulas can extend from the area around the anus to the area around the vagina. When they are particularly severe, the symptoms related to fistulas can interfere with everyday activities such as sitting, walking, exercising and riding a bike.

Extra-intestinal Manifestations

Both Crohn's disease and ulcerative colitis may be associated with inflammation of tissues outside the intestinal tract, specifically the joints, eyes, skin and liver. These extra-intestinal manifestations often occur when the intestinal disease is more active or symptomatic, but they can also occur when the bowels are not giving any trouble at all.

Unfortunately, there is no good way to predict who might get these particular complications, nor do we know how to prevent them from occurring. These extra-intestinal manifestations, of which joint problems (arthritis) are the most common, can occur at the time of first diagnosis of IBD or they can occur later on in the course of disease. In occasional cases, they can first occur months or even years before the bowel symptoms become apparent.

Bone Disease

Although bone disease is not, strictly speaking, considered to be an extra-intestinal manifestation of IBD, individuals with IBD are at higher risk of developing certain types of bone disease. In the past, osteomalacia and rickets — serious problems with bone formation — were seen as a result of severe vitamin D deficiency in patients with Crohn's disease. These conditions are now seldom seen, probably due to better medical and nutritional treatment for patients with IBD.

Osteoporosis

Osteoporosis involves a decrease in the density of bones, and is a result of a reduction in the amount of minerals, such as calcium, in the bones. The bones are not strong, and are susceptible to fracture with only minor trauma, or sometimes without any apparent cause. Osteoporosis does not produce any symptoms until a fracture occurs.

Age Factors

While osteoporosis is common in older individuals without IBD, and particularly in women, it seems to occur at an earlier age in patients with IBD. Inflammatory bowel disease, particularly Crohn's disease, and the associated inflammation appear to lead to reduced bone density, probably as a result of proteins or chemicals released into the bloodstream from the inflamed tissues. These proteins or chemicals, in turn, interfere with bone formation.

The treatment of low bone density in children and adolescents with IBD is somewhat different than in adults. Adolescents with IBD may not be able to reach their potential maximum bone density because of poor nutritional intake, because of the underlying IBD or because of medications. Special attention needs to be paid to adequately treating the IBD, to maintaining good nutrition and to minimizing the use of steroids during these critical years.

> ### ▶ Osteoporosis Risk
>
> People with IBD are at increased risk of developing osteoporosis, particularly if they have Crohn's disease or if they have received steroid medications. Some studies have indicated osteoporosis rates of 30% in IBD patients. Osteoporosis appears to be more common in Crohn's disease than in ulcerative colitis.

Q Does my diet affect my risk of developing osteoporosis if I have IBD?

A Poor intake or absorption of certain key nutrients, such as calcium and vitamin D, may play an important role in some patients with IBD and osteoporosis. In addition, a person's overall nutritional state, as reflected by body weight, is an important factor in determining bone density. In general, individuals who are underweight or malnourished tend to be more at risk of developing osteoporosis. For patients with IBD, maintaining an adequate intake of minerals and vitamins is an important means of preventing osteoporosis. This means not only good calcium and vitamin D intake, but also good overall nutrition, in terms of total calories and protein in the diet.

Medications and Nutrient Supplements

Medications are a major factor in the development of osteoporosis in IBD patients. In particular, steroid medications, such as prednisone, have been associated with an increased risk. Most doctors try to limit the duration of steroid treatment in their patients with IBD and, when starting someone on steroids, will often recommend calcium and vitamin D supplements or start the patient on bisphosphonate medications (such as etidronate, alendronate and risedronate), which can help prevent further bone density loss. Most other medications used to treat IBD do not affect bone density.

Cancer

Cancer is a common disease that can occur in many forms and degrees of seriousness. While people with IBD have an increased risk of cancer, this should not be a cause for undue concern. The increased risk appears to be limited to one or at most a handful of cancer types. The risk of colorectal cancer (cancer of the rectum or large intestine) appears to be most increased in individuals with IBD.

Q What is my risk of developing colorectal cancer if I have IBD?

A For many years, only individuals with ulcerative colitis were considered to have an increased risk of colorectal cancer, but this now appears to be true of cases of Crohn's disease where the large intestine is extensively affected. It has been estimated that people with ulcerative colitis have a 15% risk of developing colorectal cancer. While not everyone with IBD is at increased risk, some factors do seem to increase the risk. Patients who were diagnosed before 20 years of age, who have more than an 8-year history of IBD or who have associated primary sclerosing cholangitis are at increased risk. The risk appears to increase further the longer one has had IBD. Patients with a family history of colorectal cancer involving a parent, brother or sister are likely also at increased risk. It is not entirely known whether the severity of the IBD affects the cancer risk, but it is likely that longstanding uncontrolled inflammation increases the risk.

Causes and Contributing Factors

Logically, understanding the causes of a disease should lead to developing a "cure." However, the causes of inflammatory bowel disease have not been determined conclusively. There appear to be a number of causal factors — and a number of corresponding treatments.

What Causes IBD?

Although there have been huge strides in understanding Crohn's disease and ulcerative colitis, the precise causes of these disorders are not yet known. Genetic factors, passed on from parent to child, have been identified as increasing the risk of developing IBD, but these inherited factors are clearly not enough to cause the disorder. What we are exposed to in the environment, around us and inside us, can also play a role in the development of IBD. Environmental exposures could be to infections, to medications or to bacteria that normally reside in the intestinal tract — or to something in the diet. Alternatively, if a susceptible individual is not exposed to potentially protective factors in the environment, it could lead to a greater likelihood of developing IBD.

Although we have learned an enormous amount in the past decade about the genetic factors that contribute to the development of IBD, we know much less about the environmental factors that may initially trigger the disease or may result in exacerbations once the disease is established. Through ongoing research, it will be possible to identify the pieces of this complex puzzle and, ultimately, put them together to provide a complete picture of IBD and its causes.

 Unified Theory

Crohn's disease and ulcerative colitis likely develop in someone who has inherited a degree of susceptibility and then is exposed to something in the environment that triggers the onset or continuation of abnormal amounts of inflammation in the intestinal tract.

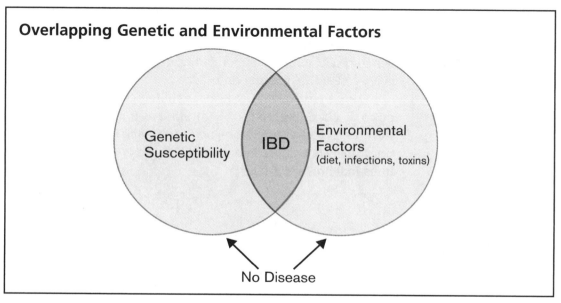

Overlapping Genetic and Environmental Factors

Genetic Susceptibility

IBD

Environmental Factors (diet, infections, toxins)

No Disease

Q **Did something I eat cause my IBD?**

A Because Crohn's disease and ulcerative colitis are disorders of the gastrointestinal tract, it would seem to make sense that your diet could cause these diseases. However, despite numerous studies, specific dietary factors have not been proven to be clear-cut causes or factors in the development of IBD in individual patients. If doctors or dietitians knew which foods, food components, food additives, food proteins, food preservatives or food contaminants contribute to the development of IBD, they would be the first to warn susceptible individuals to avoid them. However, to start avoiding foods without scientific evidence of the real cause of the disease is a risky practice because it can affect your relationship with food and eating, can leave you with limited choices and can result in serious health consequences as a result of inappropriately limited nutrients. Well-founded nutrition advice can help you achieve better health and prevent false hope without interfering with effective strategies.

Inherited (Genetic) Factors

Both Crohn's disease and ulcerative colitis tend to run in families, but this tendency is greater in Crohn's disease. Approximately 10% to 20% of individuals with IBD have another affected family member. If someone within a family has IBD, the chance of an unaffected family member developing it is as high as 10%, depending on the nature of the relationship and whether the individual has Crohn's disease or ulcerative colitis.

Although families usually have similar environmental exposures, such as living space and food, the fact that IBD tends to run in families is a strong predictor of an inherited susceptibility. This susceptibility to disease is carried within an individual's genetic code, which is present, at some point in development, in every cell of the human body.

The genetic code that leads to increased susceptibility may do so by changing a person's immune response, including how the body reacts to infection and to normal bacteria in the intestine. The genetic code may also influence the effectiveness of the intestinal lining as a barrier.

> ▶ **Susceptibility and Protection**
>
> There are several inherited susceptibility factors (genes) that, when abnormal, can increase a person's likelihood of developing IBD, and another gene that, when abnormal, can actually protect a person from developing IBD.

Q **If I have IBD, what can I do to prevent my children from developing this condition?**

A Although a family history of IBD involving a parent or a sibling is the strongest known risk factor for developing the disease, there is not much that can be done to prevent the development of the disease in a child or a sibling of a person with IBD.

This is primarily because we do not know exactly what triggers the development of IBD in a person who is at risk. We also do not know how the possible risk factors that individuals might be exposed to will interact with their genetic makeup. Some environmental factors may be protective in individuals with a certain genetic makeup, but may increase the risk of disease in other individuals with a different genetic makeup. Remember that children of a parent with IBD are much more likely *not* to develop IBD in their lifetime than they are to develop the disease. In other words, a positive genetic test or the presence of a genetic risk factor, such as a family history of IBD, does not equal the presence of IBD. Likewise, the absence of a currently known risk marker does not guarantee that IBD will not develop in the future.

Environmental Factors

Environmental factors have a significant influence on the development of IBD. We know this is true from studies of identical twins. When one twin has Crohn's disease or ulcerative colitis, it is not necessarily true that the other twin, who is genetically identical to the first, will also develop IBD. This means that, for the disease to develop, an environmental influence or exposure must interact with the genetic background that gave the individual an inherited susceptibility to IBD. Presumably, in these cases, one twin has been exposed to disease-causing environmental factors, while the other has not been exposed, has not been sufficiently exposed for long enough or has not been exposed at an opportune time in his growth and development.

Exposure to Infections

The way IBD presents in the intestines has many similarities to a number of specific infections caused by bacteria, viruses and parasites. However, these microbes typically do not produce chronic or long-lasting intestinal inflammation and have not been found in the intestines or stools of patients with IBD. The infection does not usually recur once the microbe is cleared by the immune system, unless a person is exposed to the microbe again.

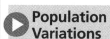
Population Variations

The prevalence of Crohn's disease and ulcerative colitis varies between countries, as well as between ethnic groups within a given country. The finding that the incidence of IBD is higher in North America and in Northern European countries and lower in countries at more southerly latitudes has spawned the theory that something we are exposed to in our day-to-day lives in a modern society contributes to the development of IBD.

Dietary Factors

Food is an environmental factor that comes into direct contact with the intestinal lining. Although no specific food or category of food has been consistently implicated as a potential triggering factor, some studies have found that a diet high in red meat or refined sugars may increase the risk of developing IBD. However, these studies have potential flaws that could have resulted in incorrect conclusions. Other studies have not identified these dietary choices as important risk factors.

INTESTINAL INFECTIONS

Well-recognized intestinal infections, caused by specific bacteria (such as *Salmonella, Campylobacter, Yersinia* and several strains of *E. coli*), by specific viruses (such as Norwalk virus and rotavirus) and by parasites (such as *Entamoeba histolytica* and *Giardia*), often produce intestinal inflammation and damage, along with the associated symptoms of abdominal pain, diarrhea and rectal bleeding, but they usually last less than a few days before they are cleared by the body's immune system.

Q **Is our Western diet a factor in the development of IBD?**

A Perhaps. In Japan, Crohn's disease was almost unheard of in the middle of the 20th century, but since then there has been a steady increase in its incidence. Similar increases have been seen in other countries. It is hard to know exactly why this is happening, but it is interesting and possibly useful to speculate. One obvious theory is a changing diet. During the time that Crohn's disease has become more common in Japan, the Japanese diet has become increasingly Westernized, with lower consumption of rice and fish and increased consumption of refined sugars and red meat. However, this is only speculation. The relationship between a change in diet and an increase in the incidence of IBD does not prove cause and effect. Many other aspects of life have also changed over this period of time in Japan and elsewhere. One could just as easily say that the increase in the prevalence of Crohn's disease is due to the introduction of color televisions or video games, something most of us would find difficult to believe.

Q **If I modify my diet, will my symptoms improve?**

A In the management of IBD, it is known that altering dietary intake may result in improvement in intestinal inflammation and symptoms of disease. This is not to say that dietary factors cause IBD, but once IBD is established, dietary modifications can improve the disease activity and symptoms. Studies have shown that, for patients with Crohn's disease of the small intestine, a liquid diet consisting of a specific and consistent source of carbohydrate, fat and protein and free of bacteria results in reduced inflammation and symptoms. Based on these findings, it seems that certain factors in the diet worsen or propagate the inflammatory reaction in the intestines of IBD patients. But it is not clear what these factors might be. Elimination diets, in which specific foods are removed from and then added back into the diet one at a time, have not identified a specific food trigger in the majority of patients.

PROTECTIVE POWER OF BREASTFEEDING

Some studies have shown that children who were breastfed as infants have a reduced risk of subsequently developing IBD. If proven to be true, this finding could mean one of two things: either there is something in breast milk that protects against IBD, or there is something in infant formula that increases an individual's chance of developing IBD later in life.

Prevention and Treatment

Can inflammatory bowel disease be prevented? Because we cannot yet predict with certainty who will suffer from IBD, and because the causes of this disease have not yet been determined conclusively, it is difficult to recommend effective prevention strategies. The best approach for now is to learn how to recognize the symptoms of the disease and bring them to the attention of your doctor for immediate diagnosis and treatment. In the next chapter, we discuss the symptoms of inflammatory bowel disease and the tests used by doctors to diagnose this condition.

What Are the Symptoms of IBD?

▶ **Flare Periods**

Crohn's disease and ulcerative colitis fluctuate in severity, and patients can experience flares and remissions. Symptoms are experienced primarily during flare periods. When the disease is in remission, patients, particularly patients with ulcerative colitis, may have no symptoms whatsoever.

Inflammatory bowel disease — and Crohn's disease in particular — can present with quite different symptoms from one person to the next, depending on many factors not always directly related to the disease, including bowel habits before developing IBD, pain tolerance, or threshold, and probably even mood. Although these individual factors may modify the symptom experience, the nature of the inflammation — its severity and location — is most important in determining the symptoms.

Crohn's disease and ulcerative colitis tend to share a number of symptoms, such as abdominal pain and diarrhea, but they can be quite different with respect to the prominence of these symptoms and their course over time. Listed below are the common symptoms of the two disorders and how they manifest.

Q Does my diet affect the seriousness of my symptoms?

A Although diet may not necessarily cause disease flares, dietary factors may influence the type of symptoms you experience. Many individuals with IBD attest to the fact that particular diets or specific foods in their diet precipitate disease flares, prevent disease flares or result in improved or worsened symptoms during a flare. In some instances, the symptoms of IBD, such as diarrhea and abdominal pain, interfere with normal eating, and the amount and types of foods eaten may need to be altered until a flare has settled down and the symptoms have improved. In most cases, once a flare has settled, individuals with IBD can resume their usual diet. During times of remission, the number and types of foods that can be eaten or tolerated without producing symptoms tend to be much greater and, in many cases, no different than for people without IBD.

Ulcerative Colitis

The symptoms of ulcerative colitis are due to inflammation, damage and ulceration of the lining of the large intestine.

Rectal Bleeding (Blood in the Stools)

The most obvious and consistent manifestation of ulcerative colitis is the presence of blood in the stools. This occurs in almost every individual with ulcerative colitis. In fact, if someone with IBD has never had blood in the stools, it is quite possible that the condition is Crohn's disease (which is not always associated with blood in the stools) rather than ulcerative colitis. Other common conditions, such as hemorrhoids, can also cause blood with stools, so not all rectal bleeding is due to ulcerative colitis. In ulcerative colitis, mucus is frequently passed along with blood.

Although this bleeding can happen with every bowel movement and can appear quite severe, it almost never results in a sudden fall in the hemoglobin (blood count); as a result, the bleeding is almost never an emergency situation. It is, however, an indication of the severity of the underlying inflammation and requires medical attention.

Rectal Urgency

Patients with rectal inflammation from ulcerative colitis experience frequent and very strong urges to move their bowels whenever there is the smallest amount of stool, blood, mucus or gas in the rectum. This urgency is often accompanied by strong lower abdominal cramping.

 Red Flags

If you experience any one or a combination of the following symptoms, consult your doctor.

- Rectal bleeding (blood in the stools)
- Rectal urgency (frequent trips to the toilet and an urgent need to move the bowels that often can't be delayed)
- Severe abdominal cramps
- Frequent diarrhea
- Weight loss

 What is the impact of rectal urgency on nutrition?

 Rectal urgency can have serious nutritional consequences if you reduce your food intake as a result. The increased bowel activity usually occurs in the early morning and soon after eating. Because of this, you may avoid going out in the morning until after the bowel movements have subsided, avoid eating before leaving the house or reduce your food intake altogether. Because bowel activity is most prominent soon after meals, many patients say their food is "going right through them." However, food intake should not be restricted. Although you have to move your bowels soon after meals, the nutrients in your diet are actually well absorbed, because the small intestine, where the vast majority of nutrient absorption takes place, is entirely normal. The frequent trips to the toilet are a reflection of inflammation of the large intestine, not of a problem with nutrient absorption.

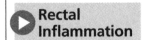

Rectal Inflammation

Inflammation of the rectum always occurs in ulcerative colitis and affects the normal ability to hold stool and gas.

When people with ulcerative colitis experience rectal urgency and are not close to a bathroom, they may not be able to control the urge long enough and may be incontinent. The fear of losing control can be the most troubling symptom for some patients with ulcerative colitis. In many cases, these individuals plan their activities so that they always have easy and quick access to a bathroom.

False Urges

False urges are another troubling symptom experienced by many patients with active ulcerative colitis. When the rectum becomes distended with gas or stool, it sends a signal to the brain indicating a need to move the bowels. When the rectum is inflamed, it becomes irritable and sends these signals to the brain with only the smallest amount of distension. In that case, the patient feels a strong urge to move the bowels and rushes to the bathroom, only to find that nothing or, at most, a small amount of blood and mucus comes out. As a result of false urges, people with ulcerative colitis may have to make countless trips to the bathroom every day, even though they may pass stool only a few times.

Constipation

Because patients pass what is recognized as stool only very infrequently, they sometimes feel as if they are constipated. When only the rectum is inflamed, the inflammation and spasm may actually block normal stool that is present in the large intestine above the rectum from getting through and being excreted.

Q **Do some foods increase bowel activity?**

A Certain foods may increase stool frequency and urgency. Fatty or greasy foods, spicy foods and foods with caffeine, such as coffee, colas and chocolate, are frequently associated with increased urgency and cramping during a flare in patients with ulcerative colitis.

Diarrhea

When the inflammation of the large intestine extends above the rectum, it can affect the normal ability of the large intestine to absorb fluid, resulting in loose or liquid stools, also known as diarrhea. The liquid stools may be mixed with variable amounts of blood and mucus.

Abdominal Pain

Abdominal pain is frequent in ulcerative colitis, but it tends to be a crampy pain experienced around the time of bowel movements. It is often associated with rectal urgency. In between these episodes, individuals with ulcerative colitis usually do not feel any pain.

Intestinal Gas

Some patients with ulcerative colitis feel that the amount of gas they produce increases or that the odor of the gas changes when they are experiencing a flare. Some even say they can tell when a flare is about to come on because of the change in the odor of the gas they produce. The amount of gas produced during a flare of colitis has never been studied, but it is likely that, even if the amount of gas produced does not increase, the inflamed rectum and large intestine are more sensitive to the presence of gas and, therefore, will pass it more frequently.

As for the changing odor of the gas, in ulcerative colitis the intestine secretes increased amounts of mucus and other protein-rich products. Bacteria metabolize these products, and some of these products have a relatively high sulfur content, thereby producing sulfur-containing gases, which can have particularly foul odors.

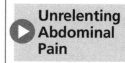

Unrelenting Abdominal Pain

If a patient with ulcerative colitis reports constant, unrelenting abdominal pain, it suggests the possibility of another diagnosis or a complication, such as bowel perforation. Be sure to consult with your doctor if your abdominal pain is unrelenting.

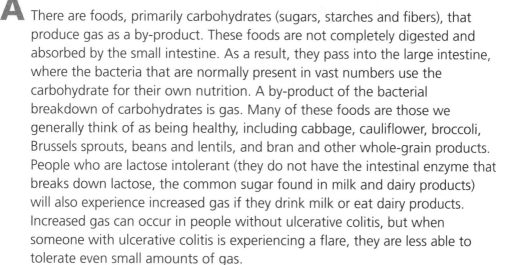

Q Do some foods cause excessive gas?

A There are foods, primarily carbohydrates (sugars, starches and fibers), that produce gas as a by-product. These foods are not completely digested and absorbed by the small intestine. As a result, they pass into the large intestine, where the bacteria that are normally present in vast numbers use the carbohydrate for their own nutrition. A by-product of the bacterial breakdown of carbohydrates is gas. Many of these foods are those we generally think of as being healthy, including cabbage, cauliflower, broccoli, Brussels sprouts, beans and lentils, and bran and other whole-grain products. People who are lactose intolerant (they do not have the intestinal enzyme that breaks down lactose, the common sugar found in milk and dairy products) will also experience increased gas if they drink milk or eat dairy products. Increased gas can occur in people without ulcerative colitis, but when someone with ulcerative colitis is experiencing a flare, they are less able to tolerate even small amounts of gas.

Fatigue and Weight Loss

When the inflammation in the colon is particularly bad, or when it involves a large portion of the colon, the patient with ulcerative colitis may suffer from fatigue and weight loss. These symptoms are most often due to the inflammation itself. Certain proteins, called cytokines, that are released from inflamed tissues can cause fatigue, loss of appetite and fever. Cytokines can also produce changes in metabolism that result in weight loss even when food intake is at a level that should be sufficient to maintain a person's nutritional state.

Fatigue can also be due to iron-deficiency anemia, which can result from chronic blood loss in the stool. When a person is anemic, blood is not able to carry oxygen to the tissues in the body as effectively, which leads to fatigue and breathlessness with minimal amounts of exertion.

Crohn's Disease

Crohn's disease can affect any part of the gastrointestinal tract. As a result, the symptoms reported by a patient with Crohn's disease can be much more varied than those reported by one with ulcerative colitis. As with ulcerative colitis, the symptoms experienced in Crohn's disease are highly dependent upon the location and severity of the inflammation within the gastrointestinal tract. Because some locations are much more commonly affected than others, some symptoms also tend to be more common than others. As a general rule, abdominal pain, diarrhea, fatigue and weight loss tend to be the most common presenting symptoms in Crohn's disease. In children, failure to grow normally, or "failure to thrive," is a common presenting symptom.

Abdominal Pain

Unlike ulcerative colitis, where the inflammation is limited to the innermost lining of the intestine, in Crohn's disease inflammation and ulcers can penetrate through all the layers of the intestinal wall. Since there are nerves that can transmit pain signals in the deeper layers of the intestine, pain may be a more consistent feature of Crohn's disease.

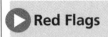

Red Flags

If you experience any one or a combination of the following symptoms, consult your doctor.

- Rectal bleeding (blood in the stools)
- Rectal urgency (frequent trips to the toilet and an urgent need to move the bowels that often can't be delayed)
- Severe abdominal cramps
- Frequent diarrhea
- Increased intestinal gas
- Weight loss
- Fistulas or abscesses around the anus or ulcers within the anal canal
- Failure to grow normally (in children)

Ulcers and Abscesses

The inflamed areas of the intestine may be tender to the touch, so that any pressure applied to the abdomen produces pain. When ulcers extend right through the intestinal wall, they can produce a reaction around the intestine, resulting in a swelling that can be felt by a physician examining the patient. Occasionally, this area can become infected by the bacteria in the intestine, which are able to penetrate through the ulcer into the area of swelling. When these abscesses occur, patients usually feel a constant pain over the affected area and may also have a fever.

Strictures and Blockages

Strictures and blockages in Crohn's disease can be experienced as a crampy abdominal pain that occurs anywhere from minutes to several hours after a meal, depending on the precise location of the narrowing. Bloating of the abdomen and, when it is particularly severe, nausea and vomiting can occur along with this pain. More complete blockages will be associated with symptoms of abdominal pain, distension, nausea and vomiting. During the episode, the person may not be able to pass any stool or gas.

Bowel Movements

As is the case in ulcerative colitis, patients with Crohn's disease may have crampy abdominal pain around the time of bowel movements. This may be due to irritability of the intestine and the associated spasm that can occur as a result of inflammation.

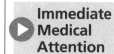

Immediate Medical Attention

Episodes of abdominal pain that last more than 4 to 6 hours without passage of gas or stool require immediate medical attention and often require hospitalization.

Diarrhea

Diarrhea is a common, but not universal, symptom of Crohn's disease. In fact, some patients with intestinal narrowing actually present with decreased bowel movements and constipation. The diarrhea that occurs in patients with Crohn's disease is usually not bloody, but when the lower part of the large intestine is inflamed, bleeding can occur.

Fatigue and Weight Loss

Fatigue is very common in patients with Crohn's disease and can be one of the most difficult symptoms to reverse completely with medical therapy. As with ulcerative colitis, fatigue and weight loss are probably caused by the release of cytokines from the inflamed intestinal tissues.

Q **Will I lose weight if I have Crohn's disease? Is this healthy?**

A Weight loss may occur in Crohn's disease because of the changes in metabolism caused by cytokines, but it can also happen when patients reduce their food intake because they experience pain after eating. In addition, patients with inflammation of the small intestine may have problems absorbing nutrients, which can lead to weight loss. This weight loss is not healthy. Depending on the part of the intestine involved, patients can develop specific nutrient deficiencies. For example, the last part of the small intestine (the terminal ileum), which is commonly affected in Crohn's disease, is also where vitamin B_{12} is absorbed. Patients with Crohn's disease of the terminal ileum may develop vitamin B_{12} deficiency even though they are eating foods that are high in this vitamin.

Anal Problems

While patients with ulcerative colitis may describe irritation of the skin around the anus and may even develop hemorrhoids (swollen veins) because of frequent bowel movements, patients with Crohn's disease are at risk of developing more serious problems: anal fissures or ulcers (painful breaks in the skin inside the anus), abscesses (painful collections of pus) and fistulas (small openings to the skin around the anus that can drain stool, pus or blood).

Extra-intestinal Symptoms

Both ulcerative colitis and Crohn's disease can present with certain associated symptoms or conditions outside of the intestine due to inflammation of other tissues — joints, eyes, skin and liver, for example. Joint manifestations (arthritis) are the most common. These extra-intestinal manifestations can occur at the time of first diagnosis of IBD, or they can occur later on in the course of disease. In occasional cases, they can first occur months or even years before the bowel symptoms become apparent. The same major extra-intestinal manifestations and symptoms can occur in both disorders.

Nutritional Assessment

A pressing concern for patients with IBD is their nutritional state. The disease may have caused them to eat less, avoid certain foods and absorb fewer nutrients from their food. Health-care professionals will assess the nutritional state of patients when IBD is detected as their first step in preparing a symptom management plan. There are several common diagnostic procedures for detecting IBD and assessing nutritional state.

Clinical Examination

The most effective, easiest and quickest way to evaluate the nutritional state of an IBD patient is to ask a few specific questions and perform a brief examination. Reduced food intake, reduced variety of foods, recent weight loss and decreased activity level can all point to malnutrition or a poor nutritional state.

People who are extremely thin or have lost a considerable amount of subcutaneous (under the skin) fat, which typically provides the normal body contours and cushions, may also be poorly nourished. These patients may also have wasting, or loss of muscle bulk, in the arms and legs that can be seen simply by looking at them. Weight and height measurements will determine if patients weigh too little for their height.

Blood Tests

Blood tests are frequently performed on patients with IBD symptoms to look for evidence of inflammation and to check for possible nutritional deficiencies that should be treated or corrected.

Albumin Test

Overall nutritional state can be assessed in a very general way by measuring certain proteins in the blood, such as with the albumin test. The albumin level in the blood tends to decrease in people who are malnourished, though it can be affected by many factors other than nutritional state.

Lymphocyte Test

The number of lymphocytes (a particular type of white blood cell that is part of the body's immune system) in the bloodstream can fall in someone who is malnourished. The lymphocyte count is easily obtained, but, like the albumin level, it can be affected by factors other than nutritional state. In addition, it falls only at a late stage in very serious instances of malnutrition, so it is not a good way to detect milder malnutrition.

Nutrient Deficiency Tests

Other blood tests can be used to detect or diagnose specific nutritional deficiencies that occur frequently in individuals with IBD. These deficiencies include iron, vitamin B_{12}, calcium and vitamin D, each of which can be tested for with relatively simple blood tests. When necessary, alterations can be made to the diet or supplements can be provided.

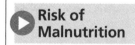

Risk of Malnutrition

Patients who experience abdominal pain after eating or diarrhea are more likely to have problems with inadequate nutrient intake or absorption and may be at greater risk of malnutrition.

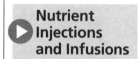

Nutrient Injections and Infusions

In some cases where a specific nutrient is not being absorbed and oral supplementation is not sufficient, other means of providing the nutrient, such as injections or intravenous infusions, may be used.

X-rays and Imaging Studies

X-rays and other imaging studies or scans provide pictures of the intestines and other internal organs without having to open up the abdomen by performing surgery. Although they are useful in diagnosing IBD and assessing the extent of the disease and possible complications, these imaging studies are not usually very helpful in evaluating nutritional status.

Q Can imaging studies help determine what diet is best for me?

A Imaging studies may be able to detect complications that could have an impact on what type of diet you can best tolerate. For example, if a barium x-ray of the small intestine (where a barium liquid is ingested or is put into the small intestine using a tube placed through the nose) or a CT or MRI scan shows a narrowing of a segment of the small intestine, you will want to avoid eating popcorn, nuts, corn or raw vegetables to prevent a bowel obstruction — or, at least, abdominal cramping and bloating — from developing.

Detecting Osteoporosis

A special type of x-ray called a dual energy x-ray absorptiometry is commonly performed to detect osteoporosis (thinning of the bones) in patients who are at risk of developing this disorder. Although it most commonly occurs in older women and men, osteoporosis can be seen in younger individuals with IBD. In some cases, it may be due to a deficiency in calcium or vitamin D intake or absorption. If not treated, osteoporosis can lead to bone fractures with little or no trauma.

Endoscopy

Endoscopy is a diagnostic procedure in which a long, narrow tube with a light and a camera chip on its tip is passed into the gastrointestinal tract. The endoscope provides detailed images of the inner lining of the gastrointestinal tract on a television monitor.

Endoscopy generally does not provide any additional information regarding a person's nutritional state, nor does it guide decisions regarding dietary management. However, it does allow the operator to perform biopsies of the lining of the small intestine, which will show whether the villi (the tiny, finger-like projections on the inner lining of the small intestine responsible for absorption of nutrients from the diet) are intact. This may provide indirect evidence that nutrient absorption is either preserved or decreased in patients with IBD, especially those with Crohn's disease, where the small intestine may be affected.

Q **Is a biopsy painful?**

A In a biopsy, small samples of the inner lining of the gastrointestinal tract are taken using a tiny instrument with small jaws that can cut or pull off pieces of the inner lining. This procedure is not painful, and the patient is not usually aware it is happening. The biopsy process is very safe, and complications, such as serious bleeding, are extremely uncommon.

Gastroscopy and Colonoscopy

When the endoscope is swallowed and the procedure examines the esophagus, stomach and duodenum, it is called an upper gastrointestinal endoscopy, or, more commonly, gastroscopy. When the instrument is inserted through the anus into the rectum and colon, it is called a colonoscopy. When doing a colonoscopy, the physician can often also examine the ileum (the last part of the small intestine), one of the areas most commonly involved in Crohn's disease.

DIAGNOSTIC EFFECTIVENESS

Colonoscopy is an extremely useful diagnostic test in IBD. It will always detect ulcerative colitis if it is present and will detect Crohn's disease in 80% to 90% of cases. In 10% to 20% of cases of Crohn's disease, the procedure is not able to examine the areas of disease because of technical factors or because the disease is beyond the reach of the colonoscope.

Q **What must I do to prepare for an endoscopy?**

A Gastroscopy requires no special preparation other than an overnight fast. Colonoscopy requires preparation of the bowel with a special diet (usually clear liquids) for 1 or more days before the procedure and a special laxative for 1 or 2 days before the procedure. This preparation is important because the presence of feces can interfere with visibility and make the procedure almost useless. In some cases, usually when the IBD is very active, the physician does not order a special laxative for the patient. However, even in these instances, a more gentle means of cleaning out the colon is probably still advisable and safe.

Wireless Capsule Endoscopy

Standard gastroscopy and colonoscopy are not able to reach large segments of the small intestine that may be affected in Crohn's disease. Wireless capsule endoscopy (WCE), also known as a PillCam, uses a capsule about the size of a large medication pill that contains a battery, a light source and a tiny lens and camera chip. The capsule is swallowed by the patient. Once ingested, it begins taking two pictures every second for 8 hours. The physician can then examine the images to look for signs of Crohn's disease. Care must be taken, because if a narrowing, or stricture, of the intestine exists, the capsule could cause a bowel obstruction.

Management Strategies

Once the diagnosis of IBD has been confirmed using one or more of the available diagnostic tools, the information gained during the tests can help the physician determine a patient's prognosis and develop a plan to manage the symptoms. The prognosis and recommended therapies can vary from person to person with the same disorder, but the primary IBD management strategies are drug therapy, surgery and dietary therapy.

▶ Detecting Impaired Absorption

The PillCam may be helpful in detecting or diagnosing subtle degrees of Crohn's disease in the small intestine when other imaging techniques have not provided a full answer to the patient's symptoms. Subtle degrees of Crohn's disease throughout the small intestine may be sufficient to impair absorption and, therefore, the patient's nutritional state.

Part 2

Managing Inflammatory Bowel Disease

Drug Therapies

Medications are commonly prescribed to manage the symptoms of IBD, and in most cases they are effective, especially in managing acute cases and flares. However, there is no standard drug treatment for IBD that is effective in all situations for all patients.

IBD is a chronic, lifelong disorder. Although some medications may be effective at controlling inflammation and symptoms for a short period of time — days or weeks — what is really needed are medications that can safely and effectively ensure that, once a disease flare is under control, the IBD patient will be less likely to experience further flares.

Medication Considerations

Making the decision to use drug therapy for IBD, and choosing what medication to take at what dose and for how long, can be very complicated. Every patient and every situation is somewhat different.

Tailored Therapy

Decisions about medical therapy need to be tailored for each person to meet the nature of the disease while taking into account personal circumstances. This typically involves consideration of the chance of improvement with therapy and the possible side effects or risks of therapy. For people in countries, states or provinces where medication is not paid for through private or public health insurance plans, the cost of the medication may also be a consideration in making treatment decisions.

Risk Tolerance

Doctor and patient should assess the risks of drug therapy, not only the common and usually less serious side effects, but also the more rare and more serious potential side effects. Patients vary widely with respect to what side effects they are willing to risk or able to tolerate. They may also have different preferences

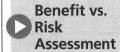

Benefit vs. Risk Assessment

Some people with IBD are not willing to risk experiencing certain rare but serious side effects associated with a given medication, even knowing that they will likely respond positively to it. Others are willing to accept a relatively high risk of side effects for the sake of receiving the most effective treatment. The final decision requires, under ideal conditions, a full discussion between the doctor and the patient — and, where necessary, the family — of all the variables involved in the medical treatment of IBD.

about how the drug is administered, whether through pills, liquid suspensions, injections under the skin, infusions into a vein, suppositories or enemas. As a result, what might be the best treatment for one patient might not be the best treatment for another with the same disease severity, location and complications.

Q **What are side effects?**

A A side effect is an unintended effect of a medication or therapy. Side effects can generally be divided into two categories: those that occur more often the higher the drug dose, and those that are unpredictable and can occur at any dose. A side effect in the first category may not occur in the majority of patients treated with the medication in the usual dose range, but becomes more common at higher doses. These side effects can sometimes be handled by reducing the dose of the drug. Side effects in the second category do not seem to occur more frequently at higher doses. These side effects appear to be similar to an allergic reaction. In most cases, use of the drug must be suspended, because the reaction may occur even at low doses.

QUESTIONS TO ASK YOUR DOCTOR ABOUT DRUG THERAPY

- Is drug treatment of my IBD necessary?
- Is the treatment intended to bring a flare under control, or is it intended to maintain a remission (that is, to prevent flares)?
- What benefits can I expect from this treatment? What symptoms will improve and what symptoms are not likely to improve?
- How quickly can I expect to see an improvement?
- What are some of the common side effects?
- What are the serious side effects that can occur on this therapy?
- Are there any other options for drug therapy in my situation?
- What is the cost of treatment?
- How long will I have to be on drug therapy?

Drug Therapy Options

In general, recommendations for drug treatment of IBD are divided into four broad categories. These categories are determined by two considerations: whether Crohn's disease or ulcerative colitis is being treated; and, within each disease, whether the aim is to bring a flare or symptoms of active disease under control or to keep a patient well once a remission has been obtained through whatever means necessary. In some instances, recommendations may be further subdivided according to the location of the disease within the gastrointestinal tract and the severity of a flare. Certain complications of the diseases, such as abscesses in Crohn's disease, may place a patient in yet another subcategory of treatment options. These categories are important because certain medications appear to be effective only in very specific situations.

PAIN RELIEF OPTIONS

NSAIDs
Non-steroidal anti-inflammatory drugs (NSAIDs) are commonly used to relieve pain and inflammation in various forms of arthritis. However, NSAIDs may result in disease flares in some people with IBD. These drugs include those with the generic names diclofenac, sulindac, naproxen and ibuprofen, to name a few. Although not every patient with IBD will run into problems when taking these drugs, some find that they produce increased abdominal pain, diarrhea and rectal bleeding. Be certain that the indication for use and the treatment goals are clear so that therapy does not go on any longer than necessary.

Acetaminophen
For relatively minor aches and pains, such as headaches, acetaminophen (Tylenol) is often effective and is perfectly safe to take if you have IBD. If your pain is more severe and you don't need an anti-inflammatory, acetaminophen with codeine (such as Tylenol #2 or Tylenol #3) will provide pain relief without risk.

Narcotics
Chronic use of codeine and other narcotic medications, such as oxycodone (a component of Percocet) or meperidine (Demerol), can lead to addiction. Narcotics should be used only for episodes of acute pain (for example, after surgery), with a definite endpoint for completing therapy.

Pain Clinics
When someone with IBD has chronic pain that is not manageable through treatment of the underlying IBD or through simple non-specific measures, such as acetaminophen, referral to a chronic pain clinic may be indicated.

COMMONLY USED IBD MEDICATIONS

Each drug or category of drugs may be used for different indications within IBD. For example, antibiotics are not typically used in ulcerative colitis because they don't appear to be effective. In patients with Crohn's disease, however, antibiotics are often used to reduce pain, improve drainage and reduce the risk of widespread infection when a complication, such as an abscess or fistula, has developed.

Mesalamine-Containing Drugs
- Delayed-release mesalamine (Asacol, Pentasa, Salofalk, Lialda, Mezavant)
- Sulfasalazine (Salazopyrin, Azulfidine)
- Balsalazide
- Olsalazine (Dipentum)

Glucocorticoids (Steroid Medications)
- Prednisone
- Budesonide (Entocort)
- Prednisolone
- Hydrocortisone
- Betamethasone (Betnesol)
- Methyl-prednisolone (Solumedrol)

Antibiotics
- Metronidazole (Flagyl)
- Ciprofloxacin (Cipro)

Immunosuppressant Medications
- Azathioprine (Imuran)
- 6-Mercaptopurine (Purinethol)
- Methotrexate
- Cyclosporine

Biologic Drugs
- Infliximab (Remicade)
- Adalimumab (Humira)
- Certolizumab (Cimzia)
- Golimumab (Simponi)

Mesalamine-Containing Drugs

Mesalamine (also known as 5-aminosalicylic acid, or 5-ASA) has a chemical structure very similar to aspirin, but its medicinal properties are somewhat different. Unlike aspirin, 5-ASA is not a pain reliever, but it does appear to have anti-inflammatory actions similar to aspirin, although these actions appear to be fairly specific to the intestinal tract. When a physician prescribes medications containing 5-ASA, the aim is to combat inflammation in the intestinal tract.

Delayed-Release Mesalamine

Taken as a pill or a powder, 5-ASA is very quickly absorbed from the upper part of the small intestine, where it enters the bloodstream. However, for this drug to be effective, it needs to be in contact with the inner lining of the intestine. It does not work if it is in the bloodstream. Mesalamine-containing drugs used in IBD therapy are designed to prevent the drug from being absorbed before it gets down to the parts of the intestine most commonly affected by IBD. Some preparations are coated in a waxy film that dissolves and releases the drug when the acid within the intestine becomes sufficiently neutralized.

Sulfasalazine

Sulfasalazine is composed of two parts — a sulfa antibiotic and 5-ASA — that are connected by a chemical bond. This bond is split by the action of an enzyme produced by the bacteria in the large intestine and the last part of the small intestine. When the bond is split, the sulfa and the 5-ASA are released into the bowel, where the 5-ASA can act on the inner lining of the intestine. The beneficial action of sulfasalazine in IBD is primarily due to the 5-ASA part of the drug, although the intact drug may also contribute to reducing inflammation.

Q I've heard that sulfa drugs can cause stomach upset. Is that true?

A In a small but significant proportion of patients, sulfasalazine has been found to have a number of troubling side effects, most commonly stomach upset, often with nausea and vomiting, especially when higher doses are used. Unfortunately, higher doses appear to be more effective than the lower doses that cause fewer problems with stomach upset.

Balsalazide

Balsalazide (Colazide) is similar to sulfasalazine in that it contains 5-ASA chemically bonded to another molecule to prevent the drug from being absorbed in the small intestine. When it reaches the large intestine, bacteria split the 5-ASA from the carrier molecule, thereby allowing the 5-ASA to act on the inner intestinal lining.

Olsalazine

Olsalazine (Dipentum) is composed of two 5-ASA molecules chemically bonded to each other. The bonded molecules cannot be effectively absorbed in the small intestine, but are split apart by the bacteria in the large intestine.

Q **Does my diet affect the action of 5-ASA-containing medications?**

A In theory, the consistent and optimal release of 5-ASA is dependent upon a number of factors that might be influenced by what you eat, when you eat it and how much you eat, because these factors could affect how quickly the medication passes through the intestine, as well as the acidity (pH) inside the intestine. For most individuals, however, the effectiveness of 5-ASA-containing medications does not appear to be dependent on what they eat or the timing of the intake of the medication relative to the intake of food.

Glucocorticoids (Steroid Medications)

Steroids have been used for decades to treat inflammatory bowel disease and, until recently, have been the most consistently effective class of medications. They generally work very quickly and can be used in a wide variety of forms of IBD. There are a number of steroids available on the market, and although they have slightly different chemical forms, they all (with the exception of budesonide) have similar actions in IBD.

Oral Steroids (Prednisone)

The oral steroid most commonly prescribed in North America is prednisone. When taken in oral form, steroids can usually be taken once a day, typically in the morning. They do not have to be taken with meals, but doing so may reduce the potential for indigestion, which some patients experience when taking higher doses of oral steroids.

Steroids are usually taken in courses of treatment lasting from 2 to 4 months. Patients who require steroid treatment for an acute flare of IBD are usually started on a relatively high dose of prednisone — 40 to 60 milligrams per day — and the dose is gradually reduced over a period of 2 to 4 months. Prednisone and other steroids cannot be stopped suddenly once they have been used for more than 10 to 14 days, because the patient becomes steroid-dependent during this time period and could become very ill or even go into shock if the medication is suddenly withdrawn.

 Anabolic Steroids

Steroid medications used to treat IBD should not be confused with anabolic steroids, used to enhance performance in athletes or body builders. In fact, the steroids used to treat IBD have the opposite effect of anabolic steroids on many aspects of the body's metabolism. For example, while anabolic steroids increase muscle bulk and strength, prednisone, if taken for long periods, can cause a loss of muscle bulk and strength.

Side Effects of Prednisone

Steroids have the potential to cause a number of side effects, some of which can be very troubling and, in some cases, irreversible. Approximately half of patients who take steroids experience at least one side effect, although most often the side effect is not serious or irreversible.

Appearance

The most common side effects of prednisone affect a person's appearance, including increased appetite and weight gain, swelling of the feet and hands, rounding of the face ("moon face"), acne and easy bruising. Fortunately, these side effects tend to go away as a person reduces the dose of prednisone and is able to discontinue it.

Q What can I do to prevent weight gain as a side effect of prednisone?

A Limiting food intake can be a challenge, because steroids, especially at high doses, can cause a large increase in your appetite. For some people with IBD, this is a welcome change from the loss of appetite they may experience during a flare of the disease, but the increase in appetite can be so great that it can make you feel as if you are hungry all the time and can result in a large amount of weight gain and increases in blood sugar levels. Here are a few suggestions for managing your appetite and weight.

- If you are on relatively high doses of prednisone, make sure the total amount of calories you consume is not more than what your body needs based on your gender, age, height, weight and activity level.
- Limit the simple sugars and starches in your diet to no more than 50% of total calories ingested.
- Snack on foods that have very few or no calories, rather than foods with high caloric density. Examples of high-calorie foods are candy bars, potato chips, french fries and most other "junk foods." Foods that have very few calories and do not tend to increase blood sugar include lettuce and celery. Be cautious, because these foods may contribute to a bowel obstruction if you have intestinal strictures (usually in Crohn's disease). In addition, some vegetables, such as carrots, may also have extra sugar, which can be a problem for people trying to control blood sugar. Check with your doctor before modifying your diet to include these types of vegetables.
- Be aware that foods labeled "low-fat" are not necessarily better. In fact, in some cases they may be worse. Certain "low-fat" foods have increased amounts of sugar or other carbohydrates in place of fat and may have just as many calories as a comparable full-fat food.

The weight gain often seen with prednisone treatment may seem like a positive effect for patients with IBD, who often have problems with weight loss. However, this weight gain is not healthy. Most of the weight gained on steroids tends to be due to an increase in fatty tissue rather than an increase in muscle or lean body mass. It may take quite some time — usually many months — to get rid of the increased body fat once the patient stops taking steroids.

Blood Sugar Levels

Steroids have a tendency to increase blood sugar levels. For people who already have diabetes, steroids can adversely affect blood sugar control. In people who develop high blood sugar while on steroids, the levels usually return to normal once steroid use has been discontinued, but developing high blood sugar while on steroids may indicate a predisposition to the development of type 2 (non-insulin-dependent) diabetes later in life. It is not routine to check blood sugar levels in all people who are on steroids. Symptoms that might suggest a problem are excessive thirst and urination, blurred vision and, in more extreme cases, drowsiness or stupor.

Bone Density

Steroids can cause a loss of bone density (osteoporosis). This is partly due to a direct effect of the steroid on the metabolism of

> ### ▶ Metabolism Changes
>
> Steroids can produce changes in the metabolism of carbohydrates and lipids and can alter the way the body handles water and electrolytes, such as sodium. Some of these changes can be counterbalanced by increasing dietary intake of certain minerals or vitamins, especially calcium, potassium and vitamin D.

STEROID SIDE EFFECTS

Common and Reversible
- Rounding of the face (moon face)
- Acne
- Easy bruising and poor wound healing
- Increased appetite
- Weight gain
- Fluid retention
- Insomnia and sleep disturbance
- Mood swings
- Increased energy

Uncommon and Possibly Irreversible
- High blood pressure
- High blood sugar
- Cataracts
- Osteoporosis
- Avascular necrosis of the hip or other joints

bone, but steroids also appear to interfere with the absorption of calcium from the food we eat and with the normal metabolism of vitamin D. Both calcium and vitamin D are important in maintaining healthy, strong bones. If you are taking steroids, be sure you are getting a sufficient amount of calcium and vitamin D in your diet. Dairy products are the main source of calcium for most people; if you, like many IBD patients, avoid dairy products, supplementation is very important.

Budesonide

Unlike other oral steroids, budesonide is very quickly broken down into a by-product that has no side effects once it is absorbed into the bloodstream. The form of budesonide (Entocort) used in IBD is encased in a special coating designed to release the drug in the last part of the small intestine (the ileum) and the first part of the colon (the ascending colon), the areas most often affected in Crohn's disease. Budesonide has also been formulated in a controlled-release preparation or coating that is effective in ulcerative colitis. In many countries, including Canada, budesonide is available as an enema for the treatment of ulcerative colitis affecting the rectum and lower part of the colon.

Antibiotics

Although the effectiveness of antibiotics in IBD is not proven or accepted by all doctors, most do believe that, for selected individuals with Crohn's disease, antibiotics can reduce pain, improve drainage and reduce the risk of widespread infection when an abscess or fistula has developed. They are not believed to be helpful for patients with ulcerative colitis. Antibiotics are not usually used for long-term maintenance treatment, but some patients have recurrent symptoms when antibiotics are

Q Will antibiotics improve my gas symptoms?

A Some people note that they produce or pass significantly less gas when they are on antibiotics. This can reduce their abdominal discomfort and can certainly reduce social embarrassment. Antibiotics probably reduce gas by changing or reducing the number of bacteria in the intestine, since it is these bacteria that produce gas. When you are on antibiotics, you may be able to eat many foods that would otherwise have caused you to experience abdominal bloating and gas.

stopped and seem to improve if they are kept on regular, some-times relatively low, doses of antibiotics.

The antibiotics most commonly used in IBD are metronida-zole (Flagyl) and ciprofloxacin. Metronidazole can produce side effects of nausea, vomiting and an unusual metallic taste in the mouth. In addition, if you drink alcohol while taking metron-idazole, you might feel quite ill and experience a reaction that may include weakness, sweating and flushing.

Immunosuppressant Medications

Immunosuppressant medications cause some suppression of the body's immune response, which may be beneficial in IBD because the disease involves overactivity or overresponse of the body's immune system to something in the body or in the sur-rounding environment. The immunosuppressant medications used most commonly to treat IBD are azathioprine, 6-mercap-topurine, methotrexate and cyclosporine. In general, the absorption, activity and potential side effects of these drugs are not affected by diet, with a few exceptions.

Methotrexate and Folic Acid

Methotrexate is taken once weekly and is usually well tolerated, although some people experience nausea and sometimes vom-iting, most often on the day of the week when the methotrexate is taken. This side effect can usually be avoided or reduced by taking the drug in the evening before bed. Taking a folic acid supplement on the day that methotrexate is taken is also advised, as methotrexate is known to interfere with the normal metabolism of folic acid.

Biologic Drugs

Biologics, or "designer drugs," are developed in the lab and are introduced to patients in a way that is different from traditional therapies. These drugs are designed to block specific molecules or receptors on cells that are important in promoting intestinal inflammation or to activate other molecules or receptors that are key players in reducing intestinal inflammation. They have the potential to provide closely targeted treatment. The hope is that, by providing targeted treatment, the overall number of side effects will be reduced when compared to traditional therapies.

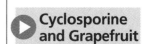
Cyclosporine and Grapefruit

Certain foods, primarily grapefruit, pomelo (a precursor to grapefruit) and tangelo (a cross between grapefruit, orange and tangerine) can increase the absorption and decrease the elimination of the oral form of cyclosporine (Neoral). Because of grapefruit's potent effects on cyclosporine absorption and elimination, it is usually recommended that individuals on cyclosporine not eat grapefruit or drink grapefruit juice.

Infliximab

Infliximab (Remicade) is an antibody that specifically attaches to and inactivates a protein called tumor necrosis factor alpha, or TNF-alpha. TNF-alpha is critical in causing inflammation; blocking its action results in improvement in intestinal inflammation and improved symptoms of IBD. Because the infliximab antibody is itself a protein, it cannot be taken orally, because it would be broken down and made inactive by the digestive enzymes in the stomach and small intestine. Instead, it is given as an intravenous infusion. Diet and dietary factors are not known to interfere with the absorption, activity or metabolism of infliximab.

Adalimumab

Another TNF-alpha blocker, adalimumab (Humira) is also an antibody, but unlike infliximab, which is given by intravenous infusion, adalimumab is given as a subcutaneous (under the skin) injection once every 1 to 2 weeks.

Certolizumab

Certolizumab (Cimzia) is a drug that was also designed to block the effect of TNF-alpha. It consists of a portion of an antibody directed against TNF-alpha and is given by subcutaneous injections every 2 to 4 weeks. Unfortunately, it appears that this drug may not be as effective as the other anti-TNF-alpha drugs and has not been approved for use in IBD in all countries.

Golimumab

Golimumab (Simponi) is another anti-TNF-alpha drug that, like adalimumab, is an antibody that is given by subcutaneous injection. However, it is usually given every 2 weeks at first and then every 4 weeks. Golimumab has not been tested in Crohn's disease.

Other IBD Management Strategies

Although many patients, families and physicians focus on medications as the primary means of treating IBD, drug therapy is just one aspect of patient care. Surgery and dietary therapies must also be considered as important strategies for the management of IBD.

Surgical Therapies

The need for surgery should not be considered a failure of the person with IBD or the health-care team. While recent advances in drug therapy may reduce the need for surgery in the future, surgery can provide patients in some situations with symptom relief that may not be possible using medications or dietary therapy.

Q What is the likelihood that I will need to have surgery?

A Approximately 70% to 80% of people suffering from Crohn's disease and about 40% of those suffering from ulcerative colitis will require surgery at some point after their diagnosis. These estimates are based on information from previous decades and do not necessarily reflect the effect of recent advances in drug therapy. Nevertheless, a significant proportion of IBD sufferers will need surgery to treat their disease.

Individualized Surgery

There is no "standard surgery" for IBD; rather, there are a small number of operations that cover most situations. The exact nature of the surgery needs to be individualized in the same way that drug therapy must be individualized, based on a patient's particular circumstances and the objectives of surgery.

Unlike drug therapy, where there is a large amount of overlap in terms of what is effective in Crohn's disease and what is effective in ulcerative colitis, the operations that can be or should be performed are often quite different for each condition. As a result, it is extremely important for the health-care team to distinguish between ulcerative colitis and Crohn's disease before embarking on most types of surgery.

Ostomy (Stoma)

One of the main concerns you may have if you are faced with the possibility of surgery for IBD is that you will end up needing to "wear a bag" on your abdomen to collect your stools. The generic term for this type of procedure is "ostomy," or "stoma." Fortunately, an ostomy procedure is not needed for most IBD patients or, if it is needed, it may be temporary. However, it is sometimes necessary for the surgeon to bring an opening in the intestine out through the layers of the abdominal wall and the skin so that intestinal contents drain into a bag placed over the external opening.

Ileostomy and Colostomy

If the small intestine (ileum) is brought out to the skin, it is called an ileostomy. If the large intestine (colon) is brought out, it is called a colostomy. An ileostomy usually sticks out several inches or centimeters from the skin, while a colostomy is usually flat or flush with the surrounding skin. Immediately after surgery, the stoma may be somewhat swollen, but the swelling will usually go down during the first 6 weeks after surgery. Because the stoma consists of the inner lining of the intestine, it is normally pink or red, but it is not painful, because the stoma has no pain-detecting nerve fibers on its surface.

Stool Consistency

The consistency of the stool coming out of the stoma varies depending on your diet, fluid intake and the time of the day. There is a period of adaptation after surgery when the stool may go from being mainly liquid to having a thicker consistency. With an ileostomy, the stool generally gets to the consistency of porridge or toothpaste after several weeks or months, but it is virtually never fully formed or solid. With a colostomy, the stool may eventually become solid.

Odor and Gas

Odor is not generally a problem as long as the appliance fits properly over the stoma and does not leak. An odor is usually noticeable only when the bag is emptied in a bathroom. Proper cleaning of the lower edge of the bag, where the stool is emptied, will help eliminate odor once the bag has been emptied. Swallowing air, breathing through the mouth, smoking, chewing gum and drinking fizzy or carbonated drinks all tend to increase the amount of gas that passes through the stoma into the appliance, which results in the bag filling up very quickly and needing more frequent emptying.

▶ Normal Lifestyle

Achieving a normal and active lifestyle with a stoma requires some adjustment and support, but it can almost always be achieved.

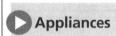

▶ Appliances

Stomas do not have a valve to control when stool or gas is excreted. As a result, patients need to wear a bag, or appliance, that fits over the stoma and collects the stool. You may need to try several different appliances before you find one that works well for your body type, stoma location and lifestyle. An enterostomal therapy (ET) nurse can help you find an appropriate appliance and teach you the proper care and maintenance of the stoma, thereby reducing the possibility of future problems.

Ileostomy, Colostomy, Diverting Loop Ileostomy

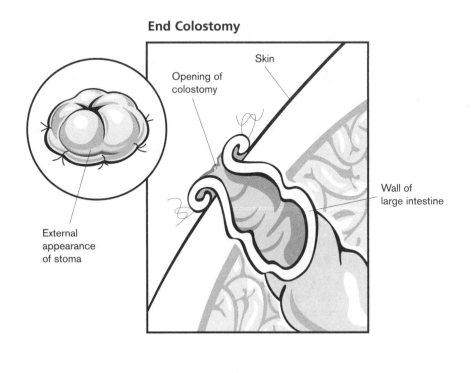

End Ileostomy

Junction of skin and bowel lining

Opening of ileostomy

Wall of small intestine

Skin

Diverting Loop Ileostomy

Opening of ileostomy

Skin

Small intestine (ileum)

End Colostomy

Skin

Opening of colostomy

Wall of large intestine

External appearance of stoma

Q **Will a stoma affect my diet and nutrition?**

A Colostomies do not usually affect nutritional requirements or require dietary restrictions. For individuals with an ileostomy there are no specific dietary restrictions long term, though you may want to limit large amounts of foods such as whole nuts and stringy vegetables because they have been known to cause blockage problems for people with stomas, particularly if not chewed well. Diet can also affect the amount of stool and gas that come out of an ileostomy. In general, low-fiber foods (see page 89) tend to minimize the amount of stool produced, thicken the consistency of the stool somewhat and reduce the amount of gas.

If you have an ileostomy, you do not have a functioning colon and, therefore, your ability to absorb water and electrolytes may be somewhat diminished. This is normally not a problem, but people who are chronically dehydrated may be at higher risk of certain types of kidney stones. During periods of hot weather, when people tend to have increased loss of fluid and electrolytes from sweat, it is important for someone with an ileostomy to maintain an adequate water intake (at least 2 to 3 quarts or liters per day) and to ingest plenty of salt with food or, if necessary, to take salt tablets. Because potassium losses may also increase, it is important to include plenty of foods and drinks containing potassium.

▶ **Successful Procedure**

The majority of ulcerative colitis patients who undergo the pelvic pouch procedure are very happy with the results. Although they may have more bowel movements than would be considered normal and the stool is often looser than normal and perhaps even smellier than normal, they can generally control the need to move their bowels, and they usually feel healthy without medications. In general, they are better off than they were before surgery.

Surgery for Ulcerative Colitis

In ulcerative colitis, the disease involves only the large intestine (colon). When the large intestine is surgically removed, the disease is effectively "cured."

Colectomy

Because the rectum is always diseased in ulcerative colitis, it has to be removed, along with the rest of the large intestine. In this operation, called a colectomy, it is not possible to reattach the lower end of the small intestine to any part of the large intestine.

At one time, having a colectomy meant that the small intestine had to be brought through an incision in the skin as an ileostomy so that fecal waste material could drain into an external appliance. For most people with ulcerative colitis, that was the end of their problems with inflammatory bowel disease. They were able to discontinue all medications and once again felt healthy, without experiencing bleeding or abdominal pain. They were also generally able to eat most foods without experiencing any unusual or unwanted symptoms.

Pelvic Pouch Procedure

In an attempt to avoid the need for an ileostomy following surgery for ulcerative colitis, surgeons now often offer a pelvic pouch procedure, also known as ileal pouch anal anastomosis (IPAA). The surgeon takes the lower end of the small intestine (the ileum), partially opens it and folds it back on itself to fashion it into a large-capacity pouch instead of a straight hose. The pouch is then attached to the remaining bottom part of the rectum, allowing patients to move their bowels in the normal fashion.

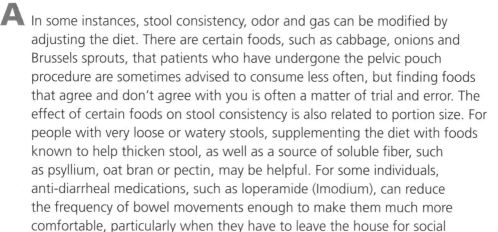

Q **What modifications to my diet can I make to improve stool consistency and reduce gas from my pelvic pouch?**

A In some instances, stool consistency, odor and gas can be modified by adjusting the diet. There are certain foods, such as cabbage, onions and Brussels sprouts, that patients who have undergone the pelvic pouch procedure are sometimes advised to consume less often, but finding foods that agree and don't agree with you is often a matter of trial and error. The effect of certain foods on stool consistency is also related to portion size. For people with very loose or watery stools, supplementing the diet with foods known to help thicken stool, as well as a source of soluble fiber, such as psyllium, oat bran or pectin, may be helpful. For some individuals, anti-diarrheal medications, such as loperamide (Imodium), can reduce the frequency of bowel movements enough to make them much more comfortable, particularly when they have to leave the house for social or work situations.

Pouchitis

A complication that occurs in approximately 10% to 15% of patients after pelvic pouch surgery is an inflammation of the inner lining of the pouch, called pouchitis. Pouchitis causes symptoms of increased stool frequency and looseness, abdominal cramping, loss of control of bowel movements, feeling unwell and blood in the stool. Pouchitis almost always responds to a 7- to 14-day course of antibiotics. While pouchitis is not caused by diet and is not cured by dietary modifications, some patients feel more comfortable if they minimize foods that tend to increase stool output and gas production. These include caffeine-containing foods and drinks, carbonated beverages and foods high in fiber.

Pelvic (Ileal) Pouch Procedure

Panel 1

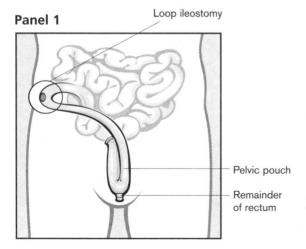

Loop ileostomy

Pelvic pouch

Remainder of rectum

The pelvic pouch procedure is usually done in two or three stages. Initially, the pouch is formed by folding the small intestine (ileum) back on itself to make a "J" shape. The bottom of the "J" is opened and sewn to the small segment of remaining rectum (detail panel). The temporary loop ileostomy is created above the pouch (panel 1), and several months later the ileostomy is closed (panel 2), thus producing an intact digestive tract (panel 3).

Panel 2

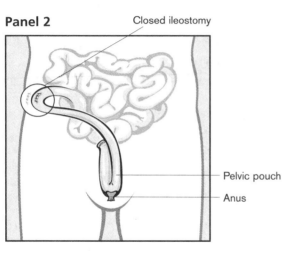

Closed ileostomy

Pelvic pouch

Anus

Detail Panel

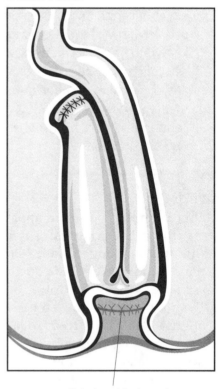

Suturing of ileal pouch to remainder of rectum

Panel 3

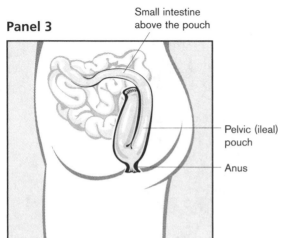

Small intestine above the pouch

Pelvic (ileal) pouch

Anus

Small and Large Intestine Resection

Small intestine resection

Resection margins

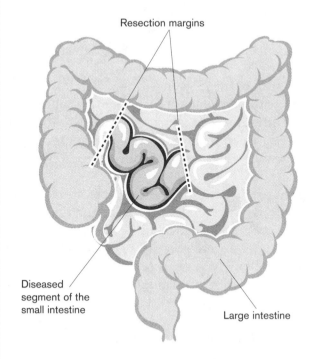

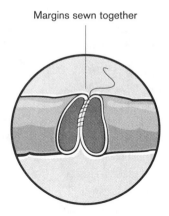

Margins sewn together

Diseased
segment of the
small intestine

Large intestine

When a resection is performed,
the diseased segment of intestine
is cut out and the remaining
margins are sewn together.

Large intestine resection

Resection margins

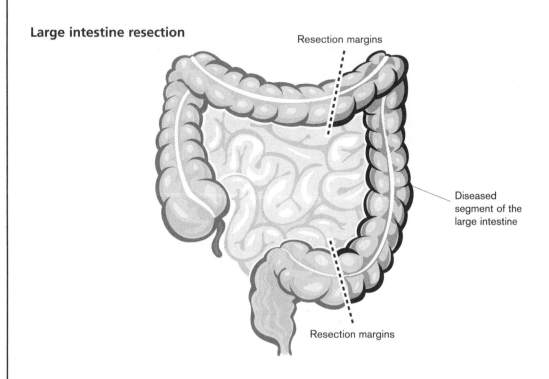

Diseased
segment of the
large intestine

Resection margins

Surgery for Crohn's Disease

Crohn's disease can affect any part of the gastrointestinal tract. As a result, a large variety of operations are possible surgical treatments of Crohn's disease. No two operations for Crohn's disease are identical. However, although there are theoretically many different types of operations that can be performed for Crohn's disease, only a handful are actually performed in the majority of cases.

Whereas removal of the large intestine in ulcerative colitis leads to a "cure," with no chance of the ulcerative colitis recurring in the small intestine or other parts of the gastrointestinal tract, Crohn's disease can recur in previously unaffected segments of intestine following surgical removal, or resection, of a diseased area.

This may lead to the need for multiple operations and the removal of additional intestinal segments at each operation, which can lead to short bowel syndrome. To avoid short bowel syndrome, there is a tendency, where it is safe, to delay surgery for Crohn's disease; when surgery is needed, the surgeon will usually try to resect the minimum amount of bowel necessary to deal with the immediate problem.

▶ Short Bowel Syndrome

Repeated resections can eventually result in short bowel syndrome, where so much of the intestine has been removed that patients are unable to keep themselves nourished or to maintain fluid and electrolyte balance through the intake of food and liquids.

Small Intestine Resection

The most common operation used to treat Crohn's disease is a small intestine resection. This operation is usually performed because an area of small intestine is affected by Crohn's disease, leading to scarring and narrowing of the intestinal opening through which food passes. Small intestine resections may also be required when a fistula or abscess has arisen from an affected segment of intestine or when symptoms of active inflammation in the small intestine (abdominal cramping, diarrhea, weight loss) do not respond to drug therapies.

The removal of a segment of intestine leaves two unattached ends of small intestine, or one end of small intestine and one of large intestine. These ends are sewn or stapled together to re-establish the continuous flow of intestinal contents through the gastrointestinal tract.

In cases where the segment is very short, resection carries very little risk of complication or of future development of short bowel syndrome.

Ileocecal Resection

In many cases, a small portion of the large intestine is resected along with the adjoining portion of the small intestine. This is called an ileocecal or ileocolic resection.

Strictureplasty

Strictureplasty is an operation that has been devised in an attempt to avoid removing segments of the intestine. Instead of resecting the small intestine, the surgeon tries to open up the narrowed segments and create a larger internal passageway, thereby allowing food to pass through more easily without causing symptoms of obstruction. By conserving the affected segments, it may be possible to reduce the future risk of short bowel syndrome.

LIMITATIONS OF STRICTUREPLASTY

In some cases, strictureplasty cannot be performed because the narrowed segment is too long, or should not be performed because only a single short segment is narrowed and the risks of the procedure (leak, infection, recurrent obstruction) are not worth the potential benefits of avoiding a resection.

Large Intestine Resection (Colectomy)

Surgery to remove all or part of the large intestine is performed when all or part of the colon is affected with Crohn's disease and the symptoms cannot be controlled with medication, or when a narrowing in the colon is causing obstructions.

If part of the colon is removed, it is called a partial colectomy; if none of the colon can be salvaged, the entire colon is removed in a total colectomy. If the operation requires removal of the rectum, a permanent ileostomy is usually required.

Perianal Procedures

Surgery for complications of Crohn's disease in the anal area (perianal disease) does not usually involve removing segments of bowel. Most operations are performed to reduce the symptoms of pain by allowing the draining of pus or infection when patients have not responded to other measures or when an acute problem, such as an abscess, has occurred.

Diverting Loop (Temporary) Ileostomy

For patients with severe perianal fistulas or with damage to the anal sphincter, a diverting loop (temporary) ileostomy may provide the best outcome. By preventing stool from passing through the anus and the area of the fistulas and abscesses, the operation may result in reduced drainage from fistulas, reduced abscess formation and, in some cases, healing of fistulas. In

 Pelvic Pouch Procedure

Patients with known Crohn's disease are not usually candidates for a pelvic pouch procedure, except in special circumstances, because the risk of complications or failure of the procedure is significantly higher than it is with ulcerative colitis.

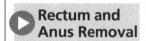

Rectum and Anus Removal

When a patient has had an end ileostomy for the treatment of rectal and perianal disease, the rectum and anus are usually removed surgically, and the area is closed up.

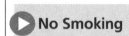

No Smoking

If you're a smoker, one of the best and safest ways to reduce the risk that Crohn's disease will recur after surgery is to quit smoking. Smokers appear to have a higher rate of recurrence after surgery than non-smokers.

these cases, the ileostomy may be reversed, or closed, and the fistulas will sometimes, but not always, remain healed.

End Ileostomy

For patients with anal sphincter damage due to perianal fistulas or abscesses, closure of the ileostomy may not be feasible, because incontinence would result. In this case, the loop ileostomy may be converted to a more permanent end ileostomy once the affected individual becomes accustomed to having a stoma.

Prognosis

Surgery can be a very effective way to manage Crohn's disease. However, the disease can recur in parts of the intestine that were previously not affected. As a result, it is not unheard of for people with Crohn's disease to require two, three, four or even more operations. Approximately one in three patients who undergo surgery for Crohn's disease will have a recurrence of symptoms within 3 to 5 years, and a portion of these will end up requiring another operation.

Recurrence

A number of different medications have been tested as a way to reduce the risk of Crohn's disease recurring after surgery. None of the currently available drugs is 100% effective. The ones most commonly used are 5-ASA-containing preparations, antibiotics and azathioprine or 6-mercaptopurine (6-MP). Preliminary studies have been done on the use of anti-TNF drugs, such as infliximab or adalimumab, after surgery, and the results appear to indicate that these drugs are effective in preventing recurrence of Crohn's disease.

People with Crohn's disease are often interested in dietary means of preventing recurrence after surgery, but no studies have been conducted to determine whether supplementing the diet with specific foods or restricting certain types of foods will prevent or delay recurrence.

Nutrient Deficiency

If you have had multiple operations and a large part of your intestine has been removed, you may not be able to adequately absorb nutrients, water, minerals and electrolytes from your diet. This can be a very serious problem — more serious than the Crohn's disease itself. Possible nutrient deficiencies need to be anticipated by your doctor, who may recommend supplements or suggest changes to your diet to compensate.

Dietary Strategies

Diet has been studied as a possible cause of Crohn's disease and ulcerative colitis and as a possible treatment for these conditions. Although no one dietary factor has been identified as a cause of IBD, certain dietary factors could play a role in triggering the disease in genetically susceptible individuals or in triggering a disease flare in someone who already has the disease. While these factors have not been identified and no one diet can cure IBD, specific foods have been identified as agents in managing some symptoms.

The Right Diet

Gaining a sense of control by changing what or how you eat can be appealing when you are living with an unpredictable disease, but you need to exercise caution in choosing the "right" diet. One diet may claim to prevent disease relapse or even cure IBD. Other diets may claim to influence your immune system positively, improve digestive health and reduce inflammation. However, just because something is in print doesn't mean it's scientifically valid. It can be difficult to sort out myth from science. A persuasive author or an anecdote from someone whose IBD responded only to the author's diet can be very convincing. But such anecdotes may provide false hope. Look for reliable, evidence-based strategies.

Individualized Diets

If you've had difficulty figuring out the "right" diet to follow, it is probably because your experience with these diets has been different from other people's experience. We each have different taste preferences, different tolerances (to spicy or gas-producing foods, for example), different budgets and even different access to foods, with limited choices in remote areas. An individual living with IBD could have additional dietary considerations, including transient intolerances to previously enjoyed foods and the need to restrict some foods temporarily and supplement others.

 There's No "IBD Diet"

There is no single diet that works for everyone with IBD. But while there is no such thing as an "IBD diet," there are many foods that can affect your symptoms adversely or positively.

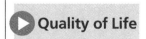
Considering these factors, it makes sense that the same food can be experienced differently by different individuals. There could be many thousand versions of the "right" diet. Remember that Crohn's disease and ulcerative colitis have different disease characteristics, different disease courses, a variety of possible symptoms and possible complications, and many variations in treatment regimens.

The Role of Nutrition

Nutrition plays an important role in the management of IBD by maintaining general health during times of disease activity and during times of remission. A person's nutritional status affects important physiological processes, such as immunity and wound healing, and as a result can contribute to the prevention of long-term complications. There are some common dietary guidelines that people with IBD can follow in the effort to manage their symptoms and improve their quality of life — and even ward off more serious complications, such as malnutrition.

Nutrition recommendations must be balanced to avoid nutrient deficiencies and individualized to specific tastes, budgets, lifestyles and, very importantly, for specific desired functional benefits (for example, regaining weight and symptom management). The diet that considers and meets these needs is the right diet for you.

Diet Modifications

If your IBD is under control and you live relatively symptom-free, there is no need to restrict foods or follow a special diet. Just follow the United States Department of Agriculture (USDA) MyPlate food guide or Eating Well with Canada's Food Guide. These reliable diet guides emphasize eating a wide variety of foods that provide the multitude of nutrients your body needs, and can be adapted for vegetarian and vegan diets. The key is to select a variety of foods from all food groups in the recommended amounts.

However, if you are experiencing acute disease activity, you may find it helpful to modify your regular diet to help minimize gastrointestinal symptoms, such as cramping, bloating, gas and diarrhea. Be sure that dietary changes for symptom management do not compromise nutritional status. For optimal well-being, your diet should allow you to maintain your weight and energy intake levels, continue enjoying food and participate in social situations involving food.

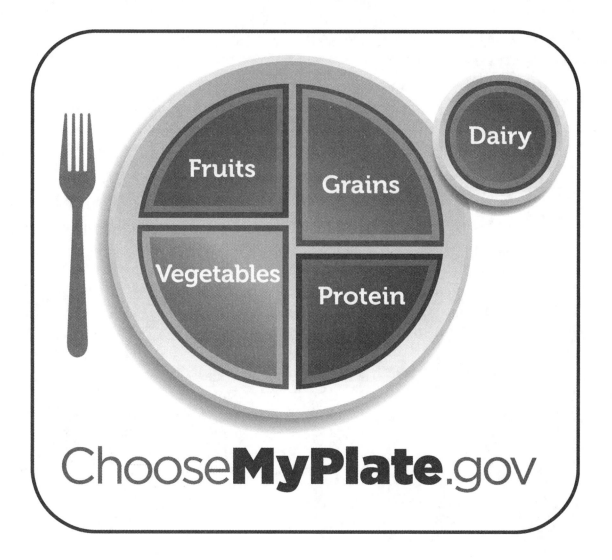

Balancing Calories
- Enjoy your food, but eat less.
- Avoid oversized portions.

Foods to Increase
- Make half your plate fruits and vegetables.
- Make at least half your grains whole grains.
- Switch to fat-free or low-fat (1%) milk.

Foods to Reduce
- Compare sodium in foods like soup, bread and frozen meals and choose the foods with lower numbers.
- Drink water instead of sugary drinks.

Eating Well with Canada's Food Guide

Recommended Number of *Food Guide Servings* per Day

	Children			Teens		Adults			
Age in Years	2-3	4-8	9-13	14-18		19-50		51+	
Sex	Girls and Boys			Females	Males	Females	Males	Females	Males
Vegetables and Fruit	4	5	6	7	8	7-8	8-10	7	7
Grain Products	3	4	6	6	7	6-7	8	6	7
Milk and Alternatives	2	2	3-4	3-4	3-4	2	2	3	3
Meat and Alternatives	1	1	1-2	2	3	2	3	2	3

What is One Food Guide Serving?
Look at the examples below.

Fresh, frozen or canned vegetables
125 mL (½ cup)

Bread
1 slice (35 g)

Bagel
½ bagel (45 g)

Milk or powdered milk (reconstituted)
250 mL (1 cup)

Cooked fish, shellfish, poultry, lean meat
75 g (2 ½ oz.)/125 mL (½ cup)

The chart above shows how many Food Guide Servings you need from each of the four food groups every day.

Having the amount and type of food recommended and following the tips in *Canada's Food Guide* will help:

• Meet your needs for vitamins, minerals and other nutrients.
• Reduce your risk of obesity, type 2 diabetes, heart disease, certain types of cancer and osteoporosis.
• Contribute to your overall health and vitality.

For a full guide, please contact Health Canada or visit their website.

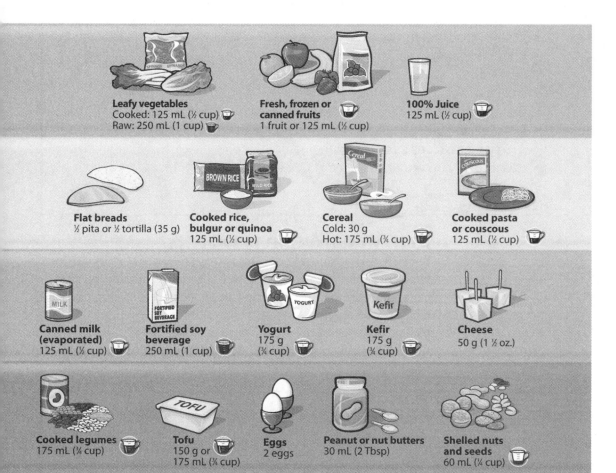

Leafy vegetables
Cooked: 125 mL (½ cup)
Raw: 250 mL (1 cup)

Fresh, frozen or canned fruits
1 fruit or 125 mL (½ cup)

100% Juice
125 mL (½ cup)

Flat breads
½ pita or ½ tortilla (35 g)

Cooked rice, bulgur or quinoa
125 mL (½ cup)

Cereal
Cold: 30 g
Hot: 175 mL (¾ cup)

Cooked pasta or couscous
125 mL (½ cup)

Canned milk (evaporated)
125 mL (½ cup)

Fortified soy beverage
250 mL (1 cup)

Yogurt
175 g
(¾ cup)

Kefir
175 g
(¾ cup)

Cheese
50 g (1 ½ oz.)

Cooked legumes
175 mL (¾ cup)

Tofu
150 g or
175 mL (¾ cup)

Eggs
2 eggs

Peanut or nut butters
30 mL (2 Tbsp)

Shelled nuts and seeds
60 mL (¼ cup)

Oils and Fats

- Include a small amount – 30 to 45 mL (2 to 3 Tbsp) – of unsaturated fat each day. This includes oil used for cooking, salad dressings, margarine and mayonnaise.
- Use vegetable oils such as canola, olive and soybean.
- Choose soft margarines that are low in saturated and trans fats.
- Limit butter, hard margarine, lard and shortening.

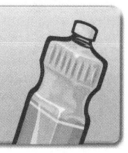

Q **Do I need to modify my diet if I have IBD?**

A By asking yourself, your doctor and your dietitian the following questions, you can determine what dietary modifications, if any, you might require.

- What is the status of my disease?
- What symptoms am I currently experiencing?
- If my disease is active, what part or parts of my bowel are affected? What nutrients are usually absorbed in this location?
- Are there any complications from my disease that I should consider — osteoporosis or strictures (narrowed bowel from scar tissue), for example?
- What effect does my treatment have on nutrient requirements?
- Do my medications interact with nutrients?
- Has surgery affected the amount of bowel available for nutrient absorption?

Diet Modification Goals

Specific goals for diet modifications should not only address symptom management, but also help you achieve better physical and emotional health. You can experience a feeling of social isolation when your food choices are limited or when you need to ask for special accommodations when eating away from home. You may not want to be asked questions about why you need a special diet. Sometimes you just want to feel "normal."

DIET MODIFICATION GOALS

1. **Prevent malnutrition.**
2. **Normalize bowel function.**
   - Decrease stool frequency.
   - Increase stool consistency.
3. **Minimize GI intolerance symptoms.**
   - Reduce gas, bloating, cramping, pain.
   - Reduce the risk of obstruction.
4. **Maintain hydration and electrolyte balance.**
5. **Maintain or improve nutritional status.**
   - Prevent further weight loss (or weight gain, if applicable).
   - Improve functional status.
   - Supplement with specific nutrients, if indicated.
6. **Continue or resume social participation and enjoyment.**
   - Normalize diet with time.
   - Improve relationship with food.

Facing the Fear of Food

If you've lived for a long time with an intestinal stricture and diet restrictions, it can be daunting to try new foods again after surgery has removed the stricture. If you've ever experienced a bowel obstruction as a result of the food you have eaten, the motivation to avoid pain and stay away from questionable foods is quite strong. It is normal to feel apprehensive about liberalizing your diet again, but with time you will feel more comfortable with the function of your gut's new anatomy and digestion. When introducing or reintroducing foods to your diet, it is important to chew slowly and thoroughly, to take small portion sizes and to try one new food at a time.

Preventing Malnutrition

Diet is the key to preventing clinical malnutrition, a condition that results when there is a deficiency or imbalance of nutrients in your body. Nutrient deficiencies can result over time from a lack of overall calories (the term "calories" can be used interchangeably with "energy") or from a lack of specific nutrients, such as protein, essential fats, vitamins, minerals or trace elements.

Malnutrition is a concern because it can affect your immune system function, leading to an increased susceptibility to infections. It can also compromise your body's normal defenses against free radicals (damaging molecules produced from pollution, radiation, stress and smoking), slow down wound healing and contribute to long-term complications, such as poor dental health and early bone loss leading to osteoporosis.

If you experience symptoms of malnutrition, see your doctor immediately. However, the fact that you have IBD does not necessarily mean you will develop malnutrition symptoms or complications.

Weight Loss

Significant loss of body weight is the most common indication of malnutrition. When people are feeling unwell, they commonly have little appetite and must force themselves to eat. Often, they lose weight despite their best efforts.

Loss of appetite and the inability to eat enough to maintain your weight are the hallmarks of a symptom called anorexia (the use of this term does not mean you have an eating disorder).

Taking Pleasure in Food

One goal of diet modifications is to facilitate an improved relationship with food and eating. All strategies that potentially restrict the types and varieties of foods you eat should be reassessed periodically so they can be adjusted and a regular diet can be resumed.

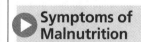

Symptoms of Malnutrition

When you are poorly nourished, your IBD symptoms are likely to become more severe or to have a more significant impact upon you. Other signs to look for include:

- Weight loss
- Loss of appetite
- Muscle weakness (from lost muscle mass)
- Changes in your skin, hair, nails, gums, eyesight or mood

Malnutrition Risk Factors

Anorexia, the medical term for loss of appetite, is one risk factor for malnutrition. Along with other symptoms, such as gastrointestinal intolerance, altered taste and dietary eliminations (due to food phobias or dependencies), anorexia can lead to inadequate nutrient intake.

Other risk factors include increased nutrient requirements, malabsorption of nutrients, and increased losses of electrolytes, minerals, trace elements and proteins. Some of these factors are specific to Crohn's disease or ulcerative colitis.

Treatment for Malnutrition

To determine whether you are malnourished, health-care professionals will evaluate your symptoms and signs, medical history, height and weight trends, diet history, social and economic circumstances, medications and laboratory tests. An appropriate nutrition plan will then be created to help manage your illness and achieve your desired health outcomes.

Your nutrition plan could include counseling for diet modifications or implementation of specialized nutrition therapies, such as supplementation with nutritional products, replacement of vitamins and minerals, provision of enteral nutrition (liquid nutrition formula delivered via a feeding tube into the stomach or small intestine) or provision of parenteral nutrition (nutrition infused through a special intravenous line).

Parenteral nutrition is usually reserved for patients who are not able to eat adequate amounts, who cannot receive tube feeding, and who do not have enough normal intestine to allow minimum amounts of absorption.

 Nutrition Support

To prevent malnutrition from developing or progressing, a more intensive and defined form of nutrition, called nutrition support, is sometimes required. There are two types of nutrition support: total enteral nutrition (tube feeding) and total parenteral nutrition (intravenous feeding).

MALNUTRITION RISK FACTORS

1. **Inadequate Intake of Nutrients**
   Anorexia
   - Decreased oral intake of food and beverages
   - Inability to tolerate solid foods and a prolonged period of consuming low-calorie and low-protein fluids

   Gastrointestinal intolerance
   - Nausea, vomiting, diarrhea, rectal urgency, cramping, bloating, pain, obstructive symptoms, pain with swallowing

   Altered taste
   - A side effect of some medications

   Dietary eliminations
   - Food phobias, food intolerances, diet experimentation
   - Dependencies (for example, substituting alcohol for nutritious foods)

2. **Increased Nutrient Requirements**
   Higher metabolic rate
   - Stress response and inflammation, infection, wound healing, fever, catabolic (breakdown) effects from steroids
   - Increased requirements for growth (children and adolescents)
   - Replete (build) body tissue stores of muscle and fat

3. **Malabsorption of Nutrients**
   Decreased absorptive surface
   - Active disease affecting bowel surface
   - Multiple surgical resections

   Nutrient bypass
   - Fistula
   - Surgically created intestinal bypass

   Drug interference
   Bile salt deficiency
   Bacterial overgrowth

4. **Increased Losses (electrolytes, minerals, trace elements, protein)**
   - Diarrhea
   - Fistula
   - Blood loss

NUTRIENT DEFICIENCY SYMPTOMS AND SUPPLEMENTS

Calories
In general, if you are not able to maintain a healthy weight, you may need to boost calories (calories come from macronutrients, namely carbohydrates, protein and fat).

Protein
You may need extra protein if you are on high-dose steroids, extra protein and iron if you have ongoing blood loss, or additional protein and zinc if you have prolonged diarrhea, a wound, or a fistula affecting your small bowel.

Fat
You may need to supplement a specific type of fat if you have extensive Crohn's disease of the ileum or have had more than 3 feet (about 100 cm) of terminal ileum surgically removed.

Iron
If you have anemia, you might require supplementation of iron.

Vitamin B$_{12}$
Vitamin B$_{12}$ is absorbed only in the terminal ileum (the last part of the small intestine), so if you have Crohn's disease in that region or have had surgical resection of your terminal ileum, you will most likely require supplements. Because the terminal ileum is diseased or removed, vitamin B$_{12}$ won't be absorbed if you take a supplement by mouth — it must be delivered by injection or, where available, by an inhalant sprayed into the nose. Vitamin B$_{12}$ absorption is also dependent on intrinsic factor (IF), which is secreted by the stomach, so if you have had surgery to remove part of the stomach, you may need vitamin B$_{12}$ supplements. Vitamin B$_{12}$ supplementation is also sometimes required if you have anemia.

Folic acid
If you are taking sulfasalazine or methotrexate, you will likely need to supplement folate, as this drug interferes with folate's metabolism. You might also require folate supplements if you have anemia. "Folic acid" is the term for a folate supplement.

Sodium and potassium
If you have had the large bowel removed, you will need to increase fluid and electrolytes (sodium and potassium) in your diet.

Calcium and vitamin D
If you are being treated with steroids, you will probably need additional calcium and vitamin D, because steroids interfere with the absorption of calcium and the metabolism of vitamin D.

Q **Can liquid supplements be used to treat IBD?**

A When some Crohn's patients drink only supplements (or receive supplements via a feeding tube), their disease often goes into remission. Some patients find that they can avoid steroid medications, which is especially important for children and adolescents who want to avoid the negative side effects of steroids, such as delayed growth. Polymeric, semi-elemental and elemental supplements all appear to provide a beneficial effect.

Different theories have been proposed to account for the effectiveness of these supplements in some patients, including the sterile properties of the supplements, the beneficial effects of specific types of fat and the simple improvement of overall nutritional status, with the consequent improvement in immunity.

Liquid Calorie Supplements

During times when you feel that you cannot get enough calories, you may want to drink commercially prepared liquid supplements. There are several different kinds designed for specific purposes, including polymeric, semi-elemental, elemental and modular supplements. Most are lactose-free. Consult your doctor or dietitian before choosing one.

Most liquid supplements have vitamins, minerals and trace elements added. To meet your nutritional requirements by drinking these supplements and eating no other foods, you must consume a specific volume. An average person might need to drink four or five units (cans, boxes, Tetra Paks or packages dissolved in water) every day. There are many different brand names, varieties and flavors.

Existing only on liquid nutritional supplements can be challenging because of the lack of variety and the lack of solid food. Different-flavor supplements can help maintain interest in drinking them.

> **▶ Balanced Nutrition**
>
> Most liquid supplements are designed to provide balanced nutrition, meaning that they provide the macronutrients (protein, carbohydrate and fat) in healthy proportions: 50% to 55% of calories from carbohydrates, 15% to 20% of calories from protein and less than 30% of calories from fat. Some specialized products may have a higher amount of protein, some may have different kinds of fat that may be more easily digested, and some may have added fiber.

Vitamin and Mineral Supplements

It may be necessary to replace or supplement nutrients if you have a problem with absorption. Nutrient absorption can be affected by disease activity, bacterial overgrowth, loss of bowel from surgical resections or interference from medications. Vitamins, minerals and trace elements are essential to your health. Because your body cannot create them, they must be consumed from a variety of foods.

KEY MICRONUTRIENTS

Water-soluble vitamins	Fat-soluble vitamins	Minerals	Trace elements
• Vitamin B_1 (thiamin) • Vitamin B_2 (riboflavin) • Vitamin B_3 (niacin) • Biotin • Pantothenic acid • Vitamin B_6 (pyridoxine) • Folic acid • Vitamin B_{12} (cyanocobalamin) • Vitamin C	• Vitamin A (precursor beta-carotene) • Vitamin D • Vitamin E • Vitamin K	• Sodium • Chloride • Potassium • Calcium • Phosphorus • Magnesium • Sulphur	• Iron • Zinc • Iodine • Selenium • Copper • Manganese • Fluoride • Chromium • Molybdenum

Q How do I know whether I need a vitamin supplement?

A The best way to determine whether you need a supplement is to identify which food groups are not well represented in your daily diet. Compare your diet to the USDA MyPlate food guide or Eating Well with Canada's Food Guide. For each food group, a set of nutrients is specified and a number of servings is recommended.

For example, grain products are significant sources of complex carbohydrates, riboflavin, thiamin, niacin, iron, protein, magnesium and fiber. If you do not eat many servings from this group, you may be deficient in these nutrients; supplementing for the missing nutrients is a good idea. There are many brands of standard adult multivitamins with minerals, and most varieties are fine for meeting general needs. Just remember that, whenever possible, eating the real thing is tastier and more filling, and provides better nutrient variety.

TIPS FOR TAKING SUPPLEMENTS

- Discuss your supplements with an expert — your pharmacist.
- Take fat-soluble vitamins with a meal. They are better absorbed with fat.
- Take fiber supplements separately. Fiber may bind to some nutrients, interfering with their absorption.
- Take calcium supplements separately from multivitamins. Many multivitamin preparations contain iron, which interferes with calcium absorption.
- Take medications cold (keep the container on ice) to ease swallowing.
- To avoid the medicine odor, mix water into the supplement and sip with a straw.
- Flavor supplements with vanilla, mint or banana extracts; decaffeinated instant coffee (dissolve in a small amount of warm water); pulp-free syrup (chocolate and other flavors used for hot beverages); or flavor packets (pudding, flavored gelatin, Crystal Light, Kool-Aid, etc.).
- Include the supplement in a milkshake or smoothie recipe.
- Substitute the supplement for milk in baking recipes.

HEALTH CANADA REGULATION OF NATURAL HEALTH PRODUCTS

In a recent survey, it was reported that more than 70% of Canadians regularly take natural health products (NHPs). NHPs refer to over-the-counter (no prescription is needed) products that are purported to have health benefits. These NHPs include vitamin and mineral supplements, herbals, probiotics, enzymes, amino acids, essential fats, traditional Chinese medicines and homeopathic medicines. Health Canada began to regulate NHPs in 2004 according to the Natural Health Products Regulations in order to recognize the unique properties of these products while having measures in place to protect consumer safety based on level of evidence.

Almost 10 years after this program started, Health Canada has authorized more than 50,000 NHPs for sale, labeled with required cautionary statements: potential adverse reactions and interactions with other products; warnings for certain populations like pregnant women; duration of use; etc. Once on the market these NHPs are monitored for situations that pose risks to the health and safety of the people taking them: poor manufacturing, adulteration (e.g., addition of prescription and non-prescription drugs to NHPs) or products making claims not substantiated by evidence. Health Canada tracks and analyzes adverse reactions to NHPs through the Canada Vigilance Program. When analysis of this adverse reaction information shows that there is a need to take action to protect the health and safety of Canadians, Health Canada can take a range of steps, such as changes to product labeling, distribution of information to consumers and health professionals and, in more serious cases, removal of a product from the market.

Maintaining Hydration and Electrolyte Balance

The more fluid you lose in stool, the more likely you are to experience dehydration. If you have had your colon removed (fluid and electrolytes are primarily absorbed in the colon), your small intestine will partially adapt to take over this function, but this takes time, and the stool will become pasty at best. When passing frequent liquid stool, be sure that you are getting adequate fluids and replacing electrolytes.

 Symptoms of Dehydration

Symptoms of dehydration and electrolyte loss include:

- Fatigue
- Feeling light-headed or faint
- Increased thirst
- Dry mouth
- Stomach cramps
- Decreased urine output
- Rapid loss in weight from day to day

Best-Absorbed Fluids

The fluids that are best absorbed match the concentration, or osmolality, of your body fluids, allowing for the best transfer of fluid across the cell membranes in your intestine. An example of a good replacement fluid would be Gastrolyte for adults or Pedialyte for children. Milk, juices and sports drinks (for example, standard formulation Gatorade or Powerade) are not absorbed as well due to their higher sugar content and consequent higher osmolality (a measure of the concentration of molecules dissolved in water).

Water may be better absorbed than the sugary drinks. When a fluid has a high sugar concentration, drinking it causes fluid to shift into the intestine from the tissues, instead of out of the intestine into the tissues and the bloodstream. Therefore, drinking

Q Can I drink coffee, cola or beer if I have IBD?

A Beware of fluids that are known to increase urine production and loss of water from the body (diuretics). Examples of diuretics include caffeinated beverages and alcohol. There is even a combination of the two — beer that has added caffeine. Caffeinated beverages include dark colas (Coke, Pepsi, house-brand colas, root beer) and some clear soft drinks (Mountain Dew), energy drinks, coffee, tea (including green tea) and hot chocolate. Guarana, added to energy drinks and teas, is a South American plant whose seeds have a higher caffeine content than coffee beans, but because guarana is a food product, the caffeine content is not required to be listed on the label. Chocolate and some medications, such as over-the-counter cold and flu remedies, also contain caffeine. Studies have demonstrated that healthy individuals who regularly consume caffeine are not at risk for dehydration; however, this conclusion cannot necessarily be applied to individuals living with IBD since caffeine and guarana stimulate bowel motility and, as a result, can lead to more frequent, liquidy bowel movements.

SOURCES OF SODIUM AND POTASSIUM

Sodium	Potassium
• Bouillon cubes • Canned fish (e.g., tuna, salmon, sardines, anchovies) and dried fish (e.g., dried cod or herring) • Canned legumes • Canned soups and vegetables • Fast foods • Processed foods (e.g., processed cheese, processed and smoked meats) • Ready-to-eat cereals (e.g., instant oatmeal) • Sauces and condiments (e.g., soy, Worcestershire and barbecue sauces, salad dressing, ketchup, relish, pickles) • Snack foods (e.g., pretzels, salted crackers, potato chips, salted popcorn, corn chips) • Table salt • Tomato sauce	• Apricots • Asparagus • Avocados • Baked beans • Bananas • Barley • Beets • Brown sugar • Chocolate • Juices (carrot, orange, passion fruit, tomato, vegetable) • Legumes (chickpeas, lentils, split peas, kidney beans, soy beans) • Mangos • Maple syrup • Melons (cantaloupe, honeydew) • Molasses • Nectarines • Okra • Oranges • Parsnips • Potatoes • Pumpkin • Salt substitute • Smooth nut butters • Strong tea and coffee • Sweet potatoes/yams • Tomato products (soup, sauce, paste) • Coconut water

fluids with a high sugar content leads to more watery stool. To avoid increased diarrhea, you can try diluting concentrated sugar sources, such as juices and sports drinks, and sipping them slowly. Some reduced-sugar sports drinks are also available, sweetened with artificial sweeteners instead of sugar.

Electrolytes

Sodium and potassium are two electrolytes critical for the regulation and balance of body fluids. They can be found in small amounts in many foods, but it is best to target higher sources on a regular basis if you are at risk of dehydration.

Elimination (Exclusion) Diets

Elimination diets that significantly restrict or exclude one or more foods or major food groups are often recommended for IBD patients. Dairy foods, wheat, red meat, yeast and refined sugars are common exclusions. However, the value of exclusion diets has not been proven effective in IBD. In studies where suspected foods were excluded, individuals did not consistently experience relapse upon reintroduction of the excluded foods.

Q Is there danger in excluding foods or food groups?

A If you choose to follow an elimination diet, be sure to consider the potential side effects. The long-term consequences of following an exclusionary diet for more than a few weeks include possible development of nutrient deficiencies, weight loss, malnutrition, food phobias or obsessions and a loss of enjoyment of eating. If you're avoiding major food groups, be sure to speak with a dietitian to learn about alternative foods or supplements for the excluded nutrients.

There is also a psychological danger. Following a diet that claims to control IBD can contribute to a feeling that you are at fault if your disease becomes active again. If they have trouble following the diet exactly, some people may feel that they are responsible for their disease coming back. This internalization of responsibility is destructive and takes strength away during a time that is difficult enough.

If you still feel it is important to try this approach, be sure to set a timeline for evaluating and stopping the dietary eliminations.

One example of a diet exclusion is gluten, a protein found in wheat, rye, triticale and barley. An individual may suspect she has non-celiac gluten sensitivity, meaning that she suspects she cannot tolerate gluten and experiences symptoms similar to those with celiac disease (yet lacks the same antibodies and intestinal damage seen in celiac disease). Often there is symptom improvement just from the change from your usual diet, as fewer processed foods are usually consumed and eating out is often reduced due to the prevalence of gluten in processed foods and in foods prepared in restaurants.

Gluten-free doesn't necessarily mean healthier. In fact, gluten-free foods tend to be lower in iron, calcium, vitamin D, folate and fiber. Many gluten-free processed foods are higher in fat and calories and can contribute to weight gain. Careful planning with the help of a registered dietitian can open options like healthier flours (sorghum, brown rice, bean) and almond meal instead of white rice flour and starches like potato and tapioca. Assistance from a dietitian can also help with evaluating symptom response, substituting for missing nutrients and planning for reintroduction if appropriate.

Q What is a low-FODMAP diet?

A The low-FODMAP diet reduces the amount of **F**ermentable **O**ligo-, **D**i-, and **M**onosaccharides **A**nd **P**olyols in the diet in order to reduce symptoms of cramping, diarrhea, constipation, gas, bloating and abdominal pain.

FODMAPs are all small carbohydrates that are poorly absorbed in the small bowel and thus highly fermentable by colonic bacteria. Examples of these carbohydrates include:

• Oligosaccharides, such as fructans and galacto-oligosaccharides (GOS)
• Disaccharides, such as lactose
• Monosaccharides, such as fructose
• Polyols, such as sorbitol, mannitol, xylitol and maltitol

The main dietary sources of fructans are wheat products (note that this diet is not the same as a gluten-free diet) and the main dietary sources of GOS are legumes. The main dietary sources of lactose are animal milks (note that this diet is not the same as a dairy-free diet) and the main dietary source of fructose is in fruits, honey and high-fructose corn syrup (note that only fructose found in higher concentrations than glucose contributes to fructose malabsorption). The main dietary source of polyols (also known as sugar alcohols) are some fruits and vegetables, as well as artificial sweeteners used in sugar-reduced foods, candies and beverages.

A low-FODMAP diet initially eliminates all FODMAP foods from the diet for a trial period of 2 to 6 weeks, or in some instances longer, while monitoring changes in the symptoms of abdominal cramping, diarrhea, constipation, bloating and gas. After 2 to 6 weeks of elimination of FODMAP-containing foods, one FODMAP class of foods is introduced into the diet at a time (rather than isolating a specific food) and the effect on the previously experienced symptoms is noted. Initially, small amounts of the FODMAP class of food are added back to the diet, then gradually larger amounts. The pace of reintroduction is patient-led, based on degree of symptom relief. Careful observation for symptoms usually involves keeping a food and symptom journal including amounts of foods and the types of symptoms experienced. It is important to note that the amount consumed, timing of the meal and other meals consumed on that day may influence any adverse reactions.

Symptoms will presumably be improved by decreasing the amount of undigestible sugars (carbohydrates) in the diet that are otherwise fermented by bacteria in the bowel. The low-FODMAP diet has been advocated for individuals suffering from irritable bowel syndrome (IBS); however, this diet has also been promoted in IBD (if symptoms of IBS are also experienced and when the inflammation is well controlled) due to the similarities in gastrointestinal intolerance symptoms. A dietary intolerance does not involve the immune system and is different from an immune-mediated reaction to a protein in a food (as is the case with a food allergy or a food hypersensitivity). While undertaking an elimination diet, caution is warranted for underweight individuals. A final word of caution involves ensuring that there is an appropriate diagnosis of GI intolerance symptoms that might result from an abnormality of the gastrointestinal tract (partial bowel obstruction, narrowing or stricture), as a low-FODMAP diet would be inappropriate and potentially harmful in that situation. The real cause of symptoms must be properly addressed and treated.

The goal of a low-FODMAP diet in IBD would be to reduce symptoms of cramping, gas and bloating. It is not intended to treat or cure the disease. Supervision by a registered dietitian familiar with the low-FODMAP diet is critical, to ensure an individualized approach that works toward the most liberal and varied diet that can be tolerated, particularly since the information available regarding the FODMAP content of various foods is constantly developing and changing.

Lactose-Restricted Diets

Is there ever a time when it may be appropriate to reduce consumption of or avoid a particular food group? When it comes to dairy products, the answer is yes. While dairy products are tasty and provide important nutrients, such as protein and calcium, there are specific situations in which it may be difficult to digest lactose, the primary sugar in milk.

Unless you have a true milk allergy (an immune reaction to the protein in milk), there is no danger of worsening your IBD by eating dairy products. However, if you have lactose intolerance, dairy products will often result in gas, bloating, cramps and diarrhea without necessarily worsening the inflammation in your intestine. Whereas lactose intolerance is relatively common, true milk protein allergy is relatively uncommon.

Lactase Deficiency

Lactose is the principal carbohydrate in dairy products. It is a disaccharide, meaning that it is a larger molecule made up of two smaller sugar molecules, which are the monosaccharides glucose and galactose. An enzyme in the small intestine called lactase is responsible for breaking lactose into glucose and galactose, which are then easily absorbed.

If the body does not have enough of the lactase enzyme available to break down lactose into its two smaller sugars, undigested lactose travels through the small intestine to the large intestine, drawing water by osmosis into the bowel, which causes bloating. This is why lactose intolerance can also be correctly called lactase deficiency.

Symptoms of Lactose Intolerance

When undigested lactose reaches the colon, bacteria ferment it, producing further bloating, cramping, gas and diarrhea. Symptoms vary among individuals, but typically appear within 30 minutes to several hours after ingestion.

Testing for Lactose Intolerance

A breath hydrogen test, which involves drinking a test dose of lactose, can help determine whether you are lactose intolerant. If you have lactase deficiency, the unabsorbed lactose will be fermented by colonic bacteria and hydrogen gas will be formed. Some of this hydrogen gas is absorbed into your bloodstream and breathed out through your lungs, where it can be measured in your breath.

If you have a breath hydrogen test, be sure to ask what dose of lactose you were tested with. Depending on the lab, doses can range anywhere from 12.5 grams of lactose (equivalent to 1 cup or 250 mL of milk) to 50 grams of lactose (equivalent to 4 cups or 1 L of milk). Many people can drink one glass of milk without difficulty, but would rarely drink a quart or liter of milk at one time, so the relevance of the test (in terms of how applicable it is to your daily life) depends on the dose administered.

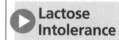

Lactose Intolerance

Dairy products do not cause IBD and generally do not result in flares, but you may experience uncomfortable symptoms if you have lactose intolerance and you drink milk or eat dairy products. "Lactose intolerance" means your body cannot adequately digest the milk sugar lactose.

Q | **What if I have an ileostomy?**

 A | If you have an ileostomy and are lactose intolerant, you can still eat dairy products. The undigested lactose will reach the ileostomy pouch instead of being fermented in the colon (which may have been surgically removed). The ileostomy pouch may develop more gas from the bacteria in the stool, but you will not experience the symptoms of cramping, bloating and diarrhea.

Q How do I know if I might be susceptible to lactose intolerance?

A There are at least two possible factors involved in causing lactose intolerance: genetics (primary lactase deficiency) and external factors (secondary lactase deficiency).

Primary Lactase Deficiency

The most common cause of lactose intolerance in adults has to do with genetics. There is a natural decline in lactase production as we age (a genetically determined rate). This decline in the amount of lactase present on the surface of the small bowel leads to progressive lactose intolerance.

Although everyone experiences a decrease in lactase production over their lifetime, the rate at which this occurs is different for different ethnic groups. Certain ethnic groups have a genetic predisposition to lactase deficiency, including individuals of African, Jewish and Asian descent. Conversely, individuals of Scandinavian and Northern European descent have the lowest prevalence of lactose intolerance. North Americans of similar ancestry have demonstrated similar prevalence rates.

Secondary Lactase Deficiency

External factors can sometimes result in a deficiency in the amount of lactase available on the surface of the small bowel. This deficiency may occur following medical treatment (for example, chemotherapy, radiation or multiple small bowel resections) or as a result of malnutrition or active disease of the small intestine, such as Crohn's disease. Once the disease or injury resolves, lactase production resumes and digestion of lactose improves.

Reducing Dairy Products

Fortunately, many individuals who develop lactose intolerance can still consume small amounts of dairy, just not as much as before. This is called a dose-dependent effect. In these cases, it is not necessary to eliminate dairy products, just to reduce the amount consumed at one time. Interestingly, some people can gradually increase their tolerance to dairy products. This has nothing to do with the amount of lactase enzyme they have; rather, their gastrointestinal bacteria are able to adapt to the lactose load without causing increased symptoms. Improved tolerance may also be experienced if lactose-containing foods are consumed with other foods. Lactose-reduced and lactose-free products may be better tolerated. The goals should be to ensure that important sources of nutrients important for bone health are met.

LACTOSE LADDER

This table lists dairy products and their lactose content. You can start climbing from the bottom (foods with the lowest amount of lactose) and make your way as far up to the top (foods with higher amounts of lactose) as you can tolerate.

Source	Serving size	Lactose
Skim milk	1 cup (250 mL)	13.3 g
2% milk	1 cup (250 mL)	11.6 g
Yogurt (with probiotics to reduce lactose)	½ cup (125 mL)	6.3–9.5 g
Ice cream	½ cup (125 mL)	4.9 g
Cottage cheese	½ cup (125 mL)	2.9–3.9 g
Cream cheese	1 oz (30 g)	0.7 g
Cream (whipping, half-and-half)	1 tbsp (15 mL)	0.6 g
Dry curd cottage cheese	½ cup (125 mL)	0.5 g
Cheese (Cheddar, Gouda, blue, Colby)	1 oz (30 g)	0.5–0.8 g
Parmesan cheese	1 tbsp (15 mL) grated	0.2 g
Cheese (Camembert, Limburger)	1 oz (30 g)	0.1 g
Butter	1 tsp (5 mL)	Trace

Hidden Sources of Lactose

If you are severely lactose intolerant, you will need to avoid all sources of lactose, including hidden sources. Lactose can be added as a filler in some medications and some foods (for example, processed meats, gravies, breads, cereals, salad dressings, breakfast drinks, cake mixes and margarine). Lactose may also be present if the label lists added milk solids, whey, curds, butter or cheese flavor. Casein does not contain lactose.

Calcium Sources and Supplements

You may limit dairy because of lactose intolerance or avoid it entirely for other reasons, such as allergy, taste, ethics, or cultural and religious traditions. Regardless of the reason, the challenge lies in getting the key nutrients provided by this food group in other ways. If you choose to restrict dairy products in your diet, you will need to consider increasing your calcium (and, perhaps, vitamin D) intake from other sources to prevent bone loss (osteopenia) and development of osteoporosis.

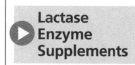

Lactase Enzyme Supplements

Commercial lactase supplements supply the body with the enzyme needed to break down lactose, allowing people with lactose intolerance to continue consuming dairy foods. These products are available as tablets, to be taken with meals, or as liquid drops, to be added to dairy products in advance of ingesting them.

Q Should I try reducing or avoiding lactose if I have IBD?

A Controversy exists regarding the clinical prevalence of secondary lactase deficiency in IBD, because lactose intolerance studies have not always taken into account age or ethnicity (factors we know affect the amount of lactase enzyme). Lactose intolerance *may* be more common in people with IBD, but this has not been definitively proven. Doctors will often ask an individual to restrict dairy temporarily to determine how the disease is responding to treatment and to prevent misdiagnosis of any lactose intolerance symptoms, such as bloating, cramping and diarrhea, as symptoms of disease activity.

If your symptoms improve while you're avoiding lactose, then a temporary restriction is right for you. If not, do not restrict dairy unnecessarily. When your flare improves, it is worthwhile to once more increase dairy in your diet, especially if you tolerated dairy products before your flare or if you miss eating dairy.

Q How do I know if I am getting enough calcium and vitamin D?

A Recommended amounts (known as Dietary Reference Intakes, or DRIs) for nutrients are based on age and gender. For adults, the DRI for calcium is generally 1,000 to 1,300 milligrams per day depending on your age, gender, if you are pregnant, if you have osteoporosis, or if you have any condition that affects metabolism or absorption of calcium and vitamin D (check with your health-care team to find the specific amount recommended for you). In 2010, the Food and Nutrition Board at the Institute of Medicine (IOM), which is the health arm of the National Academy of Sciences, published revised recommendations for the amount of recommended calcium intake. In clinical practice, doctors advise amounts that also take bone health and medication use (e.g., steroids) into consideration.

Lactose-free products (milk, yogurt, ice cream) will contain the same amount of calcium (and the same amount of vitamin D in the case of milk) as their lactose-containing versions (only the lactose content has changed). The absorption of calcium from plant-based sources is reduced due to compounds called oxalates (found in dark green leafy vegetables, such as spinach and beet greens) and phytates (found in whole grains, nuts, seeds and legumes). The oxalates and phytates in these foods bind to minerals, such as calcium, thus interfering with absorption.

If you suspect you are not meeting the recommended amounts for calcium or vitamin D, consult with your doctor or a registered dietitian.

DAIRY SOURCES OF CALCIUM

It is recommended that adults consume two to four servings of milk products per day, or 1,000 to 1,200 mg of calcium. This table lists common lactose-containing sources of calcium (milligrams of calcium rounded), approximated to typical serving sizes.

Source	Serving	Calcium
Cow's milk (skim, 1%, 2%, whole, chocolate, buttermilk) and goat's milk	1 cup (250 mL)	285–330 mg
Evaporated milk, partly skimmed	1/2 cup (125 mL)	350 mg
Powdered milk	6 tbsp (90 mL) dry	320 mg
Cream soup (made with milk)	1 cup (250 mL)	175–190 mg
Pudding (made with milk)	1/2 cup (125 mL)	105–165 mg
Yogurt (plain or flavored, or fruit bottom)	3/4 cup (175 mL)	215–325 mg
Yogurt drink	3/4 cup (175 mL)	185 mg
Frozen yogurt	1/2 cup (125 mL)	150 mg
Ice cream or ice milk	1/2 cup (125 mL)	80–90 mg
Sour cream (non-fat)	1/2 cup (125 mL)	225 mg
Cottage cheese (1% or 2%)	1/2 cup (125 mL)	70–85 mg
Processed cheese: thin slice thick slice	2 slices (42 g) 2 slices (62 g)	255 mg 385 mg
Cheese (soft) Brie Camembert Ricotta (part skim)	 50 g (1- by 1- by 3-inch piece) 50 g 1/2 cup (125 mL)	 90 mg 195 mg 340 mg
Cheese (hard) Parmesan Cheddar, Gouda, Colby, Edam, brick, Swiss Feta Mozzarella	 3 tbsp (45 mL) grated 50 g 50 g 50 g	 260 mg 350–480 mg 255 mg 270 mg

ALTERNATIVE FOOD SOURCES OF CALCIUM

If you are restricting dairy food, consider adding these alternative sources of calcium (milligrams of calcium rounded) to your diet to improve your calcium intake.

Source	Serving	Calcium
Fortified soy milk*	1 cup (250 mL)	300 mg
Fortified orange juice	1 cup (250 mL)	300 mg
Orange	1 medium	50 mg
Fortified rice beverage	1 cup (250 mL)	300 mg
Fortified plant-based beverages, such as almond, rice or cashew milk**	1 cup (250 mL)	***
Tofu (soft) set with calcium sulphate	1/3 cup (100 g)	150 mg***
Nuts and seeds Almonds Brazil nuts (dried) Sesame seeds (whole dried)	1 oz (24 nuts) 1 oz (8 medium nuts) 1 tbsp (15 mL)	75 mg 50 mg 88 mg
Legumes (cooked) Baked or refried beans Chickpeas Red kidney beans Navy, white, soybeans	1 cup (250 mL) 1 cup (250 mL) 1 cup (250 mL) 1 cup (250 mL)	130–165 mg 85 mg 50 mg 90–200 mg
Vegetables (cooked) Spinach Broccoli Bok choy, kale, Swiss chard Collard greens	1/2 cup (125 mL) 1/2 cup (125 mL) 1/2 cup (125 mL) 1/2 cup (125 mL)	130 mg 40–50 mg 50–105 mg 180 mg
Pink or sockeye salmon (with bones)	1/2 can (2/3 cup/105 g)	225–240 mg
Sardines (with bones)	1/2 can (4 pieces/55 g)	200 mg
Blackstrap molasses	1 tsp (5 mL)	60 mg
Figs	6 dried	150 mg

* Absorption of calcium may be slightly less than cow's milk.

** Nut beverages do not contain the same nutrients as cow's milk (e.g., they are lower in protein).

*** Amounts vary; check the label.

Vitamin D Sources and Supplements

Vitamin D helps your body absorb calcium. Interestingly, vitamin D is a hormone that our bodies make when sunlight shines on our skin (sunlight provides ultraviolet radiation for the body to convert vitamin D to an active form).

In northern latitudes of North America and Europe, the reduced sunshine and angle of the sun in winter months results in less vitamin D being manufactured by the skin. Similarly, people with dark skin (more pigmentation), those who are housebound or institutionalized and those who wear sunscreen at all times when outdoors are at risk of not getting enough vitamin D. Generally speaking, if you get 10 to 15 minutes of sunlight exposure (face, arms, hands), without sunscreen, twice a week, you are probably getting enough vitamin D. Your geographic location, the time of year, your age and your skin color can influence this estimate. The combination of sun exposure, food sources and supplements is thought to allow most North Americans to meet their vitamin D needs.

The importance of vitamin D relates to its well-established positive role with respect to building and maintaining healthy bones. Vitamin D has also recently been evaluated for its possible use in protecting against other chronic diseases including cancer, cardiovascular disease and diabetes; however, there has been not been enough evidence so far to be certain that a higher intake of vitamin D will protect against developing these conditions.

In 2010 the Food and Nutrition Board at the Institute of Medicine published revised recommendations for the amount of recommended vitamin D intake. In its report, commissioned by the Canadian and U.S. governments, the Daily Recommended Intake (DRI) for vitamin D for adults was raised from 200 IU up to 600 IU to 800 IU, depending on age and sex (e.g., higher amount recommended for high-risk groups such as the elderly). There has been considerable discussion following the publication of these guidelines and some public health organizations (e.g., Canadian Cancer Society, Canadian Paediatric Society and Osteoporosis Canada) have maintained recommendations for increased doses of vitamin D, anywhere from 800 to 2,000 IU per day.

Check with your health-care team to find the specific amount recommended for you. In clinical practice, doctors recommend amounts that also take bone health and medication use (e.g., steroids) into consideration.

Because of these factors that interfere with our ability to get enough, select items in our food supply are fortified with vitamin D. Milk is almost always fortified with vitamin D, but

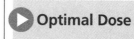

Optimal Dose

Scientific evidence now suggests that for some high-risk groups, such as the elderly, the optimal intake of vitamin D is higher than the current DRI of 200 IU. In fact, some scientists and North American osteoporosis societies recommend intakes of 800 to 2,000 IU per day.

not all dairy products are good sources. For instance, cottage cheese is not made from fortified milk, so it does not provide vitamin D. Some food manufacturers are starting to use vitamin D–fortified milk for yogurt, and they are adding vitamin D to other products, so check labels.

SOURCES OF VITAMIN D

Source	Serving	Vitamin D
Cow's milk	1 cup (250 mL)	90–100 IU
Fortified soy or almond milk, coconut milk beverage or rice beverage	1 cup (250 mL)	90–100 IU*
Fortified orange juice	1 cup (250 mL)	100 IU
Fortified margarine	1 tbsp (15 mL)	60 IU
Salmon (cooked)	3.5 oz (105 g)	360 IU
Sardines (canned)	1.75 oz (55 g)	250 IU
Tuna (canned)	3 oz (90 g)	200 IU
Egg yolk	1	20–25 IU
Cod liver oil**	1 tbsp (15 mL)	1,400 IU
Vitamin D_3–fortified tofu	3 oz	80 IU
Yogurt (made from vitamin D–fortified milk)	6 oz	80–200 IU
Vitamin D–enhanced mushrooms (wild or ultraviolet light irradiated)	Optimal levels of fortification currently under development in North America	

* Amounts vary; check the label.
** Avoid this source — it may contain contaminants, as well as high levels of vitamin A, which can weaken bones.

Low-Fiber Diets

Dietitians and physicians usually recommend increasing fiber in the diet for overall good health. Fiber is the structural part of plants (vegetables, fruits, grains and legumes).

Human digestive enzymes cannot break down fiber; however, some bacteria in the gastrointestinal tract can. Some dietary fiber can be fermented by colonic bacteria to produce short-chain fatty acids (SCFAs), which, once absorbed, provide the body with energy (used specifically by the cells that line the intestine and liver).

Soluble and Non-Soluble Fiber

Fiber is commonly classified as insoluble or soluble, according to its ability to dissolve in fluid. Insoluble fiber is best known for bulking up stool and relieving constipation. It increases the fecal weight and speeds up the passage of material through the intestines. Soluble fiber slows stomach emptying and passage of material through the intestines, helping to form, or gel, loose bowel movements. Both kinds of fiber slow the breakdown of starch, thus slowing glucose absorption into the bloodstream. Both create a full feeling, and both contribute to gas production (and thus need to be introduced and increased gradually in the diet).

Despite these clear health benefits, doctors and dietitians may ask IBD patients to limit fiber to decrease gastrointestinal intolerance symptoms from a flare or from a change in the normal anatomy after surgery. The priority when you have an IBD flare is to recover, return to better health and have improved quality of life. These goals may require adjusting or reducing fiber intake. Fiber-restricted diets are intended to be only a short-term strategy.

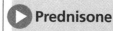 **Prednisone**

Adults on prednisone may be advised to take 1,500 mg of calcium and at least 800 IU of vitamin D a day. Vitamin D at much higher amounts can potentially lead to significant health problems, so it is important to discuss any supplementation with your physician.

Benefits of Fiber

Fiber may help manage weight gain and control blood sugar in diabetes, manage diverticulosis, reduce cholesterol and protect against some kinds of cancers.

Q Why might I need to adjust the amount of fiber in my diet?

A Both insoluble and soluble fiber are good for you, but if you are looking to reduce bowel movement frequency and thicken stool consistency, you will probably want to slowly increase your intake of soluble fiber. To avoid increased bowel movements (such as during a disease flare) and reduce stool volume, try limiting sources of insoluble fiber.

Low Residue

In clinical practice, the term "low residue" has been historically used to mean a low-fiber diet, or one that limits foods known to increase the amount of undigested food matter and the amount of stool produced. The definition of low residue is not well supported by evidence and, as such, clinicians now refer to a low-fiber diet. Low-fiber diets do allow some soluble fiber for its desirable functional effects, but limit insoluble fiber and foods that could potentially contribute to more stool production and food-related obstructions.

Low-Fiber Diet

A low-fiber diet allows some soluble fiber content but limits insoluble fiber and foods that could contribute to food-related obstructions. In clinical practice, a low-fiber diet restricts foods that increase the amount of undigested food matter and therefore the amount of stool produced. The goal is for you to return to a regular diet once your disease and symptoms have improved. In the meantime, be sure to plan meals in advance so that acceptable options are available when you are hungry.

SOURCES OF FIBER

Insoluble Fiber	Soluble Fiber
• Brown and wild rice • Membranes of fruits and vegetables (oranges, grapefruit) • Seeds of fruits and vegetables (kiwi, oranges, eggplant, field cucumbers, tomatoes) • Skins of fruits and vegetables (peppers, eggplant, tomatoes, corn, apples) • Whole-grain whole wheat breads and cereals • Whole white wheat flour (contains the bran and germ and thus the same fiber as whole wheat, but looks like refined flour)	• Banana flakes • Barley • Legumes (chickpeas, kidney beans, lentils with outer skin peeled) • Methylcellulose (Citrucel) • Oatmeal and oat bran • Pectin • Psyllium fiber (powder, biscuit or capsule, including Metamucil, Prodiem and generic brands) • Pulp of fruits (orange and grapefruit flesh, applesauce, bananas) • Tapioca • Vegetables (okra) • Chia seeds (Salba)

FOOD LABEL CAUTION

Be sure to read labels when choosing products for fiber content. For example, if a food product lists bran as a component, it is likely wheat bran, a source of insoluble fiber; however, if the product specifies oat bran, it is a source of soluble fiber.

For example, one cereal that contains bran buds with psyllium advertises one of the highest sources of fiber per serving. The label also lists "psyllium fiber," which would lead one to think the cereal is a high source of psyllium, and thus soluble fiber. Soluble fiber is good, right? The problem is that while each serving packs 3 grams of soluble fiber, it also packs a whopping 9.7 grams of insoluble fiber. If you read the ingredients list, wheat bran is the first listed ingredient, meaning that it constitutes the largest proportion of ingredients in the product.

As a source of insoluble fiber, wheat bran will promote the opposite effect you are looking for from the soluble fiber content.

Q **How can I increase soluble fiber in my diet?**

A To include more soluble fiber in your diet, try adding oat bran to moist foods, such as yogurt, pudding, sauces (e.g., spaghetti sauce) and thick-texture or puréed soups, as well as to baked goods (breads, muffins or cookies) and cereal (alongside hot cereal are many cold oat and oat-bran-containing varieties). You can even mix in oat bran when cooking your oatmeal. The same strategies work for ground chia seeds. Add chickpeas or lentils to a casserole, or include kidney beans in a stew (pinch off the clear "skin" to reduce insoluble fiber). Hummus is another good example of a healthy food option to include. Some fruits, such as avocado or the pulp of oranges, naturally contain higher amounts of soluble fiber. You can substitute applesauce for oil in a muffin recipe (this will also lower the fat). Add barley to soup, or make split pea soup. Slice bananas into Jell-O or yogurt for dessert. There are many ways to include soluble fiber in the meals you are already eating. Just be creative.

Stricture Diet

There are times when a low-fiber diet needs to be followed over a longer period of time, particularly when you have narrowing of the bowel due to scar tissue or stricturing of the intestine. In these cases, the bowels must push hard to pass undigested food matter through the narrowed area, causing cramping, pain and, in some cases, abdominal bloating and nausea.

The bowel can also be narrowed by inflammation from active Crohn's disease and bowel-wall swelling following surgery. The swelling usually decreases with treatment or time, and the bowel returns to normal. Unfortunately, scar tissue typically remains, despite treatment with medication. In that case, the narrowing is permanent unless it is surgically removed or corrected.

High Stool Output Management Diets

Sometimes, modifying fiber intake isn't enough to slow down bowel movements. This can be the case during a flare or following multiple bowel resections, if you have a high-output stoma (usually one in the upper part of the small intestine) or if you have a pelvic pouch for ulcerative colitis. It is then appropriate to try another dietary strategy, provided you are receiving appropriate medical treatment for your condition.

There are many dietary strategies that can help slow stool frequency and increase stool consistency (see table, pages 89–90). When making changes, try one strategy at a time, for a few days at a time. That way, if there is any benefit, you know what is responsible. Conversely, if you experience no positive effect from the change, you can resume your usual intake and try another strategy. Be sure to consult with your doctor or a dietitian while trying these strategies.

Anti-diarrheal Medications

Anti-diarrheal medications, such as Imodium, Lomotil and codeine phosphate, can provide some relief and help you regain better quality of life if you are experiencing high stool output. For instance, if you are unable to sleep through the night due to high stool outputs, you can use medication on a temporary basis to reduce bowel movement frequency so you can sleep a little longer. Sleeping better may, in turn, help you cope better. In some instances, particularly in people who have had the ileum (last part of the small intestine) removed surgically, cholestyramine can be very effective at improving stool consistency and frequency.

Challenges of a Low-Fiber Diet

Sticking to a low-fiber diet over an extended period brings unique challenges in terms of ensuring that vitamins, minerals and trace elements are adequate considering the many restrictions to the fruits and vegetables food group. The key is to rely on fruits and vegetables that are canned, well cooked, squeezed into juices or puréed and strained. A multivitamin and mineral supplement is sometimes needed.

DIETARY STRATEGIES TO SLOW HIGH STOOL OUTPUT

Modification	Explanations, Tips and Examples
Increase soluble fiber.	• Some people experience the most benefit from including soluble fiber at mealtime (not between meals).
Include foods known to thicken stool.	• These include applesauce (including fruit-flavored varieties), cheese, cheesecake, smooth nut butters (peanut butter, almond butter, cashew butter), pretzels, potato chips, soft cooked white rice* (especially sticky rice such as Arborio), tapioca, unleavened bread products (matzo, water crackers, flatbreads), foods containing gelatin (Jell-O, marshmallows).
Restrict lactose.	• If you reduce or eliminate lactose, be sure to consume alternative calcium sources. • Try commercial lactase enzyme products.
Reduce fat.	• Extensive ileal Crohn's disease or ileal resection of more than 3 feet (110 cm) disrupts absorption of fat and causes a greater loss of bile salts (normally reabsorbed in the ileum). • Try supplementing with MCT oil (available in specialty food shops), which is easily added to soups, beverages and salad dressings.
Reduce simple sugars.	• These are found in sweets (jams, jellies, honey, maple syrup), sweetened beverages (ice tea, fruit drinks, pop, soda, sports drinks, chocolate milk) and sweeteners, such as agave syrup and coconut sugar. • Dilute concentrated sugar sources, such as fruit juices, and sip slowly.
Reduce fructose.	• Fructose is a monosaccharide found naturally in fruits; it is also a component of high-fructose corn syrup, added to fruit drinks, soft drinks and baked goods, such as cookies. • Fructose can cause osmotic diarrhea at higher intakes (tolerance levels vary). • Fructose is fermented by bacteria in the colon, thus contributing to gas.
Reduce sugar alcohols.	• These nutritive sweeteners, found in hard candies, gum, mints, jams and jellies, have about half the calories of regular sugar. Examples include sorbitol, manitol, xylitol and hydrogenated starch hydrolysates. • Sugar alcohols are poorly absorbed and fermented in the colon, contributing to gas, cramping, bloating and diarrhea.
Try gas-reducing strategies.	• Gas is produced when fiber and residue from complex carbohydrates reach the colon.

Modification	Explanations, Tips and Examples
Try gas-reducing strategies *(continued)*.	• Plan regular snacks between meals (keep canned fruit with peel-back lids, granola bars or individually wrapped oat bran cookies in your car's glove compartment or in a desk drawer at work). • Pour carbonated beverages into a glass and let stand for 10 to 15 minutes to reduce the carbonation. • Try commercial enzyme products (Beano, Phazyme), which predigest fiber and residue without forming gas. • Avoid smoking, chewing gum and using straws. • Chew foods well.
Reduce caffeine and guarana.	• Caffeine sources include coffee (hot and cold drink varieties, e.g., iced cappuccino), canned cold coffee beverages and "refreshers," tea (including green tea), soft drinks (including dark colas and Mountain Dew), beer with added caffeine and chocolate. • Guarana seeds contain caffeine and other xanthines that stimulate bowel peristalsis. Beverages with caffeine and/or guarana include some varieties of beer and energy drinks.
Reduce alcohol.	• Beer, red wine and drinks mixed with carbonated beverages are particularly troublesome.
Modify spices and seasonings.	• Don't eliminate spices and seasonings altogether — they add flavor and keep food interesting. Instead, make some small modifications. For example, use ground pepper instead of whole peppercorns, and mild curry instead of hot.
Adjust meal sizes and timing.	• Eat three smaller meals and two to three snacks per day. • Make lunch your main meal. • Eat dinner early in the evening.
Separate solids from liquids.	• Consume solid food (e.g., a sandwich), then wait 30 to 45 minutes before consuming a beverage. • Small sips of fluid with solid food are okay.
Delay gastric emptying (provided the ileal brake mechanism is intact).	• Ileal brake is a feedback mechanism that helps slow the transit time of food through the bowel by regulating how quickly the stomach empties. • Ensure that fat and protein are components of each meal. • Focus on complex carbohydrates and include soluble fiber.

* The FDA recently identified concerns with inorganic arsenic content (found in some pesticides) in rice. Strategies to reduce risk include purchasing different varieties from different areas of the world, rinsing raw rice thoroughly prior to cooking, and using a ratio of 6 cups (1.5 L) water to 1 cup (250 mL) rice for cooking and draining the excess water afterward.

Fluid Diets

During a flare or for a short time following surgery, while you're experiencing obstructive symptoms, you may need to follow a fluid diet to relieve your symptoms by eliminating most indigestible food matter (also called residue). You might also be asked to follow a liquid diet if you have a fistula.

Even though you may not have much of an appetite under these conditions, you may find that you are able to drink fluids. However, while you're on a fluid diet, it can be difficult to consume enough calories to maintain your weight.

Clear Fluid Diet

Unfortunately, clear fluids are not a balanced source of nutrition. They are especially lacking in calories and protein. A clear fluid diet should generally be limited to no longer than several days. On this diet, you can easily develop taste fatigue and become bored with the lack of variety in texture, smell and taste.

Examples of clear fluids are strained vegetable or meat broths, tea, coffee, clear Popsicles, Jell-O, clear juices or cocktails (such as apple or cranberry), fruit punches and other sweetened drinks, soda pop and specially prepared nutritional products, such as Boost Fruit Flavored Beverage. Clear fluids flavored or sweetened with strained lemon juice, honey, sugar or artificial sweeteners are considered to be fine on this diet.

Full Fluid Diet

The full fluid diet is slightly more nutritious because of the addition of some dairy products or dairy alternatives, such as soy milk for lactose-intolerant individuals or vegans. Still, it is difficult to meet protein requirements on the full fluid diet. Supplementing with a protein powder may be a good idea if a full fluid diet is followed for a longer period of time.

Examples of full fluids are milk, cream, soy/almond/rice/coconut milk, strained hot cereals (oatmeal, cream of wheat), puddings, custard, ice cream, sorbet, gelato, strained cream soups, fruit juices, strained vegetable juices and nutritional products that are "creamier" in texture, such as Ensure, Boost, Resource and pharmacy house brands.

Synbiotic Diets

"Synbiotics" refers to both prebiotics and probiotics, which help maintain the health of intestinal bacteria and keep a sufficient number of "good" bacteria in the intestine. These good bacteria

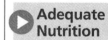

Adequate Nutrition

The challenge with fluid diets lies in getting enough nutrition, because most fluids are not balanced with adequate vitamins, minerals, protein and other essential nutrients.

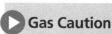

Gas Caution

To avoid gas and cramping, limit your intake of prebiotics to a few grams per day. When foods are fermented by bacteria in the intestine, gas is a normal by-product. But even though it is normal, gas may be uncomfortable and, in some situations, socially unacceptable.

may be important factors in maintaining an appropriate balance within the immune system and preventing or reducing the inflammation characteristic of IBD. There are food sources of both prebiotics and probiotics, but it is not known how much of these foods you should eat and how often you should eat them to experience benefit.

Prebiotics

Prebiotics, also known as fructo-oligosaccharides (FOS), can be found in everyday foods such as onions, bananas, tomatoes, honey, garlic, barley and wheat. These non-digestible carbohydrates are fermented by colonic bacteria. The process of fermentation provides energy for the growth of "good" bacteria, which, in turn, produce short-chain fatty acids, a fuel source for the cells lining the large intestine. Prebiotics also promote water and electrolyte reabsorption. Some food companies have been adding a prebiotic named inulin (a soluble fiber processed from chicory root) to foods such as dairy products, chocolate, and beverages. Interestingly, most soluble fibers, including psyllium fiber, are considered prebiotics, since they are fermented by bacteria in the intestine. Some of the health benefits of adding inulin, as compared with the benefits from the natural fiber in foods, are not as well supported in literature.

Probiotics

Probiotics are any number of different "good" live bacteria or yeasts that are administered by mouth, in a capsule or powder, in a drink or in food. The bacteria then establish themselves and grow within the intestine, a process called colonization. In adequate amounts, they are thought to provide immune system balance by down-regulating inflammation and may help to promote resistance against harmful strains of bacteria by improving the health of the inner lining of the intestine.

Examples of the most commonly used "families" of probiotic bacteria include *Lactobacillus* and *Bifidobacterium*. Within these families there are many, many particular species and strains of bacteria. A couple of examples of species (strains not specified) are *Lactobacillus acidophilus* and *Bifidobacterium lactis*. The different species, and the different strains within each species, may differ widely with respect to their protective or health promoting benefits. Probiotics are commonly found in yogurts to which active, or live, bacterial cultures have been added. Other examples include kefir (fermented milk drink) and tempeh (fermented soybean). Unfortunately, there is no standardization regarding the bacterial or yeast strains or the amount of bacterial colony forming units (CFUs) that are added. The manufacturers typically suggest that one should take an average dose above 100 million CFUs per day; however, suggested dosages should reflect those used in clinical studies.

To add to the complexity, invented names are sometimes used on package labels to market products — and they are not scientific names. Also, the term "live cultures" refers to live microorganisms added to foods for fermentation (a starter culture), while "probiotics" is meant to represent live microorganisms that provide a health benefit when ingested in adequate amounts.

To be sure you're getting as much live bacteria as possible, look for yogurts that "contain" active cultures, as compared to those that are "made with" active cultures. Live bacteria need to be kept refrigerated. Probiotics must also arrive alive in the gut, so they must be acid- and bile-resistant. A probiotic consumed in a food product will likely be less viable than one consumed in a capsule. A probiotic combined with a prebiotic may promote successful colonization in the bowel. Probiotics must also be taken regularly to maintain colonization.

Omega-3 Fatty Acids

The type of fat we eat is directly related to the fat that makes up our cells, which influences a cell's ability to produce eicosanoids and cytokines. These hormone-like compounds affect the body's immune response to injury and infection. By eating anti-inflammatory fats, we can encourage production of these anti-inflammatory mediators.

There are a number of different kinds of dietary fat, including trans fats, saturated fats, monounsaturated fats and the

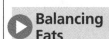

Balancing Fats

Omega-3 fats are anti-inflammatory, while omega-6 fats are pro-inflammatory. In the typical North American diet, the balance between these two essential fats is skewed; we generally consume too much omega-6 fat and not enough omega-3 fat.

essential polyunsaturated fats (omega-3 and omega-6 fatty acids). Two omega-3 fatty acids important in managing the inflammatory process are eicosapentanoic acid (EPA) and docosahexanoic acid (DHA).

Q How much omega-3 should I consume in a day?

A There is no official recommended intake for DHA and EPA, and the optimal amount of omega-3 in the diet has not yet been ascertained for people with IBD. Some experts advise those with cardiovascular disease to consume at least 500 to 1,000 milligrams of combined EPA and DHA per day, preferably from fatty fish. For the general public, some recommendations in the medical literature suggest an intake of 500 milligrams per day. This is in addition to the daily recommended intake of ALA (the World Health Organization and governmental health agencies of several countries recommend consuming 0.8 to 1.1 grams of alpha-linolenic acid daily).

To put this in perspective, one omega-3 egg has roughly 5 milligrams of EPA and 75 milligrams of DHA. Omega-3 milk has roughly 15 milligrams of DHA per cup (250 mL).

Again, to put this in perspective, 500 milligrams of EPA and DHA daily would be equivalent to 2 servings per week of fatty fish. One serving would be 2.5 oz or 75 grams or $\frac{1}{2}$ cup (125 mL). Rainbow trout is an excellent source, as one serving provides 300 milligrams of EPA and 600 milligrams of DHA (900 milligrams combined, easily meeting the American Heart Association recommendation for the general public).

Examples of ALA: One tablespoon (15 mL) of ground flax seeds would provide 1,200 milligrams ALA; 1 teaspoon (5 mL) of walnut oil provides 470 milligrams; 5 walnut halves provide 900 milligrams; and 1 tablespoon (15 mL) of chia seeds provides between 1,200 and 1,800 milligrams. Be sure to consult your doctor before supplementing your diet with omega-3 fatty acids.

Marine sources of omega-3 (e.g., fatty fish) are the best sources of EPA and DHA, the form most easily used by the body, while alpha-linolenic acid (ALA) from plant sources is only partially converted by the body to EPA and DHA. While it is important to aim to consume recommended amounts of each type of fat, it is still considered worthwhile to include plant sources of omega-3 along with marine sources, as this can better balance the ratio of omega-6 fatty acids in the diet.

SOURCES OF ESSENTIAL FATTY ACIDS (OMEGA-3 AND OMEGA-6)

Omega-3 (ALA, EPA and DHA)	Omega-6 (linoleic acid)
• Canola oil • Ground flaxseed[1] or flaxseed oil • Walnuts or walnut oil • Chia seeds (Salba) • Shelled hemp seeds • Fish oil[2] • Algae oil[3] • Krill (a shrimp-like crustacean) oil • Cold-water fatty fish: salmon, tuna,[4] trout, mackerel, anchovy, sardines, sturgeon, bluefish, mullet, herring (menhaden), Arctic char, Chilean sea bass • Functional foods: omega-3 eggs, DHA milk, cheese, yogurt, margarine, organic grain cereals (some of these foods contain only marginally higher amounts)[5]	• Corn oil • Cottonseed oil • Safflower oil • Sunflower oil • Soybean oil[6] • Processed foods and commercial baked goods

[1] Ground flaxseed can be added to baked goods and to moist foods such as yogurt, applesauce, smoothies and sauces.

[2] Fish oil supplements are often made from fish skin and liver and may contain environmental contaminants. Check the ingredients lists. Some companies now process from the fish body or choose small fish like sardines or anchovies to avoid contaminants in an unrefined supplement. Other companies remove heavy metal contaminants (mercury, cadmium, lead) and/or polychlorinated biphenyls (PCBs) during their production process. Look for products that provide information regarding testing results for environmental contaminants.

[3] Likely to contain only DHA (not EPA).

[4] To reduce mercury consumption, choose canned "light" tuna over canned albacore (white) tuna. The light tuna is produced from smaller tuna species that have not accumulated as many heavy metal contaminants as larger tuna species.

[5] While there is no universally accepted definition of a functional food, they are usually considered to be conventional foods (fish, for example) or those similar in appearance to conventional foods (omega-3 eggs, for example) that are part of a usual diet and that demonstrate a physiological health benefit.

[6] Soybean oil is considered a source of omega-6; however, soybeans and tofu do provide some ALA.

Diet Counseling

While there is no standard diet for IBD, diet modifications can help with symptom management. These modifications need to be individualized to match your condition. Diet restrictions are usually temporary measures during times of disease activity or post-operative recovery periods.

Any diet modifications should be discussed with your doctor or dietitian. The changes you make must be practical and realistic, while taking into account individual considerations of food preferences, tolerances, allergies and phobias; religious, ethnic and cultural customs and beliefs; lifestyle and activity level; and employment and finances.

Diet modifications aren't just about changing one or more elements of your diet; they are personalized recommendations that work for you as an individual living with IBD. Through diet counseling, your doctor or dietitian can help you create the dietary strategy that will work best for you.

Part 3

IBD-Friendly Meal Plans and Recipes

Introduction to the Meal Plans

Meal plans can be a helpful tool for those of you who are newly diagnosed with IBD and are unfamiliar with what diet modifications you need to make to manage your symptoms. They give you a set course of action, allowing you time to adjust to a challenging change in your life without the added pressure of trying to figure out what meals to prepare on a daily basis. They may also come in handy if the course of your illness is changing and eating is difficult for you. And meal plans provide easy-to-follow guidelines for family and friends who want to support you by preparing nutritious foods for you during times of illness.

Meal plans can also simply be a useful starting point, giving you ideas, reinforcing what foods and recipes are appropriate for your diet and providing you with a framework within which to reintroduce or try new foods, minimizing hesitation or fear. In addition, they allow you to plan in advance to ensure that you have appropriate food choices on hand for times when you feel fatigued or overwhelmed by your illness.

It is challenging to create a definitive IBD meal plan because every IBD patient is unique, with a different combination of disease location, symptoms, complications and medications. There is no one "IBD diet." In addition, of course, the meal plans in this book (pages 106–109) are not individualized to your personal taste preferences, food allergies, tolerances and intolerances, ethnic or religious considerations, cooking capabilities or budget. If you are looking for a meal plan tailored specifically to you, a nutrition professional, such as a registered dietitian, can help you create one that will not only reflect all of your needs and preferences, but will also help you meet the following diet modification goals, if appropriate for your situation:

- Normalizing bowel function
- Managing intolerance symptoms
- Minimizing obstruction risk
- Improving hydration and electrolyte balance
- Improving nutritional status

- Achieving realistic weight goals
- Targeting specific nutrients, if necessary
- Normalizing the diet as much as possible to promote enjoyment of eating, thus improving your relationship with food

The goal of a nutrition professional is not to choose foods and prescribe a diet for you, but rather to teach you what you need to know to make your own food decisions, ensuring that you are armed with enough information to make healthy food choices and, where needed, to select appropriate substitutions. You will be encouraged to trust your own judgment in creating a meal plan that will work with your tolerances and lifestyle. This approach empowers you when you are away from home and eating in a new environment, and will boost your independence, confidence and meal enjoyment. The most useful meal plan is one that is individualized for your life with IBD.

Think of the two 7-day meal plans that follow as merely an example of one way to schedule meals and to begin planning a balanced approach to eating. Review and follow the USDA's MyPlate guidelines or Eating Well with Canada's Food Guide to help you balance servings of fruits, vegetables, protein, grains

TIPS FOR EATING WELL

- Plan your grocery list in advance to include the ingredients needed for the recipes you will be preparing, as well as the snacks you like.
- Read food labels when shopping and compare products to find those that are best suited to your individual needs.
- Transport, store and prepare your food in ways that prevent food-borne illness.
- Keep your pantry well stocked.
- Incorporate leftovers into new recipes.
- Prepare large batches, divide them into single-serving portions and freeze for future meals. (This approach will save you time in the kitchen and ensure that you have easy meals on hand for times when your energy level is low.)

and dairy to meet your recommended targets. In some instances, you may need to supplement the recipes suggested in the meal plans with choices from these groups. Whenever possible, at least three food groups should be represented at *each* meal or snack. This strategy ensures better nutrient variety and, in many cases, added calories and/or protein. If you are not trying to boost your calorie intake, reduce your portion sizes rather than limiting the variety of foods you eat.

The meal plans focus on recipes that can be prepared in advance, at times when you have more energy. Breads and muffins can be frozen, then thawed the night before you want to eat them, or warmed in the microwave when desired. Soups, slow cooker dishes and casseroles can be prepared in large batches, then frozen in single-serving portions. You will also find dishes made with pantry foods such as canned seafood, for ease of preparation.

Vegetables such as kale and pumpkin — which you might be reluctant to try — are included in the meal plans in recipes where they are puréed, to minimize any negative side effects on your digestion while maximizing your intake of antioxidants and nutrients. In addition, the meal plans include recipes made with gluten-free ingredients, alternative grains such as quinoa and teff, and higher-calorie foods such as omega-3-rich salmon and tuna, as well as cheese and nuts.

The meal plans feature a variety of meat, poultry, fish, vegetarian and vegan dishes, and many more choices from each category can be found in the recipe section of this book. Where necessary, the recipes provide modifications to help you follow a low-fiber diet and/or avoid difficult-to-digest foods, to minimize the risk of obstruction.

Beverages are generally not included in these meal plans, as recommendations for amounts and types of fluids vary widely based on individual needs. Plan to supplement the meal plans with fluids such as water, juice or diluted juice, dairy or non-dairy milk (e.g., cow's milk, goat's milk, soy milk, almond milk, rice milk, hemp milk), smoothies, soup, coffee, lattes, teas (black, green and herbal), ice cream, sherbet and Jell-O.

We hope the meal plans will inspire you to try new foods or flavor combinations, and will contribute positively to your relationship with food. Remember that every recipe suggestion is just that — a suggestion. You are encouraged to substitute in your own favorites, based on your experience with IBD.

MEAL PLAN HINTS AND TIPS

- All of the recipes suggested in the meal plans appear in the recipe section of this book.
- Unless otherwise indicated, the serving size is one serving. However, you should adjust the number of servings you eat to your individual requirements.
- The recipes have been selected because they are typically well tolerated by individuals living with IBD. Because of this criteria, however, on some days the milk and alternatives food group may be underrepresented, or the grain products or meat and alternatives food groups may be overrepresented. To meet your recommended targets and ensure that you are achieving a balanced diet, adjust portion sizes as needed for overrepresented food groups and supplement underrepresented groups with your own preferred foods from that group.
- Fruit or vegetable servings may be "hidden" *within* a food (e.g., Applesauce Snack Cakes or Pumpkin Pie Smoothie).
- Because the meal plans are designed entirely of recipes, you may miss your usual choices, such as a piece of fruit, yogurt, cold breakfast cereal, eggs, toast, sandwiches, pasta with sauce, roti — meals and snacks that are staples in your diet. Substitute these choices into the meal plans as desired.
- You may not always wish to eat three snacks per day. Adjust your snacking schedule to your personal needs.
- Some recipes are repeated during the week, enabling you to cook food just once and eat it at two or three meals (storage tips are provided with many of the recipes), reducing food preparation time and minimizing food wastage.
- Certain highly perishable ingredients (e.g., avocado, watermelon) are used in different recipes within a few days, again to minimize food wastage and grocery store visits.
- You can create variety in the meal plans in following weeks by subbing in similar recipes. For example, if eating a muffin as a snack worked well for you in Week 1, try a different muffin in Week 3.

WEEK 1 MEAL PLAN

	Monday	Tuesday	Wednesday
Breakfast	• 1–2 Oatmeal Quinoa Pancakes drizzled with maple syrup or honey	• 1–2 slices Ancient Grains Bread topped with Luscious Apple Butter	• Tofu English Muffin • Spiced Carrot
Morning snack	• Apple Walnut Muffin	• 1–2 Ginger Quinoa Crinkles	• Decadent Fruit Smoothie
Lunch	• Chicken and Asparagus Salad with Lemon Dill Vinaigrette • ½ cup (125 mL) cucumber slices dipped in Avocado Dressing	• 1–2 servings Pizza with Red Peppers and Goat Cheese	• 1–2 servings Slow Cooker Squash Couscous
Afternoon snack	• Pumpkin Pie Smoothie	• 1–2 servings Lighten-Up Guacamole and Chips	• 1–2 servings Hummus with Roasted Red Peppers with ½ cup (125 mL) cucumber slices
Dinner	• Crunchy Citrus Chicken • 1–2 servings Roasted Bell Peppers	• Scandinavian Pasta Salad • 1–2 servings Green and Yellow Salad	• Creamy Onion Soup with Kale • 1–2 servings Crispy Sweet Potato Cakes
Evening snack	• Cinnamon Baked Pears	• Almond Butter on ½ cup (125 mL) chopped fruit or mixed in ¾ cup (175 mL) yogurt	• Banana Applesauce Muffin

Thursday	Friday	Saturday	Sunday
• 1–2 Oatmeal Quinoa Pancakes topped with ¾ cup (175 mL) vanilla-flavored yogurt and ½ cup (125 mL) drained canned peach slices	• Cranberry, Carrot and Apple Teff Muffin	• 1–2 slices Oat Bran Banana Bread	• 1–2 slices Ancient Grains Bread topped with Almond Butter and ½ cup (125 mL) sliced banana
• Peanut Butter Marshmallow Treat	• Almond Butter on ½ cup (125 mL) chopped fruit or mixed in ¾ cup (175 mL) yogurt	• 1–2 Original Dad's Cookies	• Banana Applesauce Muffin
• Crazy Crunch Panini • Chilled Avocado Soup	• 1–2 servings Tangerine Salmon Salad	• Tuna and Olive Rotini	• Creamy Onion Soup with Kale (leftover from Wednesday dinner) • Bannock
• 1–2 Original Dad's Cookies	• Peanut Butter Marshmallow Treat	• 1–2 servings Hummus with Roasted Red Peppers with ½ cup (125 mL) cucumber slices	• Apple Walnut Muffin
• 1–2 servings Turkey Apple Meatloaf • Stewed Okra • Cauliflower au Gratin	• Old-Fashioned Tuna Noodle Casserole • 1–2 servings Butternut Squash with Maple Syrup	• Mac and Cheese with Tomatoes	• Meat Loaf "Muffins" (without the barbecue sauce) • Curried Squash Risotto with Apricots and Dates
• 1–2 Ginger Quinoa Crinkles	• Mexican Hot Chocolate	• Cranberry, Carrot and Apple Teff Muffins	• Oat Bran Banana Bread

WEEK 2 MEAL PLAN

	Monday	Tuesday	Wednesday
Breakfast	• 1–2 Banana Cinnamon Quinoa Waffles drizzled with maple syrup or honey	• Very Lemon Muffin	• Better-Than-Instant Oatmeal
Morning snack	• Almond Butter Muffin	• Maple Barley Pudding	• Luscious Apple Butter on $\frac{1}{2}$ cup (125 mL) chopped fruit or mixed in $\frac{3}{4}$ cup (175 mL) yogurt
Lunch	• Salmon Pizza Pinwheels	• Wedding Soup	• Pumpkin and White Bean Soup
Afternoon snack	• Pumpkin Pie Smoothie	• Applesauce Snack Cake	• 1–2 servings Hummus with Roasted Red Peppers with $\frac{1}{2}$ cup (125 mL) cucumber slices
Dinner	• Terrific Chicken Burger • 1–2 servings Ginger Carrots	• 1–2 servings Ham and Cheese Quesadillas • 1–2 servings Cucumber Watermelon Salad	• Sesame Noodles with Tofu • 1–2 servings Tangy Green Beans
Evening snack	• Applesauce Snack Cake	• Lemon Mousse	• Raspberry Tapioca Pudding

Thursday	Friday	Saturday	Sunday
• Low-Fat Hash Brown Casserole	• Very Lemon Muffin	• 1–2 Banana Cinnamon Quinoa Waffles topped with ¾ cup (175 mL) vanilla-flavored yogurt and ½ cup (125 mL) sliced banana	• Applesauce Snack Cake
• Tropical Cooler	• Almond Butter Muffin	• Peanut Butter Marshmallow Treat	• Decadent Fruit Smoothie
• 1–2 servings Smoked Turkey Toss	• Low-Fat Hash Brown Casserole (leftover from Wednesday breakfast)	• Spinach Frittata	• Wedding Soup (leftover from Tuesday lunch)
• Ancient Grains Chocolate Chip Cookie	• Strawberry Orange Flaxseed Smoothie	• Tuna and Cucumber Sushi Rolls	• Pumpkin Pie Tarts with Ground Almond Crust
• Turkey Cutlets in Savory Cranberry Gravy • 1–2 servings Beet and Feta Salad	• Open Sesame Salmon Burgers with 1–2 servings Sweet Potato Fries	• Tangy Meatless Lasagna • Pumpkin and White Bean Soup (leftover from Wednesday lunch)	• Layered Beef and Noodle Bake • 1–2 servings Honey-Glazed Carrots
• Pumpkin Pie Tarts with Ground Almond Crust	• Mexican Hot Chocolate	• Maple Barley Pudding	• Banana Cream Pudding

Introduction to the Recipes

With food and drink, we satisfy our feelings of hunger and thirst, explore and enjoy the taste of new or favorite foods, and nourish our bodies with needed calories and nutrients. Our diet helps us achieve a healthy body weight and metabolic balance, which, in turn, provide us with strength and energy to participate in daily activities.

For individuals managing active IBD, however, eating can be a real challenge. If you feel tired from anemia or rapid weight loss, it might be difficult to shop for and cook a meal. If you don't have an appetite or you feel nauseated, cooking smells likely make things worse. If you dread the cramping a meal brings on, it's hard to be patient with well-intentioned family members who try to get you to eat more. You may fear that if you eat a larger meal at night, you won't be able to get to a bathroom in time once you are asleep. To avoid revisiting unpleasant past experiences, you might be eating the same foods over and over again, tired of the repetition but afraid to move outside the comfort zone of foods you know you tolerate.

Living with IBD may not be easy, but if you challenge yourself to reconsider your meal options — even during times of difficulty — you will be making a positive move toward a more healthy relationship with food. Let your preferences and appetite guide you. What are you interested in tasting that you have not tried before? Is there a food you've avoided for a long time that you used to enjoy? It might be time to try that food again. If you're apprehensive, are you willing to try it in small amounts? What do you realistically have time or energy to make?

Remember that there is no one "IBD diet" for everyone, and that everyone will have individual experiences with different foods. The diet that considers and meets your unique requirements is the right diet for you.

Just be sure that you meet your nutritional needs when selecting foods. Follow standard dietary intake recommendations, such as those found in the United States Department of Agriculture (USDA) MyPlate guidelines or Eating Well with Canada's Food Guide (see pages 65–67). These scientifically based guides will help you meet nutrient needs by recommending the *amount* and *type* of food you need based on your age. They also promote healthy eating patterns that help reduce the risk of obesity and other chronic diseases, such as heart disease and osteoporosis. Challenge yourself at each meal to eat at least three of the four food groups. This will increase the variety of nutrients your body receives.

The recipes in this book have been chosen based on these food guidelines, our clinical experience and years of feedback from individuals living with IBD. Many include suggestions on how to modify ingredients to suit different disease scenarios. All include tags in the upper corner of the page that highlight key nutritional criteria (see page 112 for a guide to these tags). Before preparing a recipe, read these tags to make sure the recipe is appropriate for your condition, situation or stage of disease. Your doctor and registered dietitian can help you determine your specific requirements or restrictions.

These recipes are not "prescribed" for you to follow; rather, they represent options you might not have considered, new ways to combine flavors and textures, choices that will bring excitement and enjoyment back to eating. Think about your specific needs, then find the recipes that suit you. Having a few new options for great-tasting food is bound to be a welcome change for you — enjoy!

About the Nutritional Analysis

The nutrient analyses for the recipes in this book were based on:

- imperial measures and weights (except for food typically packaged and used in metric);
- the larger number of servings where there is a range;
- the smaller amount where there is a range;
- the first ingredient listed where there is a choice;
- the exclusion of "optional" ingredients; and
- the exclusion of ingredients with non-specified or "to taste" amounts.

All nutrient values have been rounded to the nearest whole number.

GUIDE TO RECIPE TAGS (Based on a per-serving analysis)

Tag	Meaning
Vegetarian choice	The recipe is appropriate for a vegetarian diet. Some recipes may include eggs, dairy or fish, so stricter vegetarians should review the ingredients list carefully.
Vegan choice	The recipe is appropriate for a vegan diet. All vegan recipes are also suitable for a vegetarian diet.
Higher-calorie choice	The recipe will help you increase calories, especially if your goal is to gain weight.
Lower-calorie choice	The recipe will help you limit calories, which may be important if your goal is to maintain or lose weight, especially if you're taking steroids (which can stimulate appetite, leading to unintended weight gain).
Lower-fat choice	The recipe will help you reduce fat in your diet. This may be important after significant ileal (small intestine) resection and/or when you are experiencing diarrhea.
Lower-fiber choice	The recipe will help you reduce the amount of fiber in your diet, particularly insoluble fiber, which you may need to target if have intestinal narrowing (stricturing) due to scar tissue or inflammation during a disease flare.
Higher-protein choice	The recipe will help you increase protein, which you may need to target following periods of undernutrition and weight loss or if you're taking high-dose steroids.
Lactose-free choice	The recipe does not contain the milk sugar lactose. (Note: you may not need to avoid lactose altogether, but merely to restrict the amount you consume at one time.)
Source of soluble fiber	The recipe contains one or more sources of soluble fiber, which helps form or thicken the consistency of stool through a "gelling" effect.
Source of potassium	The recipe contains one or more sources of potassium, which you may need to target during times of frequent loose stools or if you're taking certain types of medications (e.g., some diuretics or intravenous steroids).
Source of sodium	The recipe contains one or more sources of sodium (salt), which you may need to target during times of frequent loose stools.

Breakfasts, Breads and Muffins

Breakfast is a key meal. It is important to eat something at the start of the day, as this will boost your metabolism. Skipping meals may increase gas production and may lead to increased hunger at the next meal. As a result, you'll be more likely to eat quickly, chew food inadequately or overeat, which can leave you feeling bloated, distended or unwell and can increase the risk of obstruction. To encourage yourself to eat breakfast, find foods that work for you and keep them readily available in your kitchen.

Breads and quick breads make a great part of a healthy breakfast, but they're versatile enough to be incorporated into any meal. Bread can be leavened, using a fermenting agent such as baker's or brewer's yeast, or unleavened. Quick breads such as muffins, pancakes, waffles and biscuits are prepared with baking powder as a leavening agent. The breads and muffins in this chapter can help you meet the recommendations for the grain products food group.

Plan Ahead for a Speedy Breakfast

If mornings are difficult for you and you frequently skip breakfast, try planning ahead. The night before, set the table and assemble the makings of an easy breakfast:

- Measure oatmeal or oat bran into a bowl and add sugar or cinnamon, if desired. In the morning, just add water or milk and heat your cereal in the microwave.
- Boil an egg and refrigerate it until morning. Or, if you don't like your eggs cold, you can quickly cook an egg in your microwave. Break the egg into a microwave-safe bowl and break the yolk. Cover the bowl with microwave-safe plastic wrap and pierce the plastic with a fork to allow steam to vent. Microwave on High for about 1 minute, or until desired doneness. Let stand for a minute or two before removing the plastic wrap.
- Make Jell-O with canned fruit or sliced bananas, or prepare a bowl of yogurt layered with fruit and granola. Just remove the cover in the morning and enjoy!
- Prepare one of the delicious muffin recipes in this book and then tightly wrap each muffin in foil and freeze for up to 2 weeks. Remove a muffin to defrost overnight or, in the morning, simply heat one in the microwave.

Say No to Caffeine

Starting your morning with a caffeinated beverage may stimulate increased bowel movements, resulting in diarrhea. Instead, try warm water with a slice of lemon or ginger, warm milk or decaffeinated tea or coffee.

THE NUTRITIONAL VALUE OF BREAD

Bread supplies your body with carbohydrate, B vitamins (thiamin, riboflavin, niacin and folate), iron, zinc and magnesium, and is usually low in fat. It is typically made from a blend of hard wheat flours, water and salt. Sugar (in the form of molasses or honey) and fat (such as butter) may be added. Bread products made with unrefined whole-grain flour are rich in vitamins, minerals, fiber and phytonutrients. Refined wheat flour has lost many of these nutrients because the outer grain layers are removed during milling. In the United States and Canada, wheat flour is enriched, or fortified, with B vitamins and iron to compensate for these nutrient losses, but whole-grain products still offer more nutritional value.

Store-Bought Bread Options

Buying bread can be confusing when it comes to figuring out what all the different terms mean. Here's what you need to know to make the best choice for you.

- Wheat bread is any bread made from wheat.
- White bread is made from refined wheat flour, meaning the germ and bran have been removed from the grain, resulting in a loss of some nutrients and fiber. While some refined grains are later enriched with selected vitamins and minerals, they are still less nutritious than flour made from the whole grain.
- Whole wheat bread is made from red wheat and is darker in color than white bread, thanks to the inclusion of the bran. In the U.S., the term "whole wheat" means that the whole grain was used. However, in Canada, whole wheat flour may have much of the germ removed, so "100% whole wheat" does not necessarily mean whole grain; to ensure that you're buying bread made with the whole grain, look for the words "whole-grain whole wheat" on the label.
- Whole white wheat bread looks like white bread but is nutritionally similar to whole wheat bread. It is made from white wheat, which has a bran that is lighter in color and milder in flavor than red wheat. Because the whole grain is used, none of the vitamins, minerals and fiber are lost.
- Multigrain bread (a.k.a. 7-, 9-, 12- or 15-grain bread) is made from more than one kind of grain (wheat, oats, rye, barley, millet and so on). But these grains are not necessarily whole grains, so the bread may or may not be high in fiber.

Toasting bread can reduce the enriched vitamins (thiamin, riboflavin and niacin) by up to 20%.

Commercial whole wheat bread can be made with varying proportions of white and whole wheat flour. The label "contains whole grains" can be misleading, as it does not specify *how much* whole grain is added — and the amount may be insignificant. There is also no guarantee that the bread is high in fiber.

ADD GROUND FLAXSEED TO YOUR DIET

Ground flaxseed is a fantastic addition to breads, muffins and other baked goods, and is included in several of the recipes in this book. It is a plant source of omega-3 fat, which has anti-inflammatory properties. While marine sources provide omega-3s in the forms most easily used by the body, it is still worthwhile to include plant sources of omega-3 whenever possible. Flaxseeds must be ground to access their beneficial nutrients. Consider grinding your own with a coffee grinder, then store in the freezer to delay the onset of rancidity.

Low-Fat Hash Brown Casserole

Breakfast casseroles are often loaded with fat and calories. This recipe shaves the fat by using turkey bacon and low-fat dairy products in this creamy hash brown delight.

MAKES 6 SERVINGS

IBD Tips

- Boost calories in this recipe by selecting pork bacon instead of turkey bacon, regular cream of mushroom soup, regular-fat cheese and higher-fat sour cream.

- Potatoes provide the potassium in this recipe.

- Sodium sources in this recipe include turkey bacon, cream of mushroom soup, Cheddar cheese, added salt and possibly the hash browns (depending on the brand).

- Hard cheese, such as Cheddar, is known to help thicken stool. Buy cheese when it's on sale, shred it and store it in the freezer for when you need it.

- • 11- by 7-inch (28 by 18 cm) glass baking dish, greased

6	slices turkey bacon	6
2	cloves garlic, minced	2
1 cup	chopped onion	250 mL
2 lbs	frozen hash brown potatoes	1 kg
1	can (10 oz/284 mL) reduced-sodium, fat-free condensed cream of mushroom soup	1
1 cup	shredded reduced-fat extra-sharp (extra-old) Cheddar cheese, divided	250 mL
1/2 cup	chopped green onions	125 mL
1/2 cup	fat-free sour cream	125 mL
1/2 tsp	salt	2 mL
1/2 tsp	freshly ground black pepper	2 mL

1. In a large nonstick skillet, over medium-high heat, cook bacon, turning once, until crisp. Using tongs, transfer to a plate lined with paper towels. Let cool, then crumble.

2. Drain any fat from skillet and spray with cooking spray. Reduce heat to medium; sauté garlic and onion for 5 to 7 minutes or until softened. Stir in hash browns; reduce heat to low, cover and cook, stirring occasionally, for 15 minutes.

3. In a large bowl, combine crumbled bacon, soup, 1/4 cup (60 mL) of the cheese, green onions, sour cream, salt and pepper. Gently stir in hash brown mixture. Spoon into prepared baking dish and sprinkle with remaining cheese. Cover and refrigerate for at least 6 hours or overnight.

4. Preheat oven to 350°F (180°C). Bake, covered, for 45 minutes. Uncover and bake for 15 minutes or until golden brown.

Nutrients Per Serving	
Calories	536
Fat	28 g
Fiber	6 g
Protein	15 g
Carbohydrate	55 g

IF FOLLOWING A LOW-FIBER DIET AND AVOIDING DIFFICULT-TO-DIGEST FOODS…

Finely chop onions and green onions, finely grind the pepper, and purée the cream of mushroom soup, or use a soup without chunks of mushroom. Mushrooms are surprisingly hard to digest, and although those in canned soup are chopped into small pieces, they are a potential food obstruction.

Better-Than-Instant Oatmeal

3 cups	milk or soy beverage	750 mL
1 cup	quick-cooking rolled oats	250 mL
2 tbsp	packed brown sugar or pure maple syrup	30 mL
1 tbsp	ground flaxseed	15 mL
2 tsp	wheat germ, toasted	10 mL
1 tsp	margarine or butter	5 mL
1/2 tsp	ground cinnamon (optional)	2 mL
Pinch	salt	Pinch
1/3 cup	raisins or dried cranberries (optional)	75 mL
	Toasted chopped almonds, walnuts or pecans (optional)	

1. In a large saucepan, over medium-low heat, combine milk, oats, brown sugar, flaxseed, wheat germ, margarine, cinnamon (if using) and salt. Cook, stirring often, for 10 to 15 minutes or until thick and bubbly. Remove from heat and add raisins (if using); let stand for 2 minutes. Serve topped with nuts, if desired.

> **IF YOU ARE WELL...**
> If there is no medical reason for you to avoid fiber or difficult-to-digest foods, include the optional nuts and dried fruit.

MAKES 4 SERVINGS

IBD Tips

- Oats are high in soluble fiber and may help to thicken loose stool. Therefore, despite the increased fiber content, many low-fiber diets include oats and oat products.
- Cooking the oats in milk or soy beverage rather than water increases the calories and nutrient value.
- Margarine and butter are both fats; however, non-hydrogenated margarine is considered a healthier heart choice.
- To lower the insoluble fiber content, omit the wheat germ.
- To increase your sodium intake, add more than a pinch of salt.
- If you use soy beverage and margarine, this recipe will be lactose-free.

Nutrients Per Serving	
Calories	230
Fat	7 g
Fiber	3 g
Protein	10 g
Carbohydrate	32 g

Vegetarian choice

Lower-calorie choice

Lower-fat choice

Lower-fiber choice

Higher-protein choice

Oatmeal Pancakes

These tasty pancakes are so easy to make. Maple syrup or mixed berries on the side will make this a kid favorite.

6	egg whites	6
1 cup	old-fashioned rolled oats	250 mL
1 cup	fat-free cottage cheese	250 mL
2 tsp	granulated sugar	10 mL
1 tsp	ground cinnamon (optional)	5 mL
1 tsp	vanilla	5 mL
	Vegetable cooking spray	

MAKES ABOUT 12 PANCAKES (1 per serving)

IBD Tip

• Oats are high in soluble fiber and may help to thicken loose stool. Therefore, despite the increased fiber content, many low-fiber diets include oats and oat products.

1. In blender, on medium speed, blend egg whites, oats, cottage cheese, sugar, cinnamon (if using) and vanilla until smooth.

2. Heat a griddle or large nonstick skillet over medium-low heat. Spray lightly with vegetable cooking spray. For each pancake, pour $\frac{1}{4}$ cup (60 mL) batter onto griddle and cook until bubbly around the edges, about 2 minutes. Flip and cook until golden brown, about 2 minutes. Transfer to a plate and keep warm in a low oven. Repeat with remaining batter, spraying griddle with vegetable cooking spray and adjusting heat between batches as needed.

> **IF YOU ARE WELL...**
>
> If there is no medical reason for you to avoid fiber or difficult-to-digest foods, top these pancakes with fresh berries. Look for berries in season or plan a trip to pick your own. If you are concerned about reintroducing berries into your diet, start with just a few, chew well and enjoy the taste (it's probably been a long time since you dared to try them!). And remember, while you may be modifying your diet, your family might still enjoy treats such as mixed berries.

Nutrients Per Serving	
Calories	58
Fat	1 g
Fiber	1 g
Protein	6 g
Carbohydrate	7 g

Oatmeal Quinoa Pancakes

The comfort of a warming bowl of oatmeal is captured in golden pancake form. Drizzle with warm maple syrup or honey, or top with vanilla yogurt and fresh fruit.

MAKES 14 PANCAKES (1 PER SERVING)

1 cup	quick-cooking rolled oats (certified gluten-free, if needed)	250 mL
2 cups	buttermilk, divided	500 mL
¾ cup	quinoa flour	175 mL
1½ tsp	baking powder (gluten-free, if needed)	7 mL
1 tsp	ground cinnamon	5 mL
¾ tsp	baking soda	3 mL
½ tsp	fine sea salt	2 mL
1	egg	1
2 tbsp	vegetable oil	30 mL
1 tbsp	liquid honey	15 mL
	Nonstick cooking spray	

1. In a small bowl, combine oats and half the buttermilk. Let stand for 10 minutes.

2. In a large bowl, whisk together quinoa flour, baking powder, cinnamon, baking soda and salt. Add oat mixture, the remaining buttermilk, egg, oil and honey, stirring until blended.

3. Heat a griddle or skillet over medium heat. Spray with cooking spray. For each pancake, pour about ¼ cup (60 mL) batter onto griddle. Cook until bubbles appear on top. Turn pancake over and cook for about 1 minute or until golden brown. Repeat with the remaining batter, spraying griddle and adjusting heat as necessary between batches.

Quinoa and Quinoa Flour

Quinoa (pronounced keen-wah) is a grain that provides high-quality protein, so it's a very good choice for those following a vegetarian or vegan diet. It is a higher-fiber grain, but the mechanically processed flour is not a concern for bowel obstructions. However, quinoa is not suitable for low-oxalate diets.

Tips

- An equal amount of brown rice syrup, pure maple syrup or agave nectar may be used in place of the honey.

- To store pancakes, let them cool completely on a wire rack, then wrap individually in plastic wrap and store in an airtight container in the refrigerator for up to 3 days or the freezer for up to 1 month. Reheat in the microwave on High for 45 seconds, until warmed through (no need to thaw), or toast in the toaster oven for 1 to 2 minutes or until toasted and warmed though.

IBD Tip

- When made with certified gluten-free oats and gluten-free baking powder, this recipe is gluten-free, which is important for individuals living with celiac disease or non-celiac gluten sensitivity.

Nutrients Per Serving	
Calories	93
Fat	4 g
Fiber	2 g
Protein	3 g
Carbohydrate	12 g

Finnish Apple Pancake

This is an easy recipe for a special breakfast. And it's a real hit as part of a brunch menu. Serve immediately with maple syrup or your favorite fruit preserves.

- *Preheat oven to 425°F (220°C)*
- *8-inch (20 cm) square baking pan, greased*

MAKES 2 SERVINGS

Tip

- For variety, use peaches or pears to bake this delicious breakfast dish.

IBD Tips

- Cooked apples are often better tolerated than raw apples because heating causes pectic substances (the major fiber in apples) to break down.

- Removing the core and peel of the apple is especially important for individuals following a low-fiber diet.

- Fibers can be classified according to their chemical properties (e.g., pectins, cellulose, gums and mucilages) or their solubility (soluble vs. insoluble fibers).

2 cups	thinly sliced cored peeled apples	500 mL
1 tbsp	butter, melted	15 mL
3	eggs	3
1/2 cup	milk	125 mL
1/3 cup	all-purpose flour	75 mL
1/4 tsp	baking powder	1 mL
1/8 tsp	salt	0.5 mL
Topping		
1/2 tsp	ground cinnamon	2 mL
1 tbsp	granulated sugar	15 mL

1. Place apples and butter in baking pan; toss to coat. Bake in preheated oven for 5 minutes.

2. Meanwhile, in a small bowl, whisk together eggs, milk, flour, baking powder and salt until smooth. Set aside.

3. *Prepare the topping:* In another small bowl, combine cinnamon and sugar. Set aside.

4. Pour egg mixture over cooked apples; sprinkle evenly with topping. Bake for 15 to 20 minutes or until pancake is puffed and golden brown. Serve immediately.

Nutrients Per Serving	
Calories	357
Fat	15 g
Fiber	3 g
Protein	14 g
Carbohydrate	43 g

Banana Cinnamon Quinoa Waffles

These banana and cinnamon waffles are excellent with a drizzle of maple syrup on top.

- *Preheat waffle maker to medium-high*

1¾ cups	quinoa flour	425 mL
¼ cup	ground flaxseeds	60 mL
1½ tsp	baking powder (gluten-free, if needed)	7 mL
1 tsp	ground cinnamon	5 mL
¼ tsp	fine sea salt	1 mL
2	eggs	2
1 cup	milk	250 mL
3 tbsp	unsalted butter, melted	45 mL
2 tbsp	pure maple syrup or liquid honey	30 mL
2 tsp	vanilla extract	10 mL
¾ cup	mashed ripe bananas	175 mL
	Nonstick cooking spray	

1. In a large bowl, whisk together quinoa flour, flaxseeds, baking powder, cinnamon and salt.

2. In a medium bowl, whisk together eggs, milk, butter, maple syrup and vanilla. Stir in banana.

3. Add the egg mixture to the flour mixture and stir until just blended.

4. Spray preheated waffle maker with cooking spray. For each waffle, pour about ⅓ cup (75 mL) batter into waffle maker. Cook according to manufacturer's instructions until golden brown.

Vegetarian choice

Source of potassium

MAKES 10 WAFFLES (1 PER SERVING)

Tip

- To store waffles, let them cool completely on a wire rack, then wrap individually in plastic wrap and store in an airtight container in the refrigerator for up to 2 days or the freezer for up to 1 month. Reheat in the microwave on High for 45 seconds, until warmed through (no need to thaw), or toast in the toaster oven for 1 to 2 minutes or until toasted and warmed though.

IBD Tips

- When made with gluten-free baking powder, this recipe is gluten-free, which is important for individuals living with celiac disease or non-celiac gluten sensitivity.

- Bananas boost the potassium content in this recipe and are known to thicken loose stool.

Nutrients Per Serving	
Calories	179
Fat	7 g
Fiber	4 g
Protein	6 g
Carbohydrate	24 g

Vegetarian choice

Higher-calorie choice

Higher-protein choice

Source of sodium

MAKES 4 SERVINGS

Tip

• When using margarine, choose a non-hydrogenated version to limit consumption of trans fats.

IBD Tips

• About half the calories in tofu come from fat; however, it is low in saturated fat (the type our body uses to make cholesterol) and high in polyunsaturated and monounsaturated fats (heart-healthy fats).

• If tofu was set in calcium (as the curdling agent), it will provide additional calcium. Check the label!

• If you use soy cheese, this breakfast is a lactose-free choice.

Tofu English Muffins

Whether you are vegetarian, vegan or just trying to eat less meat, these sandwiches are a great addition to your weekly breakfast menu (and kids love them)! This dish is vegan if you use soy products.

8 oz	medium tofu	250 g
2 tbsp	reduced-sodium soy sauce	30 mL
	Vegetable cooking spray	
¼ tsp	ground turmeric (optional)	1 mL
	Salt and freshly ground black pepper (optional)	
4	slices soy ham or back bacon	4
4	English muffins, halved	4
4 tsp	margarine	20 mL
4 tsp	ketchup	20 mL
4	slices (each 1 oz/30 g) soy cheese (or Cheddar, Swiss, Jack or provolone)	4

1. Break up tofu into chunks that resemble the texture of scrambled eggs.

2. In a small bowl, combine tofu and soy sauce.

3. Heat a large skillet over medium-high heat. Spray with vegetable cooking spray. Sprinkle turmeric (if using) into skillet and cook for a few seconds (this will give the tofu the yellow color of scrambled eggs). Add tofu mixture; cook, stirring occasionally, for 5 to 7 minutes or until edges of tofu are golden-brown. Season to taste with salt and pepper, if desired.

4. During the last couple of minutes of cooking the tofu, clear some space in the skillet and spray lightly with vegetable cooking spray. Add soy ham and cook, turning once, until lightly browned, about 1 minute per side.

5. Meanwhile, toast muffins. Spread each muffin bottom with 1 tsp (5 mL) margarine and each muffin top with 1 tsp (5 mL) ketchup. On each muffin bottom, place one-quarter of the scrambled tofu, 1 slice of soy cheese and 1 slice of soy ham. Top with muffin tops.

Nutrients Per Serving	
Calories	272
Fat	10 g
Fiber	5 g
Protein	17 g
Carbohydrate	33 g

Bannock

This Aboriginal favorite goes well with a hearty soup or stew. It tastes like tea biscuits, only much better.

- *Preheat oven to 350°F (180°C)*
- *Baking sheet, lightly greased*

1½ cups	all-purpose flour	375 mL
1 cup	whole wheat flour	250 mL
3 tbsp	granulated sugar	45 mL
2 tbsp	baking powder	30 mL
1 tsp	salt	5 mL
2 tbsp	margarine	30 mL
1 cup	leftover mashed potatoes	250 mL
1 cup	milk	250 mL

1. In a large bowl, combine all-purpose flour, whole wheat flour, sugar, baking powder and salt. Using a pastry cutter or two knives, cut in margarine until mixture resembles coarse crumbs. Stir in mashed potatoes and milk until a wet dough forms.

2. On a floured work surface, knead dough until smooth and elastic. Shape into a round about 1½ inches (4 cm) thick and place on prepared baking sheet. Prick the top with a fork.

3. Bake in preheated oven for about 20 minutes or until top is golden and a tester inserted in the center comes out clean. Let cool on baking sheet for 10 minutes, then remove to a wire rack to cool completely.

IF FOLLOWING A LOW-FIBER DIET AND AVOIDING DIFFICULT-TO-DIGEST FOODS...

Substitute all-purpose flour for the whole wheat flour.

Vegetarian choice

Lower-fat choice

Lower-fiber choice

Source of potassium

MAKES 1 LOAF (12 servings per loaf)

Tips

- Use mashed potatoes with your usual milk and butter added.
- If you score the top of the bannock into 12 portions with a sharp knife before baking, it is easier to cut after baking.

IBD Tips

- Potatoes are rich in potassium; milk is a source as well.
- When making mashed potatoes, butter should be used only occasionally, in small amounts, due to its high saturated fat content. Non-hydrogenated margarine is a better choice, as it is made from vegetable oils and is lower in saturated fat. It also contains more monounsaturated and polyunsaturated fat and is lower in trans fat.

Nutrients Per Serving	
Calories	148
Fat	3 g
Fiber	2 g
Protein	4 g
Carbohydrate	28 g

Vegetarian choice

Lower-fat choice

Lower-fiber choice

Lactose-free choice

**MAKES 15 SLICES
(1 PER SERVING)**

IBD Tips

- This recipe is gluten-free.
- Tapioca starch may help to thicken loose stool.
- This recipe calls for instant yeast, which doesn't need to be dissolved in water like active dry yeast. Some yeast brands are fortified with vitamin B_{12}.

To Make This Recipe Vegan

Omit eggs and egg white from the recipe. Combine $\frac{1}{3}$ cup (75 mL) flax flour or ground flaxseed with an additional $\frac{1}{2}$ cup (125 mL) warm water. Set aside for 5 minutes. Add with the liquids. You may need to increase the baking time by 5 to 10 minutes.

Nutrients Per Serving	
Calories	135
Fat	3 g
Fiber	2 g
Protein	4 g
Carbohydrate	23 g

Ancient Grains Bread

Here's a quartet of healthy grains — sorghum, amaranth, cornmeal and quinoa — combined in a soft-textured, nutritious loaf that's perfect for sandwiches.

- 9- by 5-inch (23 by 12.5 cm) loaf pan, lightly greased

1 cup	sorghum flour	250 mL
$\frac{2}{3}$ cup	amaranth flour	150 mL
$\frac{1}{2}$ cup	cornmeal	125 mL
$\frac{1}{4}$ cup	quinoa flour	60 mL
$\frac{1}{3}$ cup	tapioca starch	75 mL
$\frac{1}{3}$ cup	packed brown sugar	75 mL
1 tbsp	xanthan gum	15 mL
1 tbsp	bread machine or instant yeast	15 mL
$1\frac{1}{2}$ tsp	salt	7 mL
2	eggs	2
1	egg white	1
1 cup	water	250 mL
2 tbsp	vegetable oil	30 mL
1 tsp	cider vinegar	5 mL

1. In a large bowl or plastic bag, combine sorghum flour, amaranth flour, cornmeal, quinoa flour, tapioca starch, brown sugar, xanthan gum, yeast and salt. Mix well and set aside.

2. In a separate bowl, using a heavy-duty electric mixer with paddle attachment, combine eggs, egg white, water, oil and vinegar until well blended. With the mixer on its lowest speed, slowly add the dry ingredients until combined. Stop the machine and scrape the bottom and sides of the bowl with a rubber spatula. With the mixer on medium speed, beat for 4 minutes.

3. Spoon into prepared pan. Let rise, uncovered, in a warm, draft-free place for 60 to 75 minutes, or until dough has risen to the top of the pan. Meanwhile, preheat oven to 350°F (180°C).

4. Bake for 35 to 45 minutes, or until loaf sounds hollow when tapped on the bottom. Remove from the pan immediately and let cool completely on a rack.

> **IF FOLLOWING A LOW-FIBER DIET AND AVOIDING DIFFICULT-TO-DIGEST FOODS...**
> Use finely ground versions of each flour and the cornmeal.

Healthy Cheese 'n' Herb Bread

- *Preheat oven to 400°F (200°C)*
- *8-inch (20 cm) round pan, nonstick or lightly greased*

2 cups	all-purpose flour	500 mL
1 cup	whole wheat flour	250 mL
1/2 cup	rolled oats	125 mL
1 tbsp	granulated sugar	15 mL
2 tsp	baking powder	10 mL
1/2 tsp	baking soda	2 mL
1 tsp	dried basil	5 mL
1/2 tsp	dried oregano	2 mL
1/2 tsp	salt	2 mL
1/4 cup	cold butter or margarine	60 mL
1 cup	shredded Swiss cheese	250 mL
1	egg	1
1 cup	buttermilk	250 mL
2 tbsp	sesame seeds	30 mL

1. In a medium bowl, combine flours, oats, sugar, baking powder, baking soda, herbs and salt. Using a pastry blender, cut in butter until mixture resembles fine crumbs. Stir in cheese.

2. Beat together egg and buttermilk; add to butter mixture, stirring with fork to make a soft moist dough. Place dough in a nonstick or lightly greased 8-inch (1.2 L) round pan. Sprinkle with sesame seeds. Bake in preheated oven for 25 to 30 minutes or until tester inserted in center comes out clean. Cut into 10 wedges to serve.

> **IF FOLLOWING A LOW-FIBER DIET AND AVOIDING DIFFICULT-TO-DIGEST FOODS...**
> Substitute all-purpose flour for the whole wheat flour and omit the sesame seeds.

Vegetarian choice

Higher-calorie choice

Lower-fiber choice

Higher-protein choice

Source of sodium

MAKES 1 LOAF (10 servings per loaf)

Tip

- Containing cheese, milk and sesame seeds, this delicious bread is a great way to add calcium to your diet. Serve with a hearty soup for an easy lunch or light supper.

IBD Tips

- Oats are high in soluble fiber and may help to thicken loose stool. Therefore, despite the increased fiber content, many low-fiber diets include oats and oat products.

- Buttermilk is made commercially by adding bacterial culture to milk. It is a natural emulsifier used for many baked goods. If you don't have any handy, add 2 tsp (10 mL) of vinegar or lemon juice to 1 cup (250 mL) of milk as a replacement.

Nutrients Per Serving	
Calories	259
Fat	10 g
Fiber	2 g
Protein	10 g
Carbohydrate	33 g

Vegetarian choice

Lower-calorie choice

Lower-fat choice

Lower-fiber choice

Mixed Herb Baguette

Baguettes, immortalized in France, are long, thin loaves of crusty bread that are baked on a cookie sheet. The addition of herbs distinguishes this from the traditional version.

- *Preheat oven to 350°F (180°C)*
- *Baking sheet, greased and dusted with cornmeal*

MAKES 2 LOAVES (10 servings per loaf)

2 tsp	granulated sugar	10 mL
1⅓ cups	warm water	325 mL
1	package (¼ oz/8 g) active dry yeast (or 1 tbsp/15 mL)	1
2½ to 3 cups	all-purpose flour	625 to 750 mL
¼ cup	mixed chopped fresh herbs	60 mL
2 tsp	butter, melted	10 mL
1 tsp	salt	5 mL
1	egg	1
2 tbsp	milk	30 mL

1. In a large bowl, dissolve sugar in warm water. Sprinkle in yeast and let stand for 10 minutes or until foamy; stir well. Stir in 2 cups (500 mL) of the flour, herbs, butter and salt. Add enough of the remaining flour to make a soft dough.

2. Turn out onto floured board; knead for a few minutes or until smooth and elastic. Place in greased bowl, turning to grease all over. Cover and let rise in warm place until doubled in size, 45 to 60 minutes.

3. Punch down dough and cut in half; roll each into a long, thin cigar-shaped stick (about 15 inches/38 cm long). Place on cornmeal-dusted greased baking sheet; score tops 3 times on the diagonal. Cover and let rise in warm place until doubled in size, 30 to 45 minutes.

4. Bake in preheated oven for 30 minutes. Combine egg and milk; brush over loaves. Bake for 10 to 15 minutes longer or until loaves sound hollow when tapped on bottom. Cool on racks.

Tip

- People often purchase baking stones to use when making pizza because they promote even heating, but they improve results when baking bread, too. Heat the stone in the oven for about 45 minutes before adding the dough.

IBD Tip

- Boost calories by using higher-fat milk or cream.

IF FOLLOWING A LOW-FIBER DIET AND AVOIDING DIFFICULT-TO-DIGEST FOODS...

Finely chop the mixed fresh herbs.

Nutrients Per Serving	
Calories	37
Fat	Trace
Fiber	Trace
Protein	1 g
Carbohydrate	7 g

Orange Apricot Oatmeal Scones

These tasty scones are delicious with a relaxing cup of tea.

- *Preheat oven to 375°F (190°C)*
- *Baking sheet, greased*

2 cups	all-purpose flour	500 mL
1½ cups	quick-cooking rolled oats	375 mL
¼ cup	granulated sugar	60 mL
1 tbsp	baking powder	15 mL
2 tsp	grated orange zest	10 mL
½ tsp	baking soda	2 mL
¼ tsp	salt	1 mL
6 tbsp	butter	90 mL
½ cup	chopped apricots	125 mL
1 cup	buttermilk or sour milk (see tip, at right)	250 mL
	Milk	

1. In a bowl, combine flour, oats, all but 1 tsp (5 mL) of the sugar, baking powder, orange zest, baking soda and salt. Using a fork or pastry blender, cut in butter until mixture resembles coarse crumbs. Stir in apricots. Add buttermilk; stir until mixture is just combined.

2. On a lightly floured surface, knead dough gently 4 or 5 times. Divide into 3 pieces. Shape each piece into a round about 1 inch (2.5 cm) thick. Transfer to baking sheet.

3. Cut each round into quarters. Brush tops with milk; sprinkle with reserved sugar. Bake in preheated oven for 20 to 25 minutes or until lightly browned.

Vegetarian choice

Higher-calorie choice

Lower-fiber choice

MAKES 12 SCONES (1 per serving)

Tip

- Sour milk can be used instead of buttermilk. To prepare, combine 2 tsp (10 mL) lemon juice or vinegar with 1 cup (250 mL) milk and let stand for 5 minutes.

IBD Tips

- To reduce the insoluble fiber content of these muffins, peel the apricots before chopping.

- Soluble fibers such as oats can be incorporated into your diet in many interesting ways: in muffins, breads, cookies and cereals (hot and cold). If you don't feel like a bowl of hot oatmeal in the summer, remember great recipes like these scones! Soluble fiber helps to thicken loose stool.

Nutrients Per Serving	
Calories	205
Fat	7 g
Fiber	2 g
Protein	5 g
Carbohydrate	32 g

**MAKES 1 LOAF
(12 servings
per loaf)**

Tip

- As this loaf freezes well,
why not make an extra
one and freeze it for
later use? You can
also slice and freeze
individual servings and
have them ready to
include in lunch bags.

IBD Tips

- This recipe is suitable for
a low-fiber diet.

- Bananas are one of the
foods known to help
thicken loose stool.

- Heart-healthy canola oil
is perfect for baking and
is a source of omega-3
fatty acids. Other heart-
healthy oils, such as olive
oil, have too strong a
flavor for baked goods.

Banana Bread

For variety, try adding a handful of chocolate chips to the batter
when baking this family favorite.

- *Preheat oven to 350°F (180°C)*
- *9- by 5-inch (23 by 12.5 cm) loaf pan, greased*

1¼ cups	all-purpose flour	300 mL
1 tsp	baking soda	5 mL
½ tsp	baking powder	2 mL
¾ cup	granulated sugar	175 mL
1	egg	1
1	egg white	1
¼ cup	lower-fat plain yogurt	60 mL
¼ cup	vegetable oil	60 mL
1 tsp	vanilla	5 mL
1 cup	mashed ripe bananas (about 2 to 3 medium)	250 mL

1. In a bowl, sift together flour, baking soda and baking
powder. Set aside.
2. In a large mixing bowl, blend sugar, egg, egg white, yogurt,
oil and vanilla. Blend in bananas. Add dry ingredients; mix
until just combined. Pour batter into prepared pan. Bake in
preheated oven for 1 hour or until a tester inserted in
center of loaf comes out clean.

Variation

Banana Muffins: To make a muffin version of this recipe,
spoon batter into 12 greased or paper-lined muffin cups.
Bake at 350°F (180°C) for 18 to 22 minutes or until firm to
the touch.

IF YOU ARE WELL...

If there is no medical reason for you to avoid fiber or difficult-to-
digest foods, add a handful of fresh or frozen berries to the
batter.

Nutrients Per Serving	
Calories	165
Fat	5 g
Fiber	1 g
Protein	3 g
Carbohydrate	27 g

Oat Bran Banana Bread

This yummy bread is great for breakfast, as a snack or for dessert.

- *Preheat oven to 325°F (160°C)*
- *9- by 5-inch (23 by 12.5 cm) loaf pan, lightly greased*

1¹⁄₂ cups	whole wheat flour	375 mL
¹⁄₂ cup	oat bran	125 mL
¹⁄₃ cup	ground flaxseed	75 mL
1 tsp	baking powder	5 mL
1 tsp	baking soda	5 mL
2	egg whites	2
1	whole egg	1
¹⁄₂ cup	granulated sugar	125 mL
¹⁄₄ cup	vegetable oil or margarine	60 mL
1 tsp	vanilla	5 mL
³⁄₄ cup	low-fat plain yogurt	175 mL
3	ripe bananas, mashed (about 1¹⁄₃ cups/325 mL)	3
2 tbsp	whole flaxseed (optional)	30 mL

1. In a medium bowl, combine flour, oat bran, ground flaxseed, baking powder and baking soda.

2. In a large bowl, beat egg whites, whole egg, sugar, oil and vanilla for 3 to 4 minutes or until creamy. Stir in yogurt until well combined. Stir in bananas. Gradually fold in flour mixture.

3. Spoon batter into prepared loaf pan and smooth top. Sprinkle with whole flaxseed (if using).

4. Bake in preheated oven for 50 to 60 minutes or until top is firm to the touch and a tester inserted in the center comes out clean. Let cool in pan for 10 minutes, then remove to a wire rack to cool completely.

IF FOLLOWING A LOW-FIBER DIET AND AVOIDING DIFFICULT-TO-DIGEST FOODS...

Substitute all-purpose flour for the whole wheat flour and omit the whole flaxseed. Many individuals with IBD report that they can tolerate ground flaxseed.

Vegetarian choice

Source of soluble fiber

Source of potassium

MAKES 1 LOAF (12 servings per loaf)

Tip

- When using margarine, choose a non-hydrogenated version to limit consumption of trans fats.

IBD Tips

- Bananas are rich in potassium; yogurt contributes some as well.

- Oat bran's "gelling" properties help to thicken loose stool. Therefore, despite the increased fiber content, many low-fiber diets include oats and oat products.

- Ground flaxseed is a plant source of omega-3 fat, which has anti-inflammatory properties. Flaxseed must be ground to access the beneficial fat. At home, consider grinding your own flaxseed with a coffee grinder. Store ground flaxseed in the freezer to delay the onset of rancidity.

Nutrients Per Serving	
Calories	193
Fat	7 g
Fiber	4 g
Protein	6 g
Carbohydrate	31 g

Pumpkin Spice Nut Bread

This terrific recipe offers the benefits of pumpkin, as well as whole grains and nuts.

- *Preheat oven to 350°F (180°C)*
- *9- by 5-inch (23 by 12.5 cm) loaf pan, lightly greased*

MAKES 1 LOAF (12 servings per loaf)

IBD Tips

- Enjoy a slice of this bread, made with whole grains and nuts, when you are well and there is no medical reason for you to avoid fiber and difficult-to-digest foods.
- Pumpkin contributes potassium in this recipe.

1 cup	all-purpose flour	250 mL
³⁄₄ cup	whole wheat flour	175 mL
2 tsp	ground allspice	10 mL
1¹⁄₂ tsp	baking powder	7 mL
1 tsp	baking soda	5 mL
¹⁄₂ tsp	salt	2 mL
1 tsp	ground cinnamon	5 mL
¹⁄₂ tsp	ground nutmeg	2 mL
¹⁄₂ tsp	ground ginger	2 mL
1 cup	canned pumpkin purée (not pie filling)	250 mL
³⁄₄ cup	packed brown sugar	175 mL
¹⁄₂ cup	vegetable oil	125 mL
2	eggs, lightly beaten	2
1 tsp	vanilla	5 mL
¹⁄₃ cup	water (approx.), divided	75 mL
¹⁄₂ cup	chopped pecans or walnuts	125 mL

1. In a small bowl, combine all-purpose flour, whole wheat flour, allspice, baking powder, baking soda, salt, cinnamon, nutmeg and ginger.
2. In a large bowl, whisk together pumpkin, brown sugar and oil. Whisk in eggs, vanilla and half of the water. Fold in flour mixture (do not overmix). If batter is too thick, stir in the remaining water, a little at a time. Fold in pecans.
3. Spoon batter into prepared loaf pan and smooth top.

Nutrients Per Serving	
Calories	249
Fat	14 g
Fiber	3 g
Protein	4 g
Carbohydrate	30 g

4. Bake in preheated oven for 50 to 60 minutes or until top is firm to the touch and a tester inserted in the center comes out clean. Let cool in pan for 10 minutes, then remove to a wire rack to cool completely.

Variation

Use mini loaf pans to make 12 mini loaves. Bake at the same temperature for 25 minutes, or until a tester comes out clean. These are great for lunches or mid-morning snacks.

> **IF FOLLOWING A LOW-FIBER DIET AND AVOIDING DIFFICULT-TO-DIGEST FOODS...**
> Substitute all-purpose flour for the whole wheat flour and omit the pecans and walnuts.

IBD Tips

- Bright orange vegetables such as pumpkin are good sources of beta carotene, a powerful antioxidant. Canned pumpkin purée is convenient and can be kept in your pantry so you have it on hand whenever you wish to make this bread.

- Omega-3 fat has anti-inflammatory properties. Plant-based sources of omega-3 fat include flaxseeds, walnuts and canola oil.

Fruit and Oatmeal Muffins

These muffins, which are so moist you won't need to add butter, are chock-full of fruit. They are best eaten warm from the oven. If you must store them, do so in the freezer and thaw as needed.

MAKES 20 MUFFINS (1 per serving)

Tip

• Since these muffins freeze well, they are particularly convenient for brown baggers. Pop a frozen muffin into a lunch bag. By the time lunch rolls around, it will be defrosted and ready to eat.

IBD Tips

• To boost calories, use higher-fat milk and spread butter or non-hydrogenated margarine on the warm muffin.

• This recipe gets its potassium from the banana, orange juice and milk.

- *Preheat oven to 400°F (200°C)*
- *Two 12-cup muffin tins, greased or paper-lined*

2½ cups	all-purpose flour	625 mL
1½ cups	quick-cooking rolled oats	375 mL
1 cup	wheat germ	250 mL
¾ cup	granulated sugar	175 mL
2 tbsp	baking powder	30 mL
½ tsp	salt	2 mL
1 cup	raisins	250 mL
1	medium apple, chopped	1
⅓ cup	shelled sunflower seeds	75 mL
2	eggs	2
1 cup	mashed ripe bananas	250 mL
¾ cup	skim milk	175 mL
2 tbsp	grated orange zest	30 mL
½ cup	orange juice	125 mL
⅓ cup	vegetable oil	75 mL

1. In a large bowl, combine flour, oats, wheat germ, sugar, baking powder and salt; stir in raisins, apple and sunflower seeds.

2. In another bowl, whisk eggs lightly; blend in bananas, milk, orange zest and juice, and oil. Pour into dry ingredients, stirring just until moistened.

3. Spoon about ⅓ cup (75 mL) batter into each greased or paper-lined muffin cup. Bake in preheated oven for about 20 minutes or until firm to the touch. Cool in pans for 5 minutes. Remove from tins and cool on rack. Store in airtight container in freezer.

IF FOLLOWING A LOW-FIBER DIET AND AVOIDING DIFFICULT-TO-DIGEST FOODS...

Peel and core the apple, omit the sunflower seeds and raisins, and omit the wheat germ (or substitute oat bran).

Nutrients Per Serving	
Calories	230
Fat	7 g
Fiber	3 g
Protein	6 g
Carbohydrate	39 g

Chocolate Chip Oatmeal Muffins

- *Preheat oven to 400°F (200°C)*
- *12-cup muffin tin, lightly greased or lined with paper cups*

1½ cups	whole wheat flour	375 mL
½ cup	quick-cooking rolled oats	125 mL
¼ cup	ground flaxseed	60 mL
¼ cup	granulated sugar	60 mL
2 tsp	baking powder	10 mL
½ tsp	baking soda	2 mL
½ tsp	salt	2 mL
1	egg	1
1 cup	milk	250 mL
¼ cup	vegetable oil	60 mL
¼ cup	liquid honey	60 mL
½ cup	semisweet chocolate chips or dried fruit	125 mL
½ cup	chopped nuts (optional)	125 mL

1. In a large bowl, combine flour, oats, flaxseed, sugar, baking powder, baking soda and salt.
2. In a small bowl, whisk together egg, milk, oil and honey. Stir into flour mixture until just combined. Fold in chocolate chips and nuts (if using).
3. Divide batter evenly among prepared muffin cups.
4. Bake in preheated oven for 15 to 20 minutes or until tops are firm to the touch and a tester inserted in the center of a muffin comes out clean. Let cool in tin for 10 minutes, then remove to a wire rack to cool completely.

IF YOU ARE WELL...

If there is no medical reason for you to avoid fiber or difficult-to-digest foods, use dried fruit in this recipe.

IF FOLLOWING A LOW-FIBER DIET AND AVOIDING DIFFICULT-TO-DIGEST FOODS...

Substitute all-purpose flour for the whole wheat flour and avoid the dried fruit and chopped nuts.

Vegetarian choice

Higher-calorie choice

Source of soluble fiber

MAKES 12 MUFFINS (1 per serving)

Tip

- For the nuts, try walnuts, pecans or almonds.

IBD Tips

- Oats are high in soluble fiber and may help to thicken loose stool. Therefore, despite the increased fiber content, many low-fiber diets include oats and oat products.
- Honey is sugar made by bees and is composed of water and simple carbohydrates, namely glucose and fructose. Honey also contains trace amounts of some vitamins, minerals and antioxidants, but these amounts are very small and are not considered significant to our nutrition.
- Canola oil is a good choice for baking and is a plant source of omega-3 fat.

Nutrients Per Serving	
Calories	210
Fat	9 g
Fiber	3 g
Protein	5 g
Carbohydrate	30 g

Apple Walnut Muffins

Apples add moistness and natural sweetness to these delicious muffins. A sprinkling of toasted walnuts in the batter adds a delectable, complementary crunch.

**MAKES
12 MUFFINS
(1 PER SERVING)**

Tips

• For the apples, try Braeburn, Gala or Golden Delicious.

• Store the cooled muffins in an airtight container in the refrigerator for up to 3 days. Or wrap them in plastic wrap, then foil, completely enclosing them, and freeze for up to 6 months. Let thaw at room temperature for 2 hours before serving.

IBD Tips

• When made with gluten-free baking powder, this recipe is gluten-free, which is important for individuals living with celiac disease or non-celiac gluten sensitivity.

• Arrowroot starch may help to thicken loose stool.

• *Preheat oven to 400°F (200°C)*
• *12-cup muffin pan, sprayed with nonstick cooking spray*

2 cups	quinoa flour	500 mL
2 tbsp	cornstarch or arrowroot starch	30 mL
1 tbsp	baking powder (gluten-free, if needed)	15 mL
1/2 tsp	fine sea salt	2 mL
1/2 tsp	ground cinnamon	2 mL
1/2 cup	natural cane sugar or packed light brown sugar	125 mL
2	eggs	2
3/4 cup	buttermilk	175 mL
1/4 cup	toasted walnut oil or vegetable oil	60 mL
1 1/2 cups	chopped tart-sweet apples (unpeeled)	375 mL
1/2 cup	toasted chopped walnuts	125 mL

1. In a large bowl, whisk together quinoa flour, cornstarch, baking powder, salt and cinnamon.

2. In a medium bowl, whisk together sugar, eggs, buttermilk and oil until well blended.

3. Add the egg mixture to the flour mixture and stir until just blended. Gently fold in apples and walnuts.

4. Divide batter equally among prepared muffin cups.

5. Bake in preheated oven for 18 to 23 minutes or until tops are golden and a toothpick inserted in the center comes out clean. Let cool in pan on a wire rack for 3 minutes, then transfer to the rack to cool.

Variation

Pear Pecan Muffins: Replace the cinnamon with ground nutmeg, the apples with chopped pears (unpeeled) and the walnuts with toasted chopped pecans.

IF FOLLOWING A LOW-FIBER DIET AND AVOIDING DIFFICULT-TO-DIGEST FOODS...

Peel the apples and omit the chopped walnuts. Cooked apples are often better tolerated than raw apples. It is known that heating will cause pectic substances (the major fiber in apples) to be broken down. Ground nut butters can also be included rather than whole or chopped nuts.

Nutrients Per Serving	
Calories	216
Fat	10 g
Fiber	4 g
Protein	5 g
Carbohydrate	28 g

Banana Applesauce Muffins

- *Preheat oven to 400°F (200°C)*
- *12-cup muffin tin, lightly greased or lined with paper cups*

2 cups	whole wheat flour	500 mL
1 tbsp	baking powder	15 mL
1 tsp	baking soda	5 mL
1/2 tsp	salt	2 mL
3	ripe bananas, mashed (about 1 1/3 cups/325 mL)	3
1	egg, lightly beaten	1
1 cup	unsweetened applesauce	250 mL
1/2 cup	granulated sugar	125 mL
1/4 cup	vegetable oil	60 mL

1. In a large bowl, combine flour, baking powder, baking soda and salt.
2. In a medium bowl, combine bananas, egg, applesauce, sugar and oil. Stir into flour mixture until just combined.
3. Divide batter evenly among prepared muffin cups.
4. Bake in preheated oven for 15 to 20 minutes or until tops are firm to the touch and a tester inserted in the center of a muffin comes out clean. Let cool in tin for 10 minutes, then remove to a wire rack to cool completely.

> **IF FOLLOWING A LOW-FIBER DIET AND AVOIDING DIFFICULT-TO-DIGEST FOODS...**
> Substitute all-purpose flour for the whole wheat flour.

Vegetarian choice

Lower-fat choice

Lactose-free choice

Source of soluble fiber

Source of potassium

MAKES 12 LARGE MUFFINS (1 per serving)

IBD Tips

- Choose canola oil for its heart-healthy, anti-inflammatory omega-3 fat.
- Applesauce and banana provide soluble fiber.
- Applesauce can be used to reduce the amount of oil, and thus fat, in a recipe. Fruit-flavored varieties of applesauce make great snacks!
- Bananas and applesauce are known for their stool-thickening effect. Other helpful foods include oats, oat bran, barley, tapioca pudding, soft cooked white rice, smooth peanut butter, cheese, pretzels, potato chips, matzo and gelatin-containing foods such as marshmallows and Jell-O.

Nutrients Per Serving	
Calories	183
Fat	5 g
Fiber	3 g
Protein	4 g
Carbohydrate	32 g

Very Lemon Muffins

These light, double-lemon muffins are as good as they sound, and the recipe is gluten-free, which is important for individuals living with celiac disease or non-celiac gluten sensitivity.

**MAKES
18 MUFFINS
(1 PER SERVING)**

- *Preheat oven to 350°F (180°C)*
- *Two 12-cup muffin pans, 18 cups greased*

Tip

- When baking a batch of muffins that does not use all the cups of a muffin pan, fill the empty cups halfway with water.

IBD Tips

- This recipe is suitable for vegetarians who eat eggs.

- Xanthan gum is a corn-based binding agent crucial to gluten-free baking. It helps keep gluten-free baked goods from falling apart and provides the "chewy" texture usually supplied by wheat flour.

- Citrus juice supplies potassium, and its fresh fragrance helps stimulate interest in eating. It can usually be included in the diet of individuals living with IBD, but in times of illness or anal soreness from frequent loose stool, you may wish to select an alternative muffin recipe.

Muffins

2½ cups	Brown Rice Flour Blend (see recipe, opposite)	625 mL
1 tbsp	gluten-free baking powder	15 mL
1 tsp	salt	5 mL
½ tsp	xanthan gum	2 mL
1 cup	granulated sugar	250 mL
2	eggs	2
¾ cup	buttermilk	175 mL
½ cup	vegetable oil	125 mL
3 tbsp	finely grated lemon zest	45 mL
¼ cup	freshly squeezed lemon juice	60 mL

Glaze

1 cup	confectioners' (icing) sugar	250 mL
2 tsp	finely grated lemon zest	10 mL
1 tbsp	freshly squeezed lemon juice	15 mL

1. *Muffins:* In a large bowl, whisk together flour blend, baking powder, salt and xanthan gum.

2. In a medium bowl, whisk together sugar, eggs, buttermilk, oil, lemon zest and lemon juice until well blended.

3. Add the egg mixture to the flour mixture and stir until well blended.

4. Divide batter equally among prepared muffin cups.

5. Bake in preheated oven for 30 to 35 minutes or until tops are golden and a toothpick inserted in the center comes out clean. Let cool in pans on a wire rack for 5 minutes, then transfer to the rack to cool while you prepare the glaze.

6. *Glaze:* In a small bowl, whisk together confectioners' sugar, lemon zest and lemon juice until blended and smooth. Spoon over warm muffin tops. Let cool.

Nutrients Per Serving	
Calories	211
Fat	7 g
Fiber	1 g
Protein	2 g
Carbohydrate	37 g

Brown Rice Flour Blend

Here's an all-purpose gluten-free baking blend that can be used to replace all-purpose flour in most standard recipes.

2 cups	finely ground brown rice flour	500 mL
$\frac{2}{3}$ cup	potato starch	150 mL
$\frac{1}{3}$ cup	tapioca starch	75 mL

1. In a bowl, whisk together brown rice flour, potato starch and tapioca starch. Use as directed in recipes.

IF FOLLOWING A LOW-FIBER DIET AND AVOIDING DIFFICULT-TO-DIGEST FOODS…

Substitute white rice flour for the brown rice flour.

Tips

- You can also make the blend in smaller amounts by using the basic proportions: 2 parts finely ground brown rice flour, $\frac{2}{3}$ part potato starch and $\frac{1}{3}$ part tapioca starch.

- You can double, triple or quadruple the recipe to have it on hand. Store the blend in an airtight container in the refrigerator for up to 4 months, or in the freezer for up to 1 year. Let warm to room temperature before using.

IBD Tip

- Tapioca starch may help to thicken loose stool.

Nutrients Per Serving	
Calories	134
Fat	1 g
Fiber	1 g
Protein	2 g
Carbohydrate	31 g

**MAKES
12 MUFFINS
(1 PER SERVING)**

Tips

- Any natural nut or seed butter may be used in place of the almond butter.

- Store in an airtight container in the refrigerator for up to 3 days. Or wrap in plastic wrap, then foil, and freeze for up to 6 months. Let thaw at room temperature for 2 hours before serving.

IBD Tips

- When made with gluten-free baking powder and vanilla extract, this recipe is gluten-free.

- If you're trying to gain weight, select full-fat milk or cream.

- To make this recipe lactose-free, use non-dairy milk. Be mindful that vegetable-based milk may provide less protein than cow's milk.

Nutrients Per Serving	
Calories	236
Fat	13 g
Fiber	4 g
Protein	7 g
Carbohydrate	26 g

Almond Butter Muffins

Alternative nut butters used to be sold only at health food stores, but now they are widely available at supermarkets and superstores. Here, almond butter enriches quinoa flour, creating these hearty muffins.

- *Preheat oven to 400°F (200°C)*
- *12-cup muffin pan, sprayed with nonstick cooking spray*

1¾ cups	quinoa flour	425 mL
1 tbsp	baking powder	15 mL
½ tsp	fine sea salt	2 mL
2	eggs	2
½ cup	unsweetened natural almond butter, well stirred	125 mL
¼ cup	vegetable oil or unrefined virgin coconut oil, warmed	60 mL
¼ cup	liquid honey, brown rice syrup, pure maple syrup or agave nectar	60 mL
1 tsp	vanilla extract	5 mL
1¼ cups	milk or plain non-dairy milk (such as soy, almond, rice or hemp)	300 mL
½ cup	dried fruit (raisins, cranberries, chopped cherries or chopped apricots, or a combination)	125 mL

1. In a large bowl, whisk together quinoa flour, baking powder and salt.

2. In a medium bowl, whisk together eggs, almond butter, oil, honey and vanilla until well blended. Whisk in milk until blended.

3. Add the egg mixture to the flour mixture and stir until just blended. Gently fold in dried fruit.

4. Divide batter equally among prepared muffin cups.

5. Bake in preheated oven for 18 to 22 minutes or until tops are golden and a toothpick inserted in the center comes out clean. Let cool in pan on a wire rack for 5 minutes, then transfer to the rack to cool.

IF FOLLOWING A LOW-FIBER DIET AND AVOIDING DIFFICULT-TO-DIGEST FOODS...

Omit the dried fruit.

Cranberry, Carrot and Apple Teff Muffins

- *Preheat oven to 350°F (180°C)*
- *12-cup muffin pan, greased*

2 cups	teff flour	500 mL
½ cup	tapioca flour	125 mL
2 tsp	gluten-free baking powder	10 mL
1 tsp	pumpkin pie spice	5 mL
1 tsp	xanthan gum	5 mL
½ tsp	baking soda	2 mL
½ tsp	salt	2 mL
1	egg	1
½ cup	unsweetened apple juice	125 mL
½ cup	unsweetened applesauce	125 mL
½ cup	pure maple syrup	125 mL
⅓ cup	vegetable oil	75 mL
1 cup	finely shredded carrots	250 mL
1 cup	chopped peeled apple	250 mL
½ cup	chopped pecans, toasted	125 mL
½ cup	dried cranberries	125 mL

1. In a large bowl, whisk together teff flour, tapioca flour, baking powder, pumpkin pie spice, xanthan gum, baking soda and salt.
2. In a medium bowl, whisk together egg, apple juice, applesauce, maple syrup and oil until well blended.
3. Add the egg mixture to the flour mixture and stir until well blended. Gently fold in carrots, apple, pecans and cranberries.
4. Divide batter equally among prepared muffin cups.
5. Bake in preheated oven for 25 to 30 minutes or until a toothpick inserted in the center comes out clean. Let cool in pan on a wire rack for 5 minutes, then transfer to the rack to cool.

IF FOLLOWING A LOW-FIBER DIET AND AVOIDING DIFFICULT-TO-DIGEST FOODS...

You may need to use a different gluten-free flour blend, as teff flour is a good source of fiber. Omit the dried cranberries and chopped pecans. The finely shredded carrots and chopped peeled apple are soft after baking.

**MAKES
12 MUFFINS
(1 PER SERVING)**

Tip

- Teff, or tef, is a very tiny cereal grain native to northeastern Africa and southwestern Arabia. It has a mild, nutty, molasses-like flavor.

IBD Tips

- This recipe is suitable for vegetarians who eat eggs.
- This recipe is gluten-free, which is important for individuals living with celiac disease or non-celiac gluten sensitivity.
- Tapioca flour may help to thicken loose stool.
- Pumpkin pie spice is usually a blend of sweet spices (cinnamon, ginger, nutmeg, allspice and cloves) and can help boost the flavors in food, heightening your interest in eating.
- Applesauce and peeled apple provide soluble fiber, and applesauce is known for its stool-thickening effect.

Nutrients Per Serving	
Calories	252
Fat	11 g
Fiber	4 g
Protein	4 g
Carbohydrate	38 g

Sweet Potato Muffins

- *Preheat oven to 400°F (200°C)*
- *12-cup muffin tin, lightly greased or lined with paper cups*

**MAKES 12 MUFFINS
(1 per serving)**

1 cup	quick-cooking rolled oats	250 mL
1 cup	buttermilk (approx.)	250 mL
½ cup	all-purpose flour	125 mL
½ cup	whole wheat flour	125 mL
¼ cup	granulated sugar	60 mL
1 tbsp	wheat germ	15 mL
1 tbsp	baking powder	15 mL
1 tsp	salt	5 mL
½ tsp	baking soda	2 mL
1 cup	mixed dried fruit	250 mL
1	egg, beaten	1
½ cup	grated sweet potato	125 mL
¼ cup	lightly packed brown sugar	60 mL
¼ cup	vegetable oil	60 mL
1 tsp	grated orange zest	5 mL

IBD Tips

- Oats are high in soluble fiber and may help to thicken loose stool. Therefore, despite the increased fiber content, many low-fiber diets include oats and oat products.

- Buttermilk is made commercially by adding bacterial culture to milk. If you don't have any, add 2 tsp (10 mL) of vinegar or lemon juice to 1 cup (250 mL) of milk as a replacement.

- Sweet potato is rich in beta carotene, a powerful antioxidant that is converted to vitamin A in the body.

- Brown sugar is actually white sugar with added molasses. Molasses does contribute some nutrients, but not enough to make a difference, given the amount people usually eat.

1. Place oats in a large bowl and pour in buttermilk; stir to combine. Cover and let stand for 10 minutes.

2. Meanwhile, in a small bowl, combine all-purpose flour, whole wheat flour, granulated sugar, wheat germ, baking powder, salt and baking soda. Stir in dried fruit.

3. In another small bowl, combine egg, sweet potato, brown sugar, oil and orange zest. Stir into oatmeal mixture. Gradually fold in flour mixture until just moistened. If too stiff, add a little more buttermilk.

4. Divide batter evenly among prepared muffin cups, filling almost to the top (these muffins do not rise much).

5. Bake for 20 minutes or until a tester inserted in the center of a muffin comes out clean. Let cool in tin for 10 minutes, then remove to a wire rack to cool completely.

IF YOU ARE WELL...

If there is no medical reason for you to avoid fiber or difficult-to-digest foods, try raisins, blueberries, cherries and cranberries for the mixed dried fruit.

IF FOLLOWING A LOW-FIBER DIET AND AVOIDING DIFFICULT-TO-DIGEST FOODS...

Substitute all-purpose flour for the whole wheat flour, omit the wheat germ (or substitute oat bran), and omit the dried fruit.

Nutrients Per Serving	
Calories	194
Fat	6 g
Fiber	2 g
Protein	4 g
Carbohydrate	33 g

Snacks and Beverages

Adding snacks between smaller meals is the perfect way to "graze" — a healthy strategy for all! This chapter provides easy-to-make recipes for finger foods, dips and spreads that can be prepared in advance when you feel energetic. Simply store them in the fridge or freezer to snack on at times when you are rushed or drained of energy. For more great snack ideas, check out the breads and muffins in the previous chapter, as well as the desserts chapter, where you'll find ideas for puddings, custards and cookies, all of which make great snacks!

Beverages are the key to staying hydrated. Fluid requirements increase when the weather is warm and during times of physical activity. If you are living with a pelvic pouch and experiencing frequent loose or liquid bowel movements, are experiencing diarrhea during a disease flare or are managing high-volume liquid output from an ileostomy (or a colostomy), your fluid losses are increased, so drinking enough liquid is especially important for you. Examples of hydrating fluids include water, juice, soup, sports drinks, milk, soy milk, rice milk, almond milk, ice cream, sorbet, Jell-O, and herbal teas, as well as decaffeinated tea, coffee and carbonated beverages.

How Do I Decide Whether Snacking Is Right for Me?

Eating snacks between meals is a good strategy if you:

- are experiencing an IBD flare-up;
- have a reduced appetite;
- suffer from uncomfortable gas cramps and bloating when many hours pass between meals;
- are prone to missing meals;
- are trying to gain weight (snacking can help you add calories throughout the day);
- are trying to lose weight (snacking will help prevent hunger and overeating, but meal sizes must be adjusted accordingly);
- have had surgery recently and tolerate small amounts of food better.

SNACKS FOR A LOW-FIBER DIET

Some examples of snacks that are okay on a low-fiber diet include prepackaged containers of applesauce (including fruit-flavored applesauce), canned fruit cups (such as peaches or pears) with a peel-back lid, individual yogurts without fruits that contain seeds, cheese and crackers, hummus and pita, biscotti without nuts, potato chips or pretzels, tapioca or other puddings, Jell-O, plain cookies (such as social tea or arrowroot), nut butter (such as peanut butter) and bread sticks, and smoothies.

Dips and spreads go well with pita, crackers, melba toast, pretzels, bread sticks and sliced vegetables such as cucumber sticks (peeled and seeded, if necessary) or carrot sticks, if you can tolerate them.

Plan Ahead

Be sure to plan your snacks ahead of time. Think about what you like and make a list to shop for these foods. Prepare them in advance by making snack bags with a few cookies, or crackers and cheese, or fresh fruit cut into bite-size pieces. Store them in convenient places, such as a bar fridge at work, a snack cupboard at home, your knapsack or briefcase, or even the glove compartment of your car (be careful when outside temperatures are hot or cold).

Compact items that don't require refrigeration, such as fruit cups, pudding cups, applesauce cups, individual packages of plain cookies or crackers, granola bars and 100% juice boxes (Tetra Paks) are easy to carry with you when you're on the run.

Snack on...Potato Chips!

Potato chips are a helpful food when you have frequent, liquidy stool, as they provide salt and potassium. And if you don't have a great appetite, they pack a lot of calories into a small amount.

Snack on...Guacamole!

Avocados, the main ingredient in Lightened-Up Guacamole and Chips (page 150), are a higher-fat fruit, the majority of which is monounsaturated. They are heart-healthy and will boost calories in any recipe they are used in. Be sure to ripen them at room temperature in a cool, dark place before storing them in the refrigerator; otherwise, they will discolor and won't ripen. They are also the stars of Chilled Avocado Soup (page 172), Green and Yellow Salad (page 187) and Avocado Dressing (page 198).

Snack on...Almonds!

Almonds are a nutritious nut, packing many minerals and healthy unsaturated fats, and they boost calories. You can eat them out of hand, mix them with other nuts, seeds and dried fruits to make your own trail mix, or turn them into Almond Butter (page 149), which is appropriate for low-fiber diets and helps thicken stool. Beyond snacking, sliced almonds can be sprinkled over soups, salads or stir-fries, and ground almonds can be added to baked goods such as cookies and muffins.

Juicing raw fruits and vegetables greatly reduces the amount of fiber in them, so you can enjoy that fresh taste without experiencing discomfort. You'll consume extra calories and you won't get full as quickly, which is great if you are trying to gain weight!

Drink Your Calories

Adequate fluid intake is important to prevent dehydration, but fluids can also help you increase calories in your diet without feeling full as quickly. This is especially true during times of disease flare-up, when it may be easier to "drink calories" rather than eat. Boost calories in your drinks and smoothies by adding juice, milk, soy milk, ice cream or yogurt. Increase protein by adding tofu or a nut butter (peanut butter, almond butter, cashew butter). Silken tofu (also known as dessert tofu) may blend more smoothly in a smoothie than firm tofu. Experiment with flavor combinations: try chocolate syrup, peanut butter and a banana, or chocolate ice cream and mint or almond extract.

Maximize Your Nutrient Intake with 100% Fruit Juice

Fruit juice and fruit cocktails often contain more water and sugar than real fruit juice. Use 100% fruit juices in drinks and smoothies to maximize the vitamins, minerals and phytonutrients supplied to your body. Phytonutrients are plant chemicals that have biological activity in the body; antioxidants are one example. These nutrients are beneficial to your health and occur naturally in any food that comes from a plant.

Soy milk is fortified with calcium and vitamin D, but not all vegetable-based beverages (such as rice milk or almond milk) have this important feature. Be sure to read the label to get the most nutrition from your beverage.

The Benefits of Soy Milk

Soy milk comes in a wide selection of flavors, provides good protein, has no cholesterol and is composed of mostly unsaturated fat. Soy also supplies isoflavones, which are phytonutrients. Most varieties are fortified with calcium and vitamin D, but be sure to shake the carton, as calcium settles at the bottom. Research suggests that calcium carbonate is absorbed as well as cow's milk; however, other forms, such as tricalcium phosphate, are not. If your soy milk is fortified with tricalcium phosphate, you will need to drink more to get the same amount of calcium as from cow's milk.

Be Cautious with Drinks That Contain Lots of Sugar

Beverages with a high sugar content (sports drinks, juices, fruit punch, etc.) may need to be diluted and sipped slowly to avoid exacerbating loose stool or diarrhea. The sugar concentration (also called osmolality) draws more water into the bowel, thus contributing to a more liquidy stool.

Incorporate breakfast drinks (such as Breakfast Anytime!) or nutritional drinks (such as Boost, Ensure or Resource) to increase the calorie and protein content of your smoothies. "Plus," "1.5" and "2.0" labels usually mean more calories and protein in less fluid — another good way to optimize your intake.

BEWARE OF CAFFEINATED BEVERAGES

When selecting beverages, be wary of those containing caffeine or guarana (the seeds of this shrub contain higher levels of caffeine than coffee beans), as they stimulate gut peristalsis (movement) and cause diarrhea in some individuals. Examples include coffee, black and green tea, hot chocolate, ice tea, beer with added caffeine and energy drinks. Consuming these beverages on an empty stomach can cause cramping and loose stool, so you might want to consider forgoing that cup of coffee when you first get up in the morning. At least wait until you have some food in your stomach!

Some research has found that caffeinated beverages *do* hydrate; however, these studies were not done on individuals living with digestive disorders or who have had gastrointestinal surgery and thus should not be relied upon. As a general rule, it is best to avoid caffeinated beverages as a means of hydration.

SUGAR BY ANY OTHER NAME...

Sweeteners such as granulated sugar, brown sugar, raw sugar (also called natural brown sugar or whole cane sugar), brown rice syrup, honey, maple syrup, cane sugar, coconut sugar and agave nectar are all forms of sugar. Reducing simple sugars in your diet can help slow high stool output.

Applesauce Snack Cakes

These muffin-like cakes are a treat for kids' lunch boxes or for breakfast.

- *Preheat oven to 400°F (200°C)*
- *Two 8-cup muffin tins, greased or paper-lined*

½ cup	butter or margarine	125 mL
1½ cups	granulated sugar	375 mL
2	eggs	2
1 tsp	vanilla	5 mL
2 cups	all-purpose flour	500 mL
1 tbsp	baking powder	15 mL
1 tsp	baking soda	5 mL
1½ tsp	ground cinnamon	7 mL
1 tsp	ground allspice	5 mL
½ tsp	ground cloves	2 mL
2 cups	unsweetened applesauce	500 mL

1. In a large bowl, cream butter and sugar. Beat in eggs and vanilla until light and fluffy.

2. Sift together flour, baking powder, baking soda and spices. Add to creamed mixture alternately with applesauce, mixing well after each addition.

3. Spoon into prepared muffin cups, filling each about two-thirds full. Bake in preheated oven for about 20 minutes or until firm to the touch.

Vegetarian choice

Higher-calorie choice

Lower-fiber choice

MAKES 16 SNACK CAKES (1 per serving)

Tip

- Make your own applesauce when apples are plentiful and freeze in 2-cup (500 mL) portions.

IBD Tips

- This recipe is suitable for a low-fiber diet.
- Applesauce is known to help thicken stool. For variety, use fruit-flavored applesauce.
- Butter provides a trace of lactose; use margarine for a truly lactose-free version of this snack cake.

Nutrients Per Serving	
Calories	200
Fat	6 g
Fiber	1 g
Protein	2 g
Carbohydrate	34 g

MAKES 8 SERVINGS

IBD Tips

- To boost calories, use full-fat mayonnaise, sour cream and ham.

- Smoked meat is tasty, but consume it in moderation, as it may be a dietary risk factor for cancer.

- Buy cheese such as Cheddar when it is on sale, shred it and store it in the freezer for when you need it.

- If you're not feeling very hungry, or can't come up with an idea for dinner, prepare a light meal by choosing a snack such as this and adding a bowl of soup on the side.

Ham and Cheese Quesadillas

Your kids will love these quesadillas and the yummy dipping sauce for lunch or dinner.

- *Preheat oven to 350°F (180°C)*
- *Baking sheet, lined with parchment paper*

1 cup	shredded Cheddar cheese	250 mL
8	6-inch (15 cm) flour tortillas	8
6	slices fat-free smoked ham, chopped	6
1/4 cup	salsa	60 mL

Dipping Sauce

1/2 cup	light mayonnaise	125 mL
2 tbsp	low-fat sour cream	30 mL
2 tsp	finely chopped fresh cilantro	10 mL
2 tsp	finely chopped green onion	10 mL
2 tsp	grated lime zest	10 mL
2 tsp	freshly squeezed lime juice	10 mL

1. Sprinkle 1/2 cup (125 mL) of the cheese evenly over 4 tortillas. Sprinkle ham on top and drizzle each tortilla with 1 tbsp (15 mL) salsa. Top with the remaining cheese. Cover with the other 4 tortillas. Place on prepared baking sheet.

2. Bake in preheated oven for 10 to 12 minutes or until cheese is melted and tortillas are heated through. Let cool for a few minutes, then cut each tortilla into 4 to 6 wedges.

3. *Meanwhile, prepare the dipping sauce:* In a small bowl, combine mayonnaise, sour cream, cilantro, green onion, lime zest and lime juice.

4. Serve 2 to 3 wedges per person, with dipping sauce on the side.

> **IF FOLLOWING A LOW-FIBER DIET AND AVOIDING DIFFICULT-TO-DIGEST FOODS...**
>
> Choose tortillas made from white flour, omit the salsa and remove any tough skin or casing from the outside of the ham, if necessary.

Nutrients Per Serving	
Calories	232
Fat	12 g
Fiber	1 g
Protein	9 g
Carbohydrate	21 g

Seafood Tortilla Pinwheels

3 oz	light cream cheese, softened	75 g
½ cup	5% ricotta cheese	125 mL
2 tbsp	chopped fresh dill (or 1 tsp/5 mL dried)	30 mL
2 tbsp	chopped green onions (1 medium)	30 mL
1 tbsp	light mayonnaise	15 mL
2 tsp	freshly squeezed lemon juice	10 mL
4 oz	chopped cooked shrimp	125 g
¼ cup	chopped red bell pepper	60 mL
4	small flour tortillas	4
	Lettuce leaves (optional)	

1. Place cream cheese, ricotta, dill, green onions, mayonnaise and lemon juice in a bowl; combine thoroughly. Stir in shrimp and red pepper.

2. Divide shrimp mixture among tortillas and spread to the edges; top with lettuce leaves (if using), overlapped to cover entire tortilla. Roll up tightly, cover and refrigerate for an hour to chill.

3. Cut each roll crosswise into 6 pieces and serve.

IF FOLLOWING A LOW-FIBER DIET AND AVOIDING DIFFICULT-TO-DIGEST FOODS...

Finely chop the fresh dill (no stems) and onions, remove the skin from the red pepper before chopping, choose tortillas made with white flour and omit the lettuce leaves. If you have a new ileostomy, avoid stringy and chewy shellfish for at least 6 weeks after surgery.

Vegetarian choice

Lower-fiber choice

Higher-protein choice

MAKES 24 PINWHEELS (4 per serving)

Tips

- You may substitute crab legs (surimi, or imitation crab) for the shrimp.
- Prepare tortillas early in the day and keep tightly covered in refrigerator.

IBD Tips

- This recipe is suitable for vegetarians who eat seafood, dairy and eggs.
- To boost calories, use full-fat cream cheese, ricotta cheese and mayonnaise.

Nutrients Per Serving	
Calories	158
Fat	6 g
Fiber	1 g
Protein	11 g
Carbohydrate	15 g

**MAKES ABOUT
2 CUPS (500 ML)
(2 tbsp/30 mL per
serving)**

Tip

• Although blackstrap molasses is a good source of iron, it has a strong flavor and can be overly assertive for seasoning apples. We prefer fancy molasses from the supermarket in this recipe.

IBD Tips

• This recipe is suitable for a low-fiber diet, as the apples are peeled, cored, cooked soft and puréed.

• If you select blackstrap molasses, it will provide additional calcium and iron. Molasses provides potassium in this recipe.

Nutrients Per Serving	
Calories	70
Fat	Trace
Fiber	2 g
Protein	Trace
Carbohydrate	18 g

Luscious Apple Butter

This delicious old-fashioned spread has lots of appeal. Serve it on toast for breakfast, on nut butter sandwiches for lunch or as a snack or dessert topping. You can also forgo the puréeing and serve a warm, chunky version as an accompaniment to puddings or vanilla-flavor soy yogurt.

• *Preheat oven to 400°F (200°C)*
• *13- by 9-inch (33 by 23 cm) baking dish, ungreased*

¼ cup	water	60 mL
10	small to medium cooking apples (such as McIntosh), peeled, cored and thinly sliced	10
⅓ cup	packed dark brown sugar or other dry sweetener	75 mL
¼ tsp	ground cinnamon	1 mL
¼ tsp	ground cloves	1 mL
⅛ tsp	ground allspice	0.5 mL
Pinch	ground nutmeg	Pinch
3 tbsp	molasses (see tip, at left)	45 mL
1 tbsp	freshly squeezed lemon juice	15 mL

1. Pour water into baking dish. Add apples and brown sugar. Stir until sugar is dissolved. Sprinkle cinnamon, cloves, allspice and nutmeg over top and mix well.

2. Drizzle molasses and lemon juice over top. Stir well.

3. Bake, uncovered, in preheated oven, stirring every 20 minutes, for 1 hour or until apples are deep brown, soft and coated with syrup. Let cool in baking dish on a rack for 5 to 10 minutes.

4. Transfer cooled apple mixture to a food processor or blender and purée until smooth. Store in a glass jar or airtight container in the refrigerator for up to 6 weeks.

Variation

For convenience, make this recipe using one 26-oz (700 mL) jar unsweetened applesauce instead of the apples. Omit the water and bake at 375°F (190°C) for 1 hour. No puréeing is needed.

Almond Butter

- *Preheat oven to 350°F (180°C)*
- *Rimmed baking sheet, ungreased*

2 cups	whole raw almonds	500 mL
4 to 6 tbsp	vegetable oil	50 to 90 mL
Pinch	salt (optional)	Pinch

1. On baking sheet, spread almonds in a single layer. Bake in preheated oven for 12 to 14 minutes or until toasted and fragrant.
2. Transfer to food processor. Pulse until almonds are evenly chopped, occasionally stopping and scraping down the side of the bowl. Add 2 tbsp (30 mL) of the vegetable oil, and salt, if using. Process for 1 minute. Remove lid and scrape down the side of the bowl with a rubber spatula. Replace lid and, with motor running, slowly add remaining oil, 1 tbsp (15 mL) at a time, down the feeder tube, processing until mixture is smooth and spreadable.
3. Transfer to a glass jar or airtight container and refrigerate for up to 1 month.

Vegan choice

Higher-calorie choice

Lactose-free choice

MAKES ABOUT 1 CUP (250 ML) (2 tbsp/30 mL per serving)

Tip

- Almonds vary in moisture content, depending on how fresh they are. That's why there is a range in the amount of oil required to make the butter smooth.

IBD Tips

- This recipe is suitable for a low-fiber diet.
- Nuts are high in unsaturated fat, making them an excellent high-calorie snack. Although monounsaturated and polyunsaturated fats are considered heart-healthy, they should still be consumed in moderation.
- Smooth nut butters, including peanut butter and cashew butter, can help thicken loose stool.
- Almonds are a calcium-rich food.

Nutrients Per Serving	
Calories	265
Fat	25 g
Fiber	4 g
Protein	8 g
Carbohydrate	7 g

**MAKES 10
SERVINGS**

Tips

- The tortilla chips will keep for up to 2 weeks in an airtight plastic bag at room temperature.
- Use the baked tortillas as an inexpensive replacement for store-bought crispy flatbreads.
- Make extra tortilla chips and use for other dips or with cheese another day.

IBD Tips

- Avocados and tomatoes provide the potassium in this recipe.
- Avocados are high in unsaturated fat and will boost calories in any recipe they are used in. Be sure to ripen them at room temperature in a dark place before they are stored at a colder temperature; otherwise, they will discolor and won't ripen.

Lightened-Up Guacamole and Chips

- *Preheat oven to 350°F (180°C)*

2	ripe avocados, peeled and mashed	2
1	tomato, chopped (optional)	1
1	clove garlic, minced (or ½ tsp/2 mL garlic powder)	1
½ cup	fat-free plain yogurt	125 mL
⅓ cup	tomato salsa (mild, medium or hot)	75 mL
2 tbsp	chopped green onion (optional)	30 mL
2 tsp	freshly squeezed lemon juice	10 mL
1 tsp	ground cumin (or to taste)	5 mL
1 tsp	chili powder (or to taste)	5 mL
8 to 10	10-inch (25 cm) multigrain or whole wheat tortillas	8 to 10

1. In a large bowl, combine avocados, tomato (if using), garlic, yogurt, salsa, green onion (if using), lemon juice, cumin and chili powder.

2. In batches, place tortillas directly on the middle rack of preheated oven and toast, turning once, for 10 to 15 minutes or until golden brown and starting to crisp (check periodically to make sure they are not getting too brown). Let cool on a wire rack, then break into dipping-size pieces.

3. Serve guacamole in a dish, surrounded by toasted tortilla chips.

> **IF FOLLOWING A LOW-FIBER DIET AND AVOIDING DIFFICULT-TO-DIGEST FOODS...**
>
> Remove skin and seeds from tomato (see page 169), omit salsa and green onion, and use tortillas made with white flour.

Nutrients Per Serving	
Calories	227
Fat	10 g
Fiber	6 g
Protein	6 g
Carbohydrate	29 g

Sardine and Pesto Spread

Three simple ingredients give big taste to this chunky spread. Don't mash the sardines too much, or you'll end up with more of a paste than a spread. Serve with toasted French baguette slices.

1	can (3½ oz/106 g) sardines, drained	1
2 tbsp	basil pesto	30 mL
1 tbsp	freshly squeezed lime juice	15 mL

1. In a small bowl, mash sardines with a fork. Stir in pesto and lime juice until just blended.

IF FOLLOWING A LOW-FIBER DIET AND AVOIDING DIFFICULT-TO-DIGEST FOODS…

Select a pesto with a smooth paste texture (i.e., ingredients such as pine nuts have been finely puréed).

MAKES ½ CUP (125 ML) (2 TBSP/30 ML PER SERVING)

Tip

- Sardines are a good choice for people trying to increase their intake of vitamin B_{12}.

IBD Tips

- This recipe is suitable for vegetarians who eat seafood.

- This easy spread is a good choice when your energy is down. It packs calories and is easily added to foods like plain pasta — a helpful cooking solution during times of illness.

- Sardines packed in oil increase the calories in this recipe. Canned sardines contribute sodium.

- The oil and nuts in the pesto provide heart-healthy monounsaturated and polyunsaturated fats.

Nutrients Per Serving	
Calories	74
Fat	6 g
Fiber	0 g
Protein	6 g
Carbohydrate	2 g

Vegetarian choice

Lower-calorie choice

Lower-fat choice

Lower-fiber choice

Higher-protein choice

Source of potassium

Source of sodium

MAKES 8 SERVINGS

Tip

- White navy pea beans can also be used. If you cook your own dry beans, $\frac{1}{2}$ cup (125 mL) dry yields approximately $1\frac{1}{2}$ cups (375 mL) cooked beans.

IBD Tips

- This recipe is suitable for vegetarians who eat fish, dairy and eggs.

- Boost calories by choosing tuna packed in oil and full-fat mayonnaise and ricotta.

- Tuna provides omega-3 fats, which have anti-inflammatory properties. For more information about the safety and benefits of fish such as tuna, see page 224.

Nutrients Per Serving	
Calories	73
Fat	2 g
Fiber	2 g
Protein	8 g
Carbohydrate	7 g

Tuna and White Bean Spread

1 cup	canned, cooked white kidney beans, drained	250 mL
1	can (6$\frac{1}{2}$ oz/184 g) tuna in water, drained	1
1$\frac{1}{2}$ tsp	minced garlic	7 mL
2 tbsp	freshly squeezed lemon juice	30 mL
2 tbsp	light mayonnaise	30 mL
$\frac{1}{4}$ cup	5% ricotta cheese	60 mL
3 tbsp	minced red onion	45 mL
$\frac{1}{4}$ cup	minced fresh dill (or 1 tsp/5 mL dried)	60 mL
1 tbsp	freshly grated Parmesan cheese	15 mL
$\frac{1}{4}$ cup	diced red bell pepper	60 mL

1. Place beans, tuna, garlic, lemon juice, mayonnaise and ricotta in food processor; pulse on and off until combined but still chunky. Place in serving bowl.

2. Stir onions, dill, Parmesan and red pepper into bean mixture.

IF FOLLOWING A LOW-FIBER DIET AND AVOIDING DIFFICULT-TO-DIGEST FOODS...

Remove the skin from the outside of the beans, cook the minced onion until soft, finely mince the dill (do not include stems), and remove the skin from the red pepper before dicing.

Mediterranean Eggplant Spread

Make this creamy spread when eggplants and tomatoes are in season for maximum flavor and minimum cost. Serve with melba toast and bread sticks.

- *Preheat oven to 375°F (190°C)*
- *Baking sheet, greased*

2	medium eggplants	2
2 cups	lower-fat plain yogurt	500 mL
2 tbsp	freshly squeezed lemon juice	30 mL
1	clove garlic, minced	1
1 tbsp	red wine vinegar	15 mL
1 tbsp	olive oil	15 mL
1/2 tsp	crumbled dried oregano	2 mL
1/2 tsp	salt	2 mL
2	medium tomatoes, seeded and diced	2
1/2 cup	diced celery	125 mL

1. Cut eggplants in half lengthwise. Place on greased baking sheet, cut side down; cut 2 or 3 slits in skin. Cover with foil; bake in preheated oven for 35 to 45 minutes or until tender. Cool. Remove stalk, peel and seeds; finely chop eggplants.

2. In a bowl, combine eggplants, yogurt, lemon juice, garlic, vinegar, oil, oregano, salt, tomatoes and celery, mixing well. Cover and chill for at least 30 minutes.

> **IF FOLLOWING A LOW-FIBER DIET AND AVOIDING DIFFICULT-TO-DIGEST FOODS...**
> Purée eggplants instead of chopping them, remove skin from tomatoes (see page 145), and omit the celery.

Vegetarian choice

Lower-calorie choice

Lower-fiber choice

Higher-protein choice

Source of potassium

MAKES 5 CUPS (1.25 L) (3 tbsp/45 mL per serving)

Tip

- Choose eggplants that feel firm and have a shiny, wrinkle-free skin. The stem should look moist, as if recently cut.

IBD Tips

- This recipe is suitable for vegetarians who eat dairy.
- Boost calories by using a higher-fat yogurt.
- Use this spread instead of mayo or mustard in sandwiches and wraps.
- Tomatoes are a source of potassium; eggplant also provides some.

Nutrients Per Serving	
Calories	21
Fat	1 g
Fiber	Trace
Protein	1 g
Carbohydrate	3 g

Hummus with Roasted Red Peppers

1	can (14 to 19 oz/398 to 540 mL) chickpeas, drained and rinsed (see tips, at right), or 1 cup (250 mL) dried chickpeas, soaked, cooked and drained	1
1/4 cup	tahini	60 mL
1/4 cup	freshly squeezed lemon juice	60 mL
2	cloves garlic, minced	2
1/2	roasted red bell pepper, peeled and thinly sliced (see tip, at left)	1/2
1 tsp	ground cumin	5 mL
1/4 tsp	salt, or to taste	1 mL
	Water (optional)	

MAKES 1 1/4 CUPS (300 ML) (2 tbsp/30 mL per serving)

Tips

• Because can sizes vary, we provide a range of amounts for beans in our recipes. If you're using the larger size, you may want to adjust the seasoning by adding a pinch of cumin and salt.

• You can use bottled roasted red bell peppers in this hummus or roast your own (see Roasted Bell Peppers, page 286).

IBD Tips

• Use this spread instead of mayo or mustard.

• To boost calories, add 1 to 2 tbsp (15 to 30 mL) olive oil in step 1.

• Chickpeas and tahini are the sources of potassium in this recipe.

1. In food processor or blender, combine chickpeas, tahini, lemon juice and garlic and process until smooth.

2. Add roasted red peppers, ground cumin and salt and process until smooth. If you prefer a creamier consistency, add water, 1 tbsp (15 mL) at a time, processing until the desired texture is achieved.

3. Transfer to an airtight container and refrigerate for at least 2 hours or overnight.

Variations

Hummus with Black Olives: Substitute 1/2 cup (125 mL) chopped pitted kalamata olives for the red pepper.

Lemony Hummus: Substitute 1 tbsp (15 mL) grated lemon zest for the red pepper.

IF FOLLOWING A LOW-FIBER DIET AND AVOIDING DIFFICULT-TO-DIGEST FOODS...

Pinch off the skin from the chickpeas. The variation with black olives is allowed because this spread is puréed until smooth.

Nutrients Per Serving	
Calories	88
Fat	4 g
Fiber	2 g
Protein	3 g
Carbohydrate	11 g

Tropical Cooler

1	ripe banana	1
1 cup	diced seedless watermelon	250 mL
1 cup	pineapple juice	250 mL

1. In blender, on high speed, blend banana, watermelon and pineapple juice until smooth and creamy.

Variation

Any of your favorite fruits will work. Always use a banana for creaminess, then add 1 cup (250 mL) diced fruit and 1 cup (250 mL) fruit juice. Some fruit suggestions are: pineapple, mango, cantaloupe, honeydew, papaya, kiwi, frozen or fresh berries. Some juice suggestions are: orange, apple, cranberry, white grape, tropical blend, pomegranate, blueberry.

MAKES 2 SERVINGS

IBD Tips

- Remember that stringy fruits, such as pineapple, and fruits with seeds, such as kiwi and berries, will increase the fiber content and are not appropriate for fiber-restricted diets.

- Pomegranate juice and blueberry juice contain powerful antioxidants.

- Melons are rich in potassium, but may be gas-producing for some individuals.

- Pineapple juice is a source of potassium. It also contains the digestive enzyme bromelain, which naturally digests protein.

- Try adding soy milk for a lactose-free "creamy" version of this refreshing drink.

- Adding nutritional drinks such as Resource, Boost or Ensure will contribute calories and balanced nutrition.

Nutrients Per Serving	
Calories	145
Fat	0 g
Fiber	2 g
Protein	2 g
Carbohydrate	36 g

MAKES 2 SERVINGS

Tips

- If fresh mangos are not available, you may be able to find frozen mangos in the freezer section of your grocery store. Substitute 1 cup (250 mL) frozen mango chunks.
- This drink keeps well in the refrigerator overnight.

IBD Tips

- To enjoy a lactose-free drink, substitute soy or lactose-free versions of the milk and yogurt.
- To further reduce fat, use fat-free yogurt.
- Mangos and yogurt are sources of potassium.
- You can substitute canned mango chunks, but be sure to drain the syrup.

Nutrients Per Serving	
Calories	190
Fat	3 g
Fiber	3 g
Protein	6 g
Carbohydrate	39 g

Mango Lassi

This refreshing drink is a favorite at Indian restaurants.

1	ripe mango, peeled and chopped	1
½ cup	low-fat plain or vanilla yogurt	125 mL
½ cup	milk	125 mL
	Liquid honey	
½ cup	ice cubes	125 mL

1. In blender, on high speed, blend mango, yogurt, milk, honey to taste and ice for 2 minutes or until smooth.

Mangos

If you'll be using the mango right away, be sure to buy a ripe one. Mangoes are ripe when they can be easily indented with your thumb. Avoid mangoes that are so ripe they feel mushy.

Mangos have large, flat stones in the middle. It is a little tricky to remove the fruit, but if you follow these simple instructions, the task should be easier: Make an initial cut about ½ inch (1 cm) from the center and cut off a long slice of mango. Do the same on the other side. For each of these pieces, use a sharp knife to score the flesh in long lines, first lengthwise, then crossways, cutting almost through to the skin to create small cubes. Using a spoon, scoop cubes from skin. Peel the stone section, remove any flesh from the outside edges and cut into cubes.

Sunny Orange Shake

This shake is packed with bone-building calcium.

¾ cup	lower-fat vanilla yogurt	175 mL
2 tbsp	skim-milk powder	30 mL
½ cup	orange juice	125 mL

1. In a blender, combine yogurt, skim-milk powder and orange juice; blend until smooth.

Vegetarian choice

Higher-calorie choice

Lower-fat choice

Lower-fiber choice

Higher-protein choice

Source of potassium

MAKES 1 SERVING

Tip

- The skim milk powder adds thickness to the Sunny Orange Shake and boosts the calcium content to 353 mg per serving.

IBD Tips

- Orange juice is rich in potassium.
- Experiment with flavored yogurts, such as banana-flavored yogurt, for some tasty variations.
- To make this even higher in calories, use a higher-fat yogurt.

Nutrients Per Serving	
Calories	262
Fat	2 g
Fiber	Trace
Protein	11 g
Carbohydrate	51 g

MAKES 4 SERVINGS

Tip

• For extra frothiness, add 1 cup (250 mL) crushed ice when blending.

IBD Tips

• This recipe packs three potassium sources: banana, mango and orange juice!

• Tofu provides good-quality protein and heart-healthy polyunsaturated fat.

• Try to find tofu set with calcium sulfate or calcium chloride (check the label), as this helps to boost your calcium intake.

Nutrients Per Serving	
Calories	123
Fat	2 g
Fiber	2 g
Protein	4 g
Carbohydrate	25 g

Decadent Fruit Smoothie

This smoothie, adapted from a recipe on the back of a tofu package, tastes sweet and rich, like dessert!

1	ripe banana	1
10 oz	peach-mango-flavored dessert tofu	300 g
1 cup	frozen peach or mango slices	250 mL
1 cup	orange juice	250 mL
	Liquid honey or granulated sugar (optional)	

1. In blender, on high speed, blend banana, tofu, peach slices and orange juice until smooth.
2. Sweeten with honey to taste, if desired. Serve cold.

Strawberry Orange Flaxseed Smoothie

3	strawberries, hulled	3
1/2 cup	plain soy beverage	125 mL
1/2 cup	orange juice	125 mL
2 tbsp	vanilla-flavored soy protein powder	30 mL
1 tsp	flaxseed oil	5 mL
1 to 2	ice cubes	1 to 2

1. In blender, on high speed, blend strawberries, soy beverage, orange juice, protein powder, flaxseed oil and ice for 30 seconds or until smooth.

IF YOU ARE WELL...

If there is no medical reason for you to avoid fiber or difficult-to-digest foods, include whole fruits in your diet, even fruits with seeds, such as berries.

Flaxseed Oil

Since flaxseed oil becomes damaged if exposed to heat, it cannot be used to cook with. Instead, use cold oil in a salad dressing. Always store flaxseed oil in the refrigerator.

Vegan choice

Higher-calorie choice

Higher-protein choice

Lactose-free choice

Source of potassium

MAKES 1 SERVING

IBD Tips

- This high-protein smoothie will help you feel full longer when you're on the go.

- Flaxseed oil is an excellent way to add omega-3 fat to your diet. Omega-3 fats have anti-inflammatory properties and are considered deficient in the typical North American diet. While marine sources of omega-3 (e.g., coldwater fatty fish such as tuna, salmon, sardines and mackerel) are best, it is still worthwhile to include plant sources of omega-3 whenever possible.

Nutrients Per Serving	
Calories	228
Fat	8 g
Fiber	4 g
Protein	24 g
Carbohydrate	20 g

MAKES 2 SERVINGS

IBD Tips

- When made with gluten-free vanilla, this recipe is gluten-free, which is important for individuals living with celiac disease or non-celiac gluten sensitivity.

- To boost calories, choose full-fat milk or cream.

- To make this recipe lactose-free, use non-dairy milk. This, along with choosing maple syrup, will also make the recipe suitable for a vegan diet.

- Be mindful that vegetable-based milk may provide less protein than cow's milk.

- Banana boosts the potassium in this recipe and is known to help thicken stool.

- Don't be afraid to use spice to add flavor and appeal.

Nutrients Per Serving	
Calories	263
Fat	3 g
Fiber	5 g
Protein	9 g
Carbohydrate	52 g

Pumpkin Pie Smoothie

Full of antioxidants and vitamin A, pumpkin is an excellent food to include regularly in your diet. This sweet, creamy smoothie offers delicious proof that it deserves a place in your pantry year-round.

1 cup	sliced frozen ripe banana	250 mL
3 tbsp	quinoa flakes or flour	45 mL
1/2 tsp	pumpkin pie spice or ground cinnamon	2 mL
1 1/3 cups	milk or plain non-dairy milk (such as soy, almond, rice or hemp)	325 mL
3/4 cup	pumpkin purée (not pie filling)	175 mL
1/2 cup	ice cubes	125 mL
2 tbsp	pure maple syrup or liquid honey	30 mL
1 tsp	vanilla extract	5 mL

1. In a blender, purée banana, quinoa flakes, pumpkin pie spice, milk, pumpkin, ice cubes, maple syrup and vanilla until smooth. Pour into glasses and serve immediately.

Mega Melon Supreme

½ cup	orange juice	125 mL
½ cup	chopped seeded peeled watermelon	125 mL
½ cup	chopped seeded peeled cantaloupe	125 mL
½ cup	chopped seeded peeled honeydew melon	125 mL
½ cup	vanilla-flavored frozen yogurt	125 mL

1. In blender, combine orange juice, watermelon, cantaloupe, honeydew and frozen yogurt. Process as directed until smooth.

General Directions

Always place the lid securely on the blender before processing. Blend on Low for 30 seconds. Gradually (if possible) increase speed to High and blend an additional 30 seconds or until smooth.

Vegetarian choice

Lower-calorie choice

Lower-fat choice

Lower-fiber choice

Source of potassium

MAKES 4 SERVINGS

IBD Tips

- To enjoy a lactose-free drink, substitute soy or lactose-free versions of the frozen yogurt.
- Experiment with different flavors of frozen yogurt to create exciting new tastes!
- Melons are rich in potassium. When selecting melons, look for heaviness in relation to size, a characteristic aroma and color, and a normal shape, without any signs of spoilage. Honeydew and cantaloupe are ripe when the surface yields slightly to pressure. For watermelon, a green color with a yellowish underside is a good sign.

Nutrients Per Serving	
Calories	59
Fat	1 g
Fiber	Trace
Protein	1 g
Carbohydrate	11 g

MAKES 4 SERVINGS

Tip

- You can use fresh and frozen fruit interchangeably in most smoothies, although the results will differ. Frozen fruit not only chills a smoothie, it thickens it as well.

IBD Tips

- Apricots and peaches contribute potassium.

- Canned fruit is a good choice when you are concerned about potential food blockages or obstructions. It is also convenient when fruits are out of season.

- Whole evaporated milk and full-fat yogurt are great ways to increase the calories in this recipe. If you choose low-fat yogurt and nonfat evaporated milk, this smoothie will be a lower-fat choice.

- Ground herbs and spices, such as nutmeg, are safe for low-fiber diets and add lots of flavor.

Nutrients Per Serving	
Calories	131
Fat	3 g
Fiber	2 g
Protein	3 g
Carbohydrate	24 g

Peach Cobbler

1	can (14 oz/398 mL) halved or sliced peaches in juice	1
4	ice cubes	4
½ cup	evaporated milk	125 mL
¼ cup	peach-flavored yogurt	60 mL
2	apricots, peeled, pitted and chopped	2
⅓ cup	peach sherbet	75 mL
Pinch	ground nutmeg	Pinch

1. In blender, combine peaches with juice, ice, evaporated milk, yogurt, apricots, sherbet and nutmeg. Process as directed on page 163 until smooth.

Chocolate Peanut Butter Banana Slurry

¾ cup	milk or plain soy milk	175 mL
1	ripe banana, peeled and chopped	1
2 tbsp	peanut butter	30 mL
1 tbsp	carob powder or unsweetened cocoa powder	15 mL
2 cups	chocolate ice cream or frozen yogurt	500 mL

1. In blender, combine milk, banana, peanut butter and carob powder. Process as directed until smooth. Add ice cream and continue as directed until just mixed in.

General Directions

In blender, combine ingredients (except ice cream). Cover with lid and blend on Low for 30 seconds. Gradually (if possible) increase speed to High and blend an additional 30 seconds or until smooth. Stop motor and add ice cream. Blend on Mix or Medium speed (or Low if using a two-speed blender) for 20 to 30 seconds or until ice cream is just mixed in. Add more liquid to thin or more ice cream to thicken, if desired.

Vegetarian choice

Higher-calorie choice

Lower-fiber choice

Higher-protein choice

Source of potassium

MAKES 2 SERVINGS

IBD Tips

- Potassium is found in milk, yogurt and peanut butter. Add in banana, and this recipe packs a good dose of potassium.

- It is important to use smooth peanut butter rather than crunchy if you are living with a bowel stricture or are following post-operative diet modifications to reduce obstruction risk or intolerance symptoms.

- If chocolate syrup is handy, try it as your chocolate source.

- One hundred percent natural peanut butters or "just peanuts" versions are healthier, as they don't contain added sugars or hydrogenated oils.

- If you choose skim milk and frozen yogurt, this slurry will be a lower-fat choice.

Nutrients Per Serving	
Calories	736
Fat	45 g
Fiber	5 g
Protein	18 g
Carbohydrate	68 g

MAKES 1 SERVING

IBD Tips

- While cooked carrots still contain some fiber, in this recipe they are puréed, thus minimizing obstruction risk.

- Carrots are a good source of beta carotene, a powerful antioxidant, and contain vitamin A, a fat-soluble vitamin important for growth, healthy skin and cells, and good night vision.

- If your skin in the anal area is sore from a high stool output, omit the cayenne pepper.

- Applesauce is a good source of soluble fiber and helps to thicken stool, so consider increasing the amount in any recipe. Try using fruit-flavored applesauce, such as mango, pineapple or raspberry. Most of these products use 100% fruit juice without seeds, so they are safe for a low-fiber diet.

Nutrients Per Serving	
Calories	178
Fat	1 g
Fiber	6 g
Protein	2 g
Carbohydrate	44 g

Spiced Carrot

½ cup	apple juice	125 mL
1 cup	cooked chopped carrots	250 mL
¼ cup	applesauce	60 mL
1	piece (½ inch/1 cm) gingerroot, peeled and chopped	1
¼ tsp	ground cinnamon	1 mL
¼ tsp	salt (or to taste)	1 mL
⅛ tsp	cayenne pepper (or to taste)	0.5 mL

1. In blender, combine apple juice, carrots, applesauce, gingerroot and cinnamon. Process as directed until smooth. Season with salt and cayenne.

General Directions

Always place the lid securely on the blender before processing. Blend on Low for 30 seconds. Gradually (if possible) increase speed to High and blend an additional 30 seconds or until smooth.

Mexican Hot Chocolate

This frothy hot chocolate has subtle Mexican spice to warm you up on a chilly day.

½ cup	granulated sugar	125 mL
½ cup	water	125 mL
⅓ cup	unsweetened cocoa powder	75 mL
½ tsp	ground cinnamon	2 mL
5 cups	milk	1.25 L
½ tsp	vanilla	2 mL
½ tsp	almond extract	2 mL

1. In a large saucepan, over medium heat, heat sugar, water, cocoa powder and cinnamon until sugar dissolves. Add milk; heat until steaming (do not boil). Remove from heat and stir in vanilla and almond extract.

Vegetarian choice

Lower-fiber choice

Higher-protein choice

MAKES 6 SERVINGS

Tip

- If you have a manual frother, whirl the hot chocolate until very frothy before serving.

IBD Tips

- Extracts can add flavor variety to any beverage.

- While warm beverages are soothing and relaxing, remember that cocoa powder contains some caffeine and can stimulate the gut in very sensitive individuals.

- In comparison to "empty calorie" drinks like coffee and tea, this hot chocolate is a great way to increase calories and protein. Higher-fat milk will add more calories than skim or 1%.

Nutrients Per Serving	
Calories	178
Fat	5 g
Fiber	2 g
Protein	8 g
Carbohydrate	29 g

MAKES 2 SERVINGS

IBD Tips

- While composition and flavor may vary, honey always contains a mixture of sucrose, fructose and glucose. Research is ongoing to investigate the potential antioxidant properties of some types of honey.

- The flesh of an apple contains soluble fiber (pectin), while the skin is insoluble fiber. Peeling and coring an apple helps to reduce the amount of insoluble fiber. Some individuals tolerate cooked apple better than raw, experiencing less gas and cramping. To quickly cook an apple, heat it in your microwave; when done, it should be soft but still hold its shape.

- Ground spices and herbs are okay on a low-fiber diet and add lots of flavor.

Nutrients Per Serving	
Calories	170
Fat	Trace
Fiber	2 g
Protein	Trace
Carbohydrate	43 g

Hot Gingered Apple Cider

1 cup	apple cider or apple juice	250 mL
2 tbsp	liquid honey (or to taste)	30 mL
1	piece ($\frac{1}{2}$ inch/1 cm) candied ginger, chopped	1
$\frac{1}{8}$ tsp	ground cinnamon	0.5 mL
$\frac{1}{8}$ tsp	ground cloves	0.5 mL
Pinch	ground nutmeg	Pinch
1	apple, peeled, cored and chopped	1
1 tsp	apple cider vinegar	5 mL

1. In a medium saucepan over medium heat, bring apple cider, honey, ginger, cinnamon, cloves and nutmeg just to a boil.
2. In blender, combine half of the cider mixture, the apple and cider vinegar. Process as directed.

General Directions

Place required amount of hot liquid in the blender with the other ingredients. Place the lid securely on the jug. Blend on Low for 30 seconds. With blender still running, add the remaining hot liquid gradually through the opening in the center of the lid. Replace center cover securely, increase speed to High and process for 30 seconds or until smooth.

Soups

When asked to think of comfort foods, many people agree that soup makes it to the top of the list. For individuals who struggle with illness, however, soup is often a reminder of times when they are not well. Before you skip this chapter, look through the selected recipes and open your mind to a variety of soup ingredients and flavors you haven't tried before. Consider including soups made with foods you've avoided because you worry they may not be tolerated. Some of these soups are puréed, which is a perfect way to avoid the risk of obstruction that might occur with certain foods, especially if you are living with a stricture, have narrowing due to inflammation or are following a post-operative fiber-restricted diet. While the puréed soups still contain fiber, its properties are somewhat altered by the mechanical breakdown from puréeing. So plan to expand your soup repertoire and stimulate your taste buds with the following exciting soups!

Drink Your Calories

Like beverages, soups are an easy way to "drink" calories without feeling as full as you would from eating solids. Soups may be easier to swallow when you don't feel good or have mouth sores, and they pack a good dose of nutrients. In fact, many soups are an easy way for you to work toward your recommended daily servings of fruits and vegetables. Use soups to accompany a meal, as a meal in themselves or as a handy snack when you're hungry after school or work. Consider buying a thermos and taking soup with you on your travels, or make a large batch and freeze individual portion sizes in your freezer for busy times.

Boost Your Calories and Protein

Boost calories in soups by making them with higher-fat milk, adding skim milk powder or cream, topping with shredded cheese or adding butter, margarine or a heart-healthy oil. Boost protein by adding chicken, turkey, fish, beef, veal or pork. You could also try adding tofu and puréeing the soup for a creamy texture.

Boosting calories in soup can be easy when you remember that a balanced meal contains foods from each of the four food groups. For example, if you have a meat- or soy-based soup with vegetables, add milk to make it a creamy soup and serve oat bran bread as an accompaniment. Now you have a more interesting meal, and all four food groups are represented!

Boost Your Soluble Fiber

Add a handful of barley to ready-made or commercial soup to add a good dose of soluble fiber. Remember to add more fluid while cooking and to cook long enough to make the barley soft and not too chewy.

Boost Your Sodium and Potassium

Sodium and potassium are the two electrolytes that are depleted during times of excessive sweating, vomiting and liquidy stool losses. Canned products such as canned vegetables and soups are high in sodium (salt). Including these foods in your diet can be a good way to boost salt intake when you are experiencing high stool outputs. Choose soups that contain tomatoes, as they will also be high in potassium.

> Always use iodized salt, as the added iodine is essential for thyroid health and mental development.

Rinse Canned Beans to Reduce Indigestible Carbohydrates

To reduce the gas-producing compounds (indigestible carbohydrates) present in canned beans, it is very important to rinse them. Once the "bubbles" are gone, the beans are rinsed properly.

Legumes Are Worth Including in Your Diet

Legumes (peas and beans) contain protein, iron and soluble fiber. However, many people with IBD believe they cannot consume them because they are gas-producing. Soaking or rinsing legumes removes much of their gas-forming compounds. You should also be aware that the outside "skin" of a bean is insoluble fiber, while the inside contains more soluble fiber. Some people "pinch" or peel off the outside skin to target the soluble fiber. Start with small portions if you are worried about cramps from gas.

> Brightly colored vegetables provide an array of phytonutrients, including antioxidants.

PEEL AND SEED TOMATOES TO REDUCE INSOLUBLE FIBER

To remove the skin and seeds from a tomato:

1. Fill a saucepan three-quarters full of water and bring to a boil over high heat.

2. Blanch the tomato in the boiling water for 1 minute. Remove and set aside to cool.

3. Gently pierce the skin of the tomato with the tip of a sharp knife. Loosen the skin with the knife and peel the skin away. If the tomato doesn't peel well, return it to the boiling water for 30 seconds and cool again.

4. Cut the peeled tomato in half and squeeze gently so that the seeds drip out.

To help with peeling, you can cut a small X in the base of the tomato before blanching it. The skin will split slightly around the X, making it easier to peel back the corners to remove the skin.

Boost Your Interest in Eating

Herbs, spices and other seasonings and flavorings are a fantastic, easy way to add flavor and aroma to your meals, which may heighten your interest in eating. Here are tips on some of our favorite flavor-boosters.

- Parsley is considered helpful to digestion and, for some, may improve appetite. To avoid the risk of obstruction, finely chop parsley leaves without the stems.
- Ginger aids digestion and, for some, may improve appetite and reduce nausea. Pre-minced gingerroot is available at most grocery stores and is a great time-saver. If mincing gingerroot yourself, use the side of a spoon to scrape off the skin first. Gingerroot keeps well in the freezer for up to 3 months and can be grated from frozen.
- Citrus juice (such as orange, lime or lemon juice) supplies potassium, and its fresh fragrance stimulates interest in eating. Citrus juice can usually be included in the diet of individuals living with IBD. In times of illness or anal soreness from frequent loose stool, you may choose to limit the amount in a recipe.
- Sea salt is distilled from ocean water and is sold fine- or coarse-grained. It retains minerals, such as magnesium and potassium, but in amounts that are considered insignificant to our nutrition. Iodized varieties are recommended.
- Paprika is a powdered red spice made from ground dried bell peppers, sometimes mixed with ground dried chile peppers. If you don't like heat, look for sweet paprika rather than hot paprika.
- Turmeric is a bright yellow-orange powdered spice that contains curcumin, which is thought to have antioxidant and anti-inflammatory properties.
- Curry powder adds great flavor, but you may want to avoid it during times of illness or when you're experiencing anal soreness from frequent loose stools.

Onions add a tremendous amount of flavor, and offer the added benefits of prebiotics. If following a low-fiber diet, make sure to always finely chop onions. To help prevent them from making you cry, try using a sharp knife, setting up a fan to blow the fumes away, placing the onion in the freezer for 10 minutes beforehand or even wearing goggles!

Garlic is a member of the Allium family, which includes onions, leeks, shallots and chives. Garlic contains many chemicals, including allicin, which provides the strong taste and smell. It is not known for sure which chemicals provide the health benefits.

Basic Vegetable Stock

If you're looking for a snack to keep you going until dinner, try heating a mug of broth.

8 cups	fresh water or cooking water	2 L
2	stalks celery, chopped	2
2	large onions, chopped	2
2	large carrots, washed and chopped	2
4	cloves garlic, chopped	4
4	bay leaves	4
4	whole cloves (or pinch ground)	4
10	peppercorns, crushed	10
$\frac{1}{4}$ cup	chopped fresh parsley (or $\frac{1}{4}$ tsp/1 mL dried)	60 mL
$\frac{1}{4}$ tsp	salt (optional)	1 mL

1. Combine all ingredients in a large pot. Bring to a simmer and cook, uncovered, for 45 minutes.
2. Remove from heat; let cool. Strain, discarding solids. Store in a container with tight-fitting lid. Stock will keep 1 week in refrigerator and several months if frozen.

Vegan choice

Lower-calorie choice

Lower-fat choice

Lower-fiber choice

Lactose-free

MAKES 8 CUPS (2 L)

Tips

- Use vegetable bouillon cubes, powder or canned vegetable bouillon.
- Freeze in 1-cup (250 mL) portions; label and date.
- Substitute other vegetables of your choice. Try fennel, mushrooms, leeks, potatoes, yams or lettuce.

IBD Tip

- Boost sodium in this recipe by adding salt liberally or adding a packaged soup base, such as onion soup mix (strain out the rehydrated onion pieces with the rest of the solids).

Nutrients Per Serving	
Calories	36
Fat	Trace
Fiber	Trace
Protein	1 g
Carbohydrate	8 g

Chilled Avocado Soup

Rich and creamy avocados make a wonderful base for this summer soup.

MAKES 4 SERVINGS

IBD Tips

- If you experience frequent loose bowel movements and anal soreness, consider omitting the cayenne pepper, white pepper and hot pepper sauce. Otherwise, enjoy the kick these spices provide.

- If you're trying to increase sodium intake, be liberal with the "pinch" of salt.

- Avocados are a higher-fat fruit, the majority of which is monounsaturated. This means they are heart-healthy and can help boost calories when added to salads, soups and other dishes. They are also rich in potassium.

Garnish

1	tomato, peeled and diced	1
1 tbsp	chopped chives	15 mL
2 tsp	freshly squeezed lime or lemon juice	10 mL
1/4 tsp	cayenne pepper	1 mL
Pinch	salt	Pinch

Soup

2 cups	chilled defatted chicken stock	500 mL
1/2 cup	chopped sweet onion	125 mL
1/4 tsp	ground cumin	1 mL
1/4 tsp	salt	1 mL
Pinch	freshly ground white pepper	Pinch
Dash	hot pepper sauce	Dash
2	avocados, halved, pitted and peeled	2
1/2 cup	chilled whipping (35%) cream, table (18%) cream or sour cream	125 mL

1. *Prepare the garnish:* In a small bowl, mix together tomato, chives, lime juice, cayenne and salt; cover and chill for at least 2 hours or for up to 2 days.

2. *Prepare the soup:* In blender, on high speed, purée stock, onion, cumin, salt, pepper and hot pepper sauce. Add avocado and purée on high speed. On low speed, blend in cream.

3. Ladle soup into bowls and garnish with tomato mixture.

Variation

Chilled Avocado and Basil Soup: Replace whipping (35%) cream with 1/3 cup (75 mL) extra-virgin olive oil, increase lemon juice in garnish to 4 tsp (20 mL) and top with 12 shredded basil leaves.

IF FOLLOWING A LOW-FIBER DIET AND AVOIDING DIFFICULT-TO-DIGEST FOODS...

Remove the seeds from the tomato and omit the chives from the garnish. When making the variation, use finely chopped or dried flaked basil leaves.

Nutrients Per Serving	
Calories	316
Fat	27 g
Fiber	6 g
Protein	6 g
Carbohydrate	15 g

Chilled Melon Soup with Mango

2 cups	cubed cantaloupe	500 mL
1 cup	diced mango	250 mL
¾ cup	orange juice	175 mL
½ cup	lower-fat plain yogurt	125 mL
2 tbsp	lime juice	30 mL
2 tbsp	liquid honey	30 mL
	Chopped fresh mint (optional)	

1. In a food processor or blender, combine fruit; purée until smooth. Add orange juice, yogurt, lime juice and honey. Blend until combined. Chill. Serve sprinkled with mint, if desired.

Honey

Honey is sugar made by bees and is composed of water and simple carbohydrates, namely glucose and fructose. Honey also contains trace amounts of some vitamins, minerals and antioxidants, but these amounts are very small and are not considered significant to our nutrition.

Vegetarian choice

Lower-fat choice

Lower-fiber choice

Source of potassium

MAKES 4 SERVINGS

IBD Tips

- Chilled soups are refreshing in the warmer months and are a great way to avoid using the oven or stove.

- This recipe contains orange juice, mango and melon, all rich sources of potassium. Remember that melon can make some individuals gassy; consume a moderate amount to start.

- This recipe packs a beta carotene antioxidant punch with the orange fruits cantaloupe, mango and orange juice!

Nutrients Per Serving	
Calories	131
Fat	1 g
Fiber	2 g
Protein	3 g
Carbohydrate	30 g

MAKES 4 TO 6 SERVINGS

IBD Tips

- To boost calories, use higher-fat milk or cream instead of the soy milk.

- Certain fruits, such as pears, contain higher amounts of fructose, which may contribute to osmotic diarrhea when eaten in large amounts. However, the 3 pears in this recipe are divided into 4 to 6 servings, so you shouldn't have a problem.

- Parsnips, carrots and fresh pears are sources of potassium.

- If you use vegetable stock, this recipe is appropriate for vegetarian and vegan diets.

- To avoid the risk of obstruction, finely chop parsley leaves without the stems.

Nutrients Per Serving	
Calories	196
Fat	5 g
Fiber	5 g
Protein	8 g
Carbohydrate	31 g

Pear and Parsnip Soup

Very ripe pears are essential for bringing out the earthiness of parsnips. Salty garnishes such as sliced dry-roasted almonds, garlic croutons or crispy bacon best complement the soup's sweet flavors.

1 tbsp	vegetable oil	15 mL
1	clove garlic, minced	1
3 cups	chopped peeled parsnips (about 1 lb/500 g)	750 mL
¾ cup	chopped onion	175 mL
¾ cup	chopped peeled carrots	175 mL
1 tsp	dried thyme	5 mL
¼ tsp	salt	1 mL
¼ tsp	freshly ground black pepper	1 mL
2 tbsp	all-purpose flour	30 mL
3	very ripe pears, peeled, cored and chopped	3
4 cups	chicken or vegetable stock	1 L
1 cup	plain soy milk	250 mL
	Chopped fresh parsley	

1. In a large saucepan, heat oil over medium-high heat. Add garlic, parsnips, onion, carrots, thyme, salt and pepper; cook, stirring, until vegetables are soft and slightly browned, about 8 minutes. Stir in flour and cook, stirring, until flour no longer smells raw, about 2 minutes. Add pears and stock; bring to a boil. Cover, reduce heat to low and simmer until vegetables are very tender, about 15 minutes. Stir in soy milk.

2. Transfer to blender in batches and purée on high speed.

3. Pour into clean saucepan and simmer until heated through.

4. Ladle into bowls and sprinkle with parsley.

Carrot and Ginger Soup

Ginger has a great affinity for carrots, and this soup, with its appetizing color, is a sweet treat that both children and adults will love.

3 cups	water	750 mL
2	cloves garlic, crushed	2
4 cups	sliced carrots	1 L
1/2 cup	chopped onion	125 mL
1 tbsp	vegetable bouillon powder	15 mL
2 tsp	pure maple syrup	10 mL
1 tsp	curry powder	5 mL
1/2 tsp	grated gingerroot	2 mL
1 1/2 cups	milk	375 mL

1. In a large saucepan, bring water to a boil. Add garlic, carrots, onion, bouillon powder, maple syrup, curry powder and ginger; return to a boil. Reduce heat, cover and simmer for 40 to 45 minutes or until carrots are tender. Remove from heat.

2. Working in batches, transfer soup to blender and purée on high speed until smooth.

3. Return soup to saucepan and add milk. Heat over low heat (do not boil or milk will curdle).

Gingerroot

Use the side of a spoon to scrape off the skin before chopping or grating. Gingerroot keeps well in the freezer for up to 3 months and can be grated from frozen.

Vegetarian choice

Lower-calorie choice

Lower-fiber choice

Higher-protein choice

MAKES 6 SERVINGS

IBD Tips

- Small amounts of soft cooked carrots are considered okay for a low-fiber diet; in this recipe, they are puréed, thus minimizing the risk of obstruction.

- Don't be afraid to experiment with herbs, seasonings and spices. Garlic, curry powder and gingerroot add great flavor to this recipe. Avoid them only if you are certain you will experience difficulties after eating them. Remember that these foods may be better tolerated as your disease status changes and you feel better.

- To boost calories, use higher-fat milk.

Nutrients Per Serving	
Calories	66
Fat	2 g
Fiber	2 g
Protein	3 g
Carbohydrate	11 g

Vegetarian choice

Higher-calorie choice

Lower-fiber choice

Source of potassium

MAKES 6 SERVINGS

Tip

• Use frozen cauliflower florets and/or diced onion in this recipe for convenience. If you run out, 1 medium onion produces about 1 cup (250 mL) diced onion.

IBD Tips

• Potatoes are rich in potassium. Canned potatoes save time and add sodium.

• Canned broth and liberal salt use will up the sodium content.

• Small amounts of soft cooked cauliflower are considered okay for a low-fiber diet; in this recipe, the cauliflower is puréed, so the risk of obstruction is minimal. Remember that cauliflower is a gas-producing food and consume it in moderation.

• Butter and whipping cream boost the calories in this soup.

Nutrients Per Serving	
Calories	239
Fat	14 g
Fiber	2 g
Protein	8 g
Carbohydrate	21 g

Creamy Cauliflower Soup

2 tbsp	butter	30 mL
1 cup	diced onion (see tip, at right)	250 mL
1 tsp	salt	5 mL
	Freshly ground black pepper	
1	can (19 oz/540 mL) sliced potatoes, drained, or 2 cups (500 mL) chopped cooked potatoes	1
4 cups	cauliflower florets (see tip, at left)	1 L
6 cups	vegetable or chicken stock	1.5 L
1/2 cup	whipping (35%) cream	125 mL
2 tbsp	prepared sun-dried tomato pesto	30 mL

1. In a large saucepan, melt butter over medium heat. Add onion and cook, stirring, until softened, about 3 minutes. Add salt, and black pepper to taste, and cook, stirring, for 1 minute.

2. Add potatoes, cauliflower and stock. Bring to a boil. Reduce heat to low. Cover and cook until cauliflower is tender and flavors are combined, about 15 minutes.

3. Using a slotted spoon, transfer solids to a food processor or blender. Add 1/2 cup (125 mL) of the cooking liquid and process until smooth. (You can also do this in the saucepan, using a hand-held blender.)

4. Return mixture to saucepan over low heat. Add cream and pesto and heat gently until mixture almost reaches a simmer. Ladle into bowls and serve immediately.

Variations

Mulligatawny Soup: Add 1 tbsp (15 mL) curry powder along with the salt. Eliminate the pesto and stir in 2 cups (500 mL) chopped cooked chicken and/or 1/4 cup (60 mL) mango chutney along with the cream.

Creamy Cauliflower Soup with Smoked Salmon: Garnish the finished soup with 2 oz (60 g) chopped smoked salmon and, if desired, 2 tbsp (30 mL) chopped green onion, chives or dill.

Creamy Onion Soup with Kale

There is no cream in this delicious soup — unless you decide to drizzle a bit over individual servings as a finishing touch. The creaminess is achieved with the addition of potatoes, which are puréed into the soup, providing it with a velvety texture.

- *Medium to large (3 1/2- to 5-quart) slow cooker*

1 tbsp	olive oil	15 mL
4	onions, thinly sliced	4
2	cloves garlic, minced	2
4	whole allspice	4
1	bay leaf	1
1 tsp	grated lemon zest	5 mL
1/2 tsp	cracked black peppercorns	2 mL
4 cups	vegetable stock	1 L
3	potatoes, peeled and diced	3
1 tsp	paprika dissolved in 2 tbsp (30 mL) freshly squeezed lemon juice (see tip, at right)	5 mL
4 cups	chopped kale	1 L

1. In a skillet, heat oil over medium heat. Add onions and cook, stirring, until softened, about 5 minutes. Add garlic, allspice, bay leaf, lemon zest and peppercorns and cook, stirring, for 1 minute. Transfer to slow cooker stoneware. Stir in stock.

2. Add potatoes and stir well. Cover and cook on Low for 8 hours or on High for 4 hours, until potatoes are tender. Discard allspice and bay leaf. Stir in paprika solution and add kale, in batches, stirring after each to submerge the leaves in the liquid. Cover and cook on High for 20 minutes, until kale is tender.

3. Purée using an immersion blender. (You can also do this in batches in a food processor or stand blender.) Serve immediately.

IF FOLLOWING A LOW-FIBER DIET AND AVOIDING DIFFICULT-TO-DIGEST FOODS...

Finely chop the onions, and add all spices (allspice, bay leaf, peppercorns) in finely ground form. Because the kale is cooked and puréed, the risk of food obstruction is minimized.

Vegan choice

Lower-calorie choice

Lower-fat choice

Lactose-free choice

Source of potassium

Source of sodium

MAKES 6 SERVINGS

Tips

- You can use any kind of paprika in this recipe: regular or sweet; hot, which produces a nicely peppery version; or smoked, which adds a delicious note of smokiness to the soup.

- If you are halving this recipe, be sure to use a small (approx. 2-quart) slow cooker.

IBD Tips

- Commercial vegetable stock provides sodium (unless it is labeled "no-salt-added").

- Potatoes provide the potassium in this recipe, with a small amount added from the lemon juice.

Nutrients Per Serving	
Calories	128
Fat	3 g
Fiber	4 g
Protein	4 g
Carbohydrate	25 g

MAKES 4 SERVINGS

IBD Tips

- To reduce insoluble fiber and the risk of obstruction, use seeded tomatoes and omit the sesame seeds.

- Tofu contains high-quality protein and is high in heart-healthy polyunsaturated fat. Puréeing it in this recipe creates a creamy effect.

- Use vegetable stock instead of chicken stock to create a vegetarian soup.

- Up the sodium in this soup by using additional salt.

- Tomatoes and tomato paste are rich in potassium; tofu also supplies some.

- Brightly colored vegetables (such as green, red and yellow bell peppers) provide an array of phytonutrients, including antioxidants.

Nutrients Per Serving	
Calories	140
Fat	6 g
Fiber	4 g
Protein	8 g
Carbohydrate	17 g

Creamy Roasted Sweet Pepper Soup

2 tsp	olive oil	10 mL
1	medium onion, chopped	1
1	clove garlic, minced	1
1	each large red, yellow and green bell pepper, roasted and peeled (see box, below)	1
2 cups	chicken broth	500 mL
1	can (10 oz/284 mL) regular or seasoned tomatoes, drained	1
2 tbsp	tomato paste	30 mL
1 tsp	ground cumin	5 mL
6 oz	soft tofu	175 g
½ tsp	salt	2 mL
¼ tsp	freshly ground white pepper	1 mL
	Black sesame seeds or toasted white sesame seeds	

1. In a large saucepan, heat oil over medium heat; cook onion and garlic, stirring, for 2 to 3 minutes or until softened. Add peppers, broth, tomatoes, tomato paste and cumin; bring to a boil. Cover, reduce heat and simmer for 30 minutes. Cool slightly.

2. In a blender, purée pepper mixture with tofu in batches. Strain through sieve into saucepan; season with salt and pepper. Reheat over low heat. Garnish with sesame seeds.

To Roast Peppers

Heat barbecue or broiler; place peppers on grill or broiling pan and cook until skins turn black. Keep turning peppers until skins are blistered and black. Place roasted peppers in large pot with lid. Steam will make them sweat and skin will be easier to peel off. Let peppers cool. Remove stems, seeds and skin.

Save yourself time and money by buying a large quantity of red peppers at the end of the season when they are plentiful. Roast them, remove the skins and freeze in small amounts so they are ready to use throughout the winter.

Pumpkin and White Bean Soup

2 tsp	vegetable oil	10 mL
2 tsp	minced garlic	10 mL
1 cup	chopped onions	250 mL
½ cup	chopped carrots	125 mL
½ cup	chopped celery	125 mL
3½ cups	Basic Vegetable Stock (see recipe, page 171)	875 mL
1	can (14 oz/398 mL) pumpkin (not pie filling)	1
1	can (19 oz/540 mL) white kidney beans, rinsed and drained	1
1	bay leaf	1
1 tsp	ground ginger	5 mL
¼ cup	maple syrup	60 mL

1. In a nonstick saucepan sprayed with vegetable spray, heat oil over medium-high heat. Add garlic, onions, carrots and celery; cook 4 minutes or until onions and celery are softened.

2. Stir in stock, pumpkin, beans, bay leaf and ginger. Bring to a boil; reduce heat, cover, and cook 15 to 20 minutes or until vegetables are tender.

3. Stir in maple syrup. Serve immediately.

IF FOLLOWING A LOW-FIBER DIET AND AVOIDING DIFFICULT-TO-DIGEST FOODS...

Small amounts of soft cooked chopped onions and carrots are fine; however, you may wish to remove the celery. It can be placed in cheesecloth and added to the soup for flavor while the soup is cooking, then removed before you eat the soup.

Vegan choice

Lower-fat choice

Higher-protein choice

Lactose-free choice

Source of soluble fiber

Source of potassium

Source of sodium

MAKES 4 TO 6 SERVINGS

Tip

- In season, use fresh pumpkin. Bake for approximately 1 hour at 375°F (190°C) or until tender.

IBD Tips

- Squash and pumpkin are good sources of beta carotene.

- Kidney beans contribute protein, iron and soluble fiber. Rinse them well to reduce the gas-forming compounds. To reduce insoluble fiber, "pinch" the skin from the bean before using.

- The beans and pumpkin (especially if using fresh) provide potassium. Canned goods provide sodium.

- Canola oil and olive oil are heart-healthy choices.

Nutrients Per Serving	
Calories	175
Fat	2 g
Fiber	6 g
Protein	7 g
Carbohydrate	34 g

Higher-calorie choice

Lower-fat choice

Lower-fiber choice

Higher-protein choice

Lactose-free choice

Source of potassium

MAKES 6 SERVINGS

Tip

• When buying ham, make sure it's "fully cooked" or "ready-to-eat."

IBD Tip

• Sweet potatoes are a source of potassium and beta carotene.

• Many individuals with IBD avoid legumes; however, split peas provide some soluble fiber and, when eaten in moderate amounts, do not appear to have a significant gas-producing effect.

• Ham provides high-quality protein and heme iron, which is more bioavailable than iron from legumes, vegetables and grains.

• Canned stock boosts sodium.

Nutrients Per Serving	
Calories	289
Fat	2 g
Fiber	2 g
Protein	17 g
Carbohydrate	41 g

Sweet Potato Soup with Split Peas and Ham

¾ cup	chopped onions	175 mL
¾ cup	chopped carrots	175 mL
1½ tsp	minced garlic	7 mL
6½ cups	chicken or beef stock	1.625 L
1½ cups	diced sweet potatoes	375 mL
¾ cup	dried yellow split peas	175 mL
⅓ cup	small soup pasta (such as orzo or ditali)	75 mL
1 cup	diced cooked ham	250 mL

1. In a nonstick saucepan sprayed with vegetable spray, cook onions, carrots and garlic over medium-high heat for 3 minutes or until softened. Add stock, sweet potatoes and split peas; bring to a boil. Reduce heat to medium-low; cook, covered, for 40 minutes or until split peas are tender.

2. Transfer mixture to a food processor; purée until smooth. Return soup to saucepan. Add pasta and ham; cook over medium heat, covered, for 8 minutes or until pasta is tender.

Wedding Soup

Many individuals with IBD report that they can tolerate ground meat well, especially small, moist meatballs cooked in soup.

• *Baking sheet, lined with parchment paper*

2	slices white bread, crusts removed, shredded	2
¼ cup	milk	60 mL
1	egg, beaten	1
4 oz	lean ground beef	125 g
4 oz	regular or lean ground pork	125 g
4 oz	lean ground veal	125 g
⅓ cup	freshly grated Parmesan cheese	75 mL
2 oz	prosciutto, finely chopped	60 g
¼ cup	minced fresh flat-leaf (Italian) parsley	60 mL
2	cloves garlic, minced	2
1	small onion, minced	1
½ tsp	salt	2 mL
Pinch	ground nutmeg	Pinch
	Freshly ground black pepper	
10 cups	chicken stock	2.5 L
1	head escarole, thinly sliced	1
¾ cup	acini di pepe pasta	175 mL
	Additional freshly grated Parmesan cheese (optional)	

1. In a large bowl, combine bread and milk; let soak for 2 minutes. Add egg, beef, pork, veal, cheese, prosciutto, parsley, garlic, onion, salt, nutmeg and pepper to taste; mix with your hands until well combined.

2. In a small skillet, sauté a small spoonful of the meat mixture over medium heat until no longer pink. Taste and adjust the seasoning of the meat mixture with salt and pepper, if necessary. Roll meat mixture into small balls, about 1 inch (2.5 cm) in diameter, and place on prepared baking sheet.

3. In a large pot, bring stock to a simmer over medium heat. Slowly add meatballs, keeping liquid at a simmer so that the meatballs are moving and don't stick together. Add escarole and simmer until meatballs are cooked through and escarole is tender, about 10 minutes. Add pasta and simmer until tender to the bite, about 4 minutes. Taste and adjust seasoning with salt and pepper, if necessary.

4. Ladle into heated bowls and garnish with cheese, if desired.

Higher-protein choice

Lower-fiber choice

Source of sodium

MAKES 6 SERVINGS

IBD Tips

• Sodium sources in this recipe include prosciutto, commercial chicken stock (unless it is labeled "no-salt-added"), Parmesan cheese and added salt.

• If you are sensitive to the milk sugar lactose, you may still be able to tolerate aged hard cheeses such as Parmesan and Romano, as they have relatively small amounts of lactose.

IF FOLLOWING A LOW-FIBER DIET AND AVOIDING DIFFICULT-TO-DIGEST FOODS...

Make sure the nutmeg and black pepper are finely ground, and the escarole is finely chopped or minced.

Nutrients Per Serving	
Calories	398
Fat	16 g
Fiber	4 g
Protein	32 g
Carbohydrate	32 g

Lower-fat choice

Higher-protein choice

Lactose-free choice

Source of soluble fiber

Source of potassium

Source of sodium

Beef Barley Soup

Here's a delicious rib-sticking soup for a cold winter's day.

3½ cups	water	875 mL
¾ cup	tomato sauce	175 mL
¾ cup	dried soup mix (lentils, split peas, barley)	175 mL
1	beef bouillon cube	1
1	medium carrot, diced	1
1	medium potato, diced	1
2 tsp	dried basil	10 mL
½ tsp	salt	2 mL
¼ tsp	freshly ground black pepper	1 mL
½ cup	cubed cooked lean beef	125 mL

1. In a large stockpot, combine water, tomato sauce, dried soup mix, bouillon cube, carrot, potato and seasonings; bring to a boil. Reduce heat and simmer, covered, for about 1 hour. Add beef. Cook for 30 minutes longer.

MAKES 4 SERVINGS

Tips

• Dried soup mix is available in bulk or health food stores, as well as in the supermarket. If desired, replace with an equal quantity of barley.

• For a more robust broth, eliminate the bouillon cube and substitute 1 can (10 oz/284 mL) condensed beef broth. Reduce the quantity of water to 3 cups (750 mL).

IBD Tips

• Legumes and beef add protein and iron to this recipe; tomato sauce and potato add potassium.

• Tomato sauce and bouillon cubes are rich in sodium.

• Barley is a rich source of soluble fiber.

Nutrients Per Serving	
Calories	194
Fat	2 g
Fiber	5 g
Protein	13 g
Carbohydrate	33 g

Salads

Y ou might be thinking that this is the forbidden chapter, but we encourage you to read on. "Salad" does not need to be synonymous with "difficult to digest." Here you'll find ideas that will expand your salad repertoire beyond the usual lettuce, with appropriate modifications if you are following a low-fiber diet. Pasta or potato salads are excellent choices when you are concerned about your tolerance to fibrous foods. If you are well, and there is no medical reason for you to avoid fiber or difficult-to-digest foods, traditional raw vegetable and lettuce leaf salads provide a fresh, crisp, flavorful snack or side dish. In fact, many salads, particularly those made with fish, meat or eggs, can be meals on their own.

Individuals with IBD *do* eat salad, and living with a chronic disease is reason enough to ensure that you are well nourished. The more often you eat fruits and vegetables, the more often your body will benefit from the many vitamins, minerals, trace elements and phytonutrients provided by these foods. Thanks to complex food distribution systems, most of us have access to fruits and vegetables year-round and can count on including many combinations of colors, tastes and nutrients in our diet on a regular basis. There may be times when you simply cannot tolerate raw vegetables and need to take vitamin and mineral supplements, drink juices or make ingredient modifications, but be sure to take advantage of the times when you are well to enjoy salads!

Boost Your Calories and Protein

Enhance your salads by adding cottage cheese, feta or mozzarella cubes, chopped herbed tofu or canned salmon, tuna or sardines. When preparing meat for a meal, cook an extra chicken breast or boil another egg to keep in the fridge and later add to a salad.

Boost Your Soluble Fiber

Looking to add some fiber to your salad? Simply open a can of chickpeas, kidney beans or black beans, rinse well, pinch off the skins to reduce the insoluble fiber, and combine with your other salad ingredients. Legumes provide a good dose of fiber, as well as protein, iron and potassium, and they're low in fat.

Indigestible carbohydrate in beans causes bacterial fermentation in the intestine — that's why you get gassy. If using dried beans, soak them first and then discard the water. If using canned beans, rinse well until all the bubbles are gone. If you are not in the habit of eating legumes, start with a small amount. Your body will get used to them if you eat them regularly.

Experiment with Salad Fixings!

When you are well, try fresh vegetables such as snow peas, broccoli, bok choy, celery, spinach, bean sprouts, corn and carrots; nuts such as pecans or walnuts; and grains such as wild rice, couscous, bulgur, quinoa, kasha, millet, cornmeal and barley. The combinations are endless!

The Facts About Olive Oil

Olive oil is flavorful and contains a high percentage of oleic acid, a monounsaturated fat. Good grades of olive oil are those that have not been processed, deodorized or refined. "Virgin olive oil" is obtained from the first pressing of the olives, without further processing. Top-grade olive oil with very low acidity may be labeled "extra virgin." "Pure" can mean a blend of virgin and refined oils.

Even though the fat in olive oil is monounsaturated, fat provides a higher amount of calories per gram than do protein or carbohydrate. If you're trying to maintain or lose weight, use this oil in moderation. If you're trying to gain weight, use this oil more liberally. Like all vegetable products, olive oil contains no cholesterol.

PLAN AHEAD

Preparing vegetables does require some work and time, but plan ahead. Store cleaned and cut vegetables in Tupperware containers so you can quickly throw together a salad when your time is limited. Having ingredients prepared in advance may also encourage you to bring salads to work or school.

The Facts About Added Fats

- There are many healthy vegetable oils, including canola, olive, flaxseed and avocado oils. Some have distinct flavors that can enhance the taste of your recipe. They also have different smoke points (the temperature at which the oil will start to smoke when heated). Choose the oil that's most suitable for your recipe.

- Walnut oil is a plant source of omega-3 fat, which has anti-inflammatory properties. While marine sources provide omega-3s in the forms most easily used by the body, it is still worthwhile to include plant sources of omega-3 whenever possible.

- Sesame oil is a healthy polyunsaturated vegetable oil with a distinct flavor. Because it is stable at room temperature (thanks to its natural preservatives), it is an excellent addition to your pantry.

- Grapeseed oil is available in various flavors, including butter flavor. It has a high smoke point, so it is suitable for cooking at high temperatures.

- Coconut oil may have health benefits related to its medium-chain fat content. It has a high saturated fat content (which raises total cholesterol and bad LDL cholesterol), but also appears to increase good HDL cholesterol. Unsaturated oils like canola, olive and grapeseed oil are better options for heart health, but coconut oil is a reasonable choice in place of butter.

- Butter gives good flavor when added during cooking, but use it only occasionally and in small amounts, as it is high in saturated fat, which your liver uses to make cholesterol.

- Margarine is higher in monounsaturated and polyunsaturated fats and lower in saturated fat than butter. As an added benefit, margarine is fortified with vitamin D. For heart health, choose a non-hydrogenated margarine as often as possible. Avoid hydrogenated margarines, which are higher in unhealthy trans fat.

- Nonstick cooking sprays are useful for limiting the amount of added fat when cooking, a big help if you are trying to reduce calories from fat for heart health and weight goals.

Try adding kale to your salads. Kale is a nutritious dark green vegetable, full of vitamins, minerals and phytochemicals. Its flavor becomes stronger the longer you store it (unwashed kale will keep up to a week in your refrigerator crisper). Kale tastes sweeter if it is harvested after a light frost and during mid-winter to early spring.

Bell peppers, also known as sweet peppers, can be peeled after they are roasted (see recipe, page 286), to make them easier to digest. Red bell peppers have a higher beta carotene and vitamin C content than yellow or green bell peppers.

Vegetarian choice

Lower-calorie choice

Lower-fiber choice

Source of potassium

Source of sodium

Cucumber Watermelon Salad

Salad is a food that individuals living with IBD often feel more comfortable avoiding. This one can be well tolerated and adds a crisp texture and fresh taste.

½	seedless watermelon, rind removed, flesh cut into 1-inch (2.5 cm) chunks (4 to 6 cups/1 to 1.5 L)	½
1	English cucumber, quartered lengthwise, seeds removed and cut into ¼-inch (0.5 cm) slices	1
1 tbsp	canola or extra virgin olive oil	15 mL
½ cup	finely chopped fresh basil	125 mL
½ cup	crumbled feta cheese	125 mL

1. In a large bowl, combine watermelon and cucumber. Drizzle with oil. Add basil and cheese; gently toss to combine.

Variation

For a twist, drizzle with 1 tbsp (15 mL) balsamic vinegar.

MAKES 8 SERVINGS

Tips

- This salad becomes very liquidy if left overnight.

- Feta cheese is a soft cheese made predominantly from goat's or sheep's milk (or a blend), though it may also contain cow's milk. It has a mild and creamy taste, and is high in salt.

IBD Tips

- This recipe is suitable for vegetarians who eat dairy.

- Cold foods may be better tolerated during times of nausea.

- Watermelon provides the potassium in this recipe, and is also a good source of the antioxidant lycopene.

IF FOLLOWING A LOW-FIBER DIET AND AVOIDING DIFFICULT-TO-DIGEST FOODS...

Peel and seed the cucumber and finely chop the basil leaves (do not include stems).

Nutrients Per Serving	
Calories	64
Fat	4 g
Fiber	1 g
Protein	2 g
Carbohydrate	7 g

Green and Yellow Salad

Parrot green and mellow yellow, this refreshing concoction successfully combines the al dente crunch of fresh beans with the rich smoothness of ripe avocado.

8 oz	fresh green beans, trimmed	250 g
8 oz	fresh yellow beans, trimmed	250 g
1 tbsp	lime juice	15 mL
1	ripe avocado	1
	Salt and freshly ground black pepper	
3 tbsp	olive oil	45 mL
3	green onions, finely chopped	3
4 oz	feta cheese, crumbled into large chunks	125 g
	Few sprigs fresh cilantro, roughly chopped	

MAKES 4 TO 6 SERVINGS

IBD Tips

- Substitute canned green and yellow beans if you are running short on time.
- Avocado provides the potassium in this recipe. Avocados should be ripened at room temperature in a dark place before they are stored at a colder temperature; otherwise, they will discolor and won't ripen.

1. Boil green and yellow beans over high heat for 5 to 7 minutes. Drain and immediately refresh in a bowl of ice-cold water. Drain, and put in a wide salad bowl.

2. Put lime juice in a bowl. Peel avocado and cut into slices (or scoop out with a small spoon), and add to the lime juice. Fold avocado into the juice until well coated. Scatter avocado slices (or scoops) decoratively over the beans, along with any leftover lime juice. Season to taste with salt and pepper.

3. Drizzle olive oil over salad, and garnish with chopped green onions. Distribute feta over the salad, and top with a scattering of the chopped coriander. The salad can wait up to 1 hour, covered and unrefrigerated.

IF FOLLOWING A LOW-FIBER DIET AND AVOIDING DIFFICULT-TO-DIGEST FOODS...

Trim the ends off the green and yellow beans and pull off stringy veins, then boil until soft (or use canned beans). Finely grind the pepper, sauté the green onions until soft, and finely chop the cilantro (do not include stems).

Nutrients Per Serving	
Calories	448
Fat	17 g
Fiber	20 g
Protein	23 g
Carbohydrate	56 g

Beet and Feta Salad

1	can (14 oz/398 mL) sliced beets or whole baby beets, drained	1
½ cup	finely chopped celery	125 mL
¼ cup	bottled oil and vinegar dressing	60 mL
½	bag (10 oz/300 g) washed salad greens or 2 cups (500 mL) torn lettuce, washed and dried	½
2 oz	crumbled feta cheese	60 g

MAKES 4 SERVINGS

1. In a salad bowl, combine beets, celery and dressing. Cover and refrigerate for at least 1 hour or overnight.
2. Add salad greens and toss well. Sprinkle feta over top and serve immediately.

Variation

Beet and Avocado Salad: Substitute ¼ cup (60 mL) finely chopped green onion for the celery and 1 avocado, cut into ½-inch (1 cm) cubes, for the feta. Cut avocado and add to greens just before tossing.

IF FOLLOWING A LOW-FIBER DIET AND AVOIDING DIFFICULT-TO-DIGEST FOODS...

Omit celery and use only a small amount of iceberg lettuce. Canned beets are okay on a low-fiber diet, but if you prefer to use whole fresh beets, cook them until soft (30 to 60 minutes, depending on size), then place under cold water and peel.

Tips

- If you don't have time to chill the beet mixture, keep the canned beets refrigerated so they will be cold when you're ready to use them.
- If using whole baby beets, halve before using.

IBD Tips

- Be sure to remember when you ate beets so you are not alarmed when their characteristic color darkens your stool, resembling blood.
- If you are looking to decrease calories from saturated fat, choose reduced-fat feta cheese (usually 17% M.F.). Always read the label carefully, as "light" or "lite" can refer to color, flavor or texture, not necessarily to calories or fat.
- Beets and avocados are rich in potassium; canned beets and feta provide sodium in this recipe.

Nutrients Per Serving	
Calories	168
Fat	10 g
Fiber	6 g
Protein	4 g
Carbohydrate	18 g

Mediterranean Lentil and Rice Salad

This salad travels well, making it a great lunchbox choice.

2	roasted red bell peppers, patted dry and julienned	2
1	can (19 oz/540 mL) lentils, drained and rinsed	1
3 cups	cooked brown rice	750 mL
1 cup	chopped fresh Italian (flat-leaf) parsley	250 mL
1/2 cup	thinly sliced green onions	125 mL
1/4 cup	slivered dried apricots	60 mL
Dressing		
1/4 cup	olive oil	60 mL
2 tbsp	freshly squeezed lemon juice	30 mL
2 tbsp	balsamic vinegar	30 mL
1 tsp	liquid honey	5 mL
1 tsp	ground cumin	5 mL
1/2 tsp	ground coriander	2 mL
	Salt and freshly ground black pepper	

1. In a large bowl, combine red peppers, lentils, rice, parsley, green onions and apricots.

2. *Prepare the dressing:* In a small bowl, whisk together olive oil, lemon juice, vinegar, honey, cumin, coriander, and salt and pepper to taste.

3. Pour dressing over salad and toss to coat.

IF FOLLOWING A LOW-FIBER DIET AND AVOIDING DIFFICULT-TO-DIGEST FOODS...

Remove the skin from the roasted red peppers, use white rice instead of brown, finely chop the parsley (do not include stems), sauté the green onions until soft, substitute peeled ripe fresh apricots for dried, and finely grind the black pepper. Dried ground or flaked spices and seasonings are okay to use.

Vegetarian choice

Lactose-free choice

Source of soluble fiber

Source of potassium

MAKES 10 SERVINGS

Tips

- For 3 cups (750 mL) cooked brown rice, cook 1 cup (250 mL) rice with 2 cups (500 mL) water.

- If you serve this as a main course instead of as a side salad, it serves 6.

- This salad keeps well for up to 1 week in the refrigerator.

IBD Tips

- Cumin is considered helpful for digestion. Also consider commercial enzyme products such as Beano or Phazyme to reduce gas.

- Lentils and apricots provide potassium in this recipe.

Nutrients Per Serving	
Calories	182
Fat	6 g
Fiber	3 g
Protein	6 g
Carbohydrate	27 g

Vegetarian choice

Higher-calorie choice

Higher-protein choice

Source of soluble fiber

Source of potassium

Source of sodium

MAKES 8 SERVINGS

IBD Tips

- The dressing in this recipe calls for pine nuts, Parmesan and basil leaves. These flavorful ingredients are puréed until smooth and are thus not a concern for a food-related obstruction.

- If you are trying to gain weight, use full-fat Parmesan, yogurt and mayonnaise.

- Aged hard cheeses have relatively small amounts of lactose, and Parmesan is generally well tolerated by those with lactose intolerance.

- Tomatoes and legumes are rich sources of potassium; yogurt also supplies some.

- The canned legumes and the Parmesan provide the sodium in this recipe.

Nutrients Per Serving	
Calories	456
Fat	10 g
Fiber	7 g
Protein	18 g
Carbohydrate	75 g

Pasta and Bean Salad with Creamy Basil Dressing

Dressing

1½ cups	tightly packed fresh basil leaves	375 mL
3 tbsp	freshly grated low-fat Parmesan cheese	45 mL
2 tbsp	toasted pine nuts	30 mL
1½ tsp	minced garlic	7 mL
⅓ cup	low-fat yogurt	75 mL
3 tbsp	freshly squeezed lemon juice	45 mL
3 tbsp	light mayonnaise	45 mL
3 tbsp	water	45 mL
1 tbsp	olive oil	15 mL
¼ tsp	freshly ground black pepper	1 mL

Salad

12 oz	medium shell pasta	375 g
¾ cup	canned black beans, rinsed and drained	175 mL
¾ cup	canned chickpeas, rinsed and drained	175 mL
¾ cup	canned red kidney beans, rinsed and drained	175 mL
¾ cup	diced red onions	175 mL
½ cup	shredded carrots	125 mL
2 cups	diced ripe plum tomatoes	500 mL

1. *Prepare the dressing:* In a food processor or blender, combine basil, Parmesan cheese, pine nuts and garlic; process until finely chopped. Add yogurt, lemon juice, mayonnaise, water, olive oil and pepper; purée until smooth. Set aside.

2. *Prepare the salad:* In a large pot of boiling water, cook pasta for 8 to 10 minutes or until tender but firm; drain. Rinse under cold running water; drain.

3. In a serving bowl, combine pasta, black beans, chickpeas, kidney beans, red onions, carrots and plum tomatoes. Pour dressing over salad; toss to coat well. Serve immediately.

IF FOLLOWING A LOW-FIBER DIET AND AVOIDING DIFFICULT-TO-DIGEST FOODS...

Remove the stems from the basil leaves, finely grind the black pepper, pinch skins from legumes, finely dice the red onion and sauté until soft, use soft cooked carrots, and remove the skin and seeds from the plum tomatoes (see page 169).

Scandinavian Pasta Salad

2 cups	rotini or fusilli pasta, preferably tricolor	500 mL
1/2 cup	mayonnaise	125 mL
1/2 cup	sour cream	125 mL
1 tbsp	Dijon mustard	15 mL
1/2 tsp	salt	2 mL
	Freshly ground black pepper	
8 oz	shredded smoked deli ham, such as Black Forest ham or diced cooked ham	250 g
1	roasted red bell pepper, diced	1
2	hard-cooked eggs, thinly sliced	2
	Dill or parsley sprigs for garnish (optional)	

1. In a pot of boiling salted water, cook pasta until tender to the bite, about 8 minutes. Drain and rinse under cold running water.
2. In a serving bowl, mix together mayonnaise, sour cream, Dijon mustard, salt, and black pepper to taste. Add cooked pasta, ham and roasted red pepper. Toss to combine. Chill thoroughly. Garnish with sliced egg, and dill, if using, just before serving.

IF FOLLOWING A LOW-FIBER DIET AND AVOIDING DIFFICULT-TO-DIGEST FOODS...

Finely grind the black pepper, remove any casing from the deli meat, remove the skin from the roasted red pepper, and finely chop the dill or parsley (do not include stems).

Hard-Cooked Eggs

Hard-cooked eggs, sliced or quartered, are an easy way to add nutrients, substance and variety to salads. They can also make an attractive garnish. I prefer to use the cold-water cooking method, which is foolproof.

To make hard-cooked eggs: Place eggs in a saucepan and add cold water to cover. Bring to a boil and cook vigorously for 2 minutes. Remove from heat and let stand for 15 minutes. Drain and immediately plunge eggs into a bowl of cold water. Refrigerate until ready to use.

MAKES 4 SERVINGS

IBD Tips

- Tricolor pasta is okay for a low-fiber diet. The dehydrated spinach and tomato powder used to color the pasta are not difficult to digest.
- Ham provides high-quality protein and heme iron.
- Smoked meat adds distinctive flavor to this dish, but eat it in moderation, as it is considered a modifiable risk factor for cancer.
- To boost the anti-inflammatory omega-3 fats in your diet, try omega-3 eggs!
- Sodium is provided by the mustard, added salt, mayonnaise and deli meat.

Nutrients Per Serving	
Calories	778
Fat	33 g
Fiber	4 g
Protein	28 g
Carbohydrate	90 g

Vegetarian choice

Lower-fat choice

Lower-fiber choice

Higher-protein choice

Lactose-free choice

Source of sodium

MAKES 8 SERVINGS

IBD Tips

- This recipe is suitable for vegetarians who eat fish.
- When asparagus is out of season, use green beans or broccoli instead, provided you are well and there is no medical reason for you to avoid fiber or difficult-to-digest foods.
- Fish is an excellent source of protein, vitamins and minerals. Cold-water fatty fish are the best sources of omega-3 fat, which has anti-inflammatory properties.
- Choose light tuna, which has lower mercury levels than white tuna.
- If your goal is to gain weight, use tuna packed in oil.

Nutrients Per Serving	
Calories	223
Fat	5 g
Fiber	2 g
Protein	14 g
Carbohydrate	31 g

Penne Salad with Asparagus and Tuna

3 cups	penne (about 10 oz/300 g)	750 mL
3 cups	fresh asparagus, trimmed and cut into bite-size pieces (about 1 lb/500 g)	750 mL
2	cans (each 5.7 oz/170 g) water-packed tuna, drained	2
1 cup	diced red bell peppers	250 mL
2 tbsp	chopped chives or green onions	30 mL
2 tbsp	capers, drained (optional)	30 mL
Dressing		
2 tbsp	balsamic vinegar or red wine vinegar	30 mL
2 tbsp	olive oil	30 mL
2 tsp	Dijon mustard	10 mL
1 tsp	brown sugar	5 mL
1/2 tsp	minced garlic	2 mL
1/2 tsp	minced gingerroot	2 mL
	Salt and freshly ground black pepper	

1. In a large pot of boiling water, cook penne according to package directions or until tender but firm, adding asparagus during last 2 minutes of cooking time; drain. Rinse under cold water; drain. Transfer to a large bowl. Add tuna, red peppers, chives and, if using, capers. Set aside.

2. *Prepare the dressing:* In a small bowl or measuring cup, whisk together vinegar, oil, mustard, sugar, garlic and ginger. Season with salt and pepper to taste. Pour over salad; toss gently to combine. Serve immediately.

> **IF FOLLOWING A LOW-FIBER DIET AND AVOIDING DIFFICULT-TO-DIGEST FOODS...**
>
> Use canned asparagus tips, remove the skin of the red peppers before dicing, finely chop the chives or green onions and sauté until soft, and omit the capers.

Tangerine Salmon Salad

Dressing

6 tbsp	freshly squeezed tangerine juice	90 mL
¼ cup	extra virgin olive oil	60 mL
1	small clove garlic, minced	1
1 tsp	Dijon mustard	5 mL
½ tsp	finely grated tangerine zest	2 mL
¼ tsp	salt	1 mL
⅛ tsp	freshly ground black pepper	0.5 mL

Salad

4 cups	mixed baby greens	1 L
1	can (7½ oz/213 g) sockeye salmon, drained, deboned and broken into chunks	1
2	green onions (white and light green parts), thinly sliced	2

1. *Dressing:* In a small bowl, whisk together tangerine juice, oil, garlic, mustard, tangerine zest, salt and pepper.
2. *Salad:* Arrange the greens on serving plates, dividing equally. Scatter salmon overtop. Drizzle about 2 tbsp (30 mL) dressing over each. Sprinkle with onions.

Variation

Substitute tuna for the salmon

> ### IF FOLLOWING A LOW-FIBER DIET AND AVOIDING DIFFICULT-TO-DIGEST FOODS…
> Select smooth (not coarse or grainy) Dijon mustard, finely grind the black pepper (larger pieces can increase the risk of a food-related obstruction), use only a small amount of iceberg or Boston lettuce (and chew it well), and finely mince the green onions.

Vegetarian choice

Higher-calorie choice

Higher-protein choice

Lactose-free choice

Source of potassium

Source of sodium

MAKES 2 SERVINGS

Tip

- This recipe makes about ⅔ cup (150 mL) dressing. Use the leftover portion on other salads, or drizzle it on steamed fish or poached chicken.

IBD Tips

- This recipe is suitable for vegetarians who eat seafood.
- Recipes using canned ingredients may be easier to prepare during times of illness.
- Boost calories by selecting canned salmon packed in oil.
- Crush the bones of the salmon for added calcium and vitamin D.
- Sodium is provided by the canned salmon and mustard, and some potassium is provided by the tangerine juice.

Nutrients Per Serving	
Calories	468
Fat	36 g
Fiber	2 g
Protein	26 g
Carbohydrate	8 g

MAKES 4 SERVINGS

Tips

- For a change, replace the salmon with canned tuna packed in water.
- If desired, make your own vinaigrette rather than using the bottled variety.

IBD Tips

- This recipe is suitable for vegetarians who eat fish.
- You can crush and eat the bones in canned salmon for additional calcium. One can contains the same amount of calcium as a cup (250 mL) of milk.
- Salmon contains significant amounts of omega-3 fat, which has anti-inflammatory properties.
- Potatoes, tomatoes and salmon provide potassium.

Nutrients Per Serving	
Calories	295
Fat	13 g
Fiber	2 g
Protein	19 g
Carbohydrate	25 g

Salmon, Potato and Green Bean Salad

This main-meal salad makes a great summer supper when fresh vegetables and herbs are in season.

1 lb	small new white potatoes, halved or quartered	500 g
1 cup	green beans, cut into 2-inch (5 cm) pieces	250 mL
1	green onion, chopped	1
1 cup	halved cherry tomatoes or diced tomatoes	250 mL
2 tbsp	chopped fresh basil (or 1 tsp/5 mL dried)	30 mL
$\frac{1}{3}$ cup	bottled oil-and-vinegar-type dressing	75 mL
2	cans (each $7\frac{1}{2}$ oz/213 g) salmon, drained, bones and skin removed	2
	Salt and freshly ground black pepper	

1. In a medium saucepan, gently boil potatoes for 10 to 15 minutes or until tender but firm, adding beans during last 4 minutes of cooking time. Drain and transfer vegetables to a large bowl.

2. Add green onion, tomatoes and basil. Add dressing; toss gently to combine. Gently stir in salmon. Season with salt and pepper to taste. Chill until serving.

IF FOLLOWING A LOW-FIBER DIET AND AVOIDING DIFFICULT-TO-DIGEST FOODS...

Peel the potatoes, trim the ends off the green beans and pull off stringy veins, then boil until soft (or use canned beans), finely chop the green onion and sauté until soft, remove the skin and seeds from the tomatoes (see page 169; you may need to use a larger size than cherry tomatoes), and finely chop the basil (do not include stems).

Chicken and Asparagus Salad with Lemon Dill Vinaigrette

12	baby red potatoes (or 4 small white)	12
8 oz	boneless skinless chicken breasts, cubed	250 g
1/4 cup	water	60 mL
1/4 cup	white wine	60 mL
8 oz	asparagus, trimmed and cut into small pieces	250 g
2	small heads Boston lettuce, torn into pieces	2

Lemon Dill Vinaigrette

3 tbsp	balsamic vinegar	45 mL
2 tbsp	freshly squeezed lemon juice	30 mL
1 tbsp	water	15 mL
1	large green onion, minced	1
3/4 tsp	garlic	3 mL
2 tbsp	chopped fresh dill (or 1 tsp/5 mL dried dillweed)	30 mL
3 tbsp	olive oil	45 mL

1. In saucepan of boiling water, cook potatoes until just tender. Peel and cut into cubes. Place in salad bowl and set aside.

2. In saucepan, bring chicken, water and wine to boil; reduce heat, cover and simmer for approximately 2 minutes or until chicken is no longer pink. Drain and add to potatoes in bowl.

3. Steam or microwave asparagus until just tender-crisp; drain and add to bowl. Add lettuce.

4. *Prepare the vinaigrette:* In bowl, whisk together vinegar, lemon juice, water, onion, garlic and dill; whisk in oil until combined. Pour over chicken mixture; toss to coat well.

IF FOLLOWING A LOW-FIBER DIET AND AVOIDING DIFFICULT-TO-DIGEST FOODS...

Peel the potatoes, use canned asparagus tips, use only a small amount of iceberg or Boston lettuce, finely mince the green onion and sauté until soft, and finely chop the dill (do not include stems) or use dried.

MAKES 4 TO 6 SERVINGS

IBD Tips

- You can substitute broccoli or fresh green beans for the asparagus, provided you are well and there is no medical reason for you to avoid fiber or difficult-to-digest foods.

- Many individuals with IBD report that they find poultry and fish easier to digest than red meat.

- Potatoes are a rich source of potassium; chicken and asparagus also contribute some.

- While it is not rich in vitamins and minerals, garlic does contain many chemicals that are thought to have health benefits.

- The alcohol content of wine evaporates with cooking.

Nutrients Per Serving	
Calories	199
Fat	8 g
Fiber	3 g
Protein	11 g
Carbohydrate	19 g

Higher-calorie choice

Lower-fat choice

Higher-protein choice

Source of potassium

Source of sodium

MAKES 6 SERVINGS

IBD Tips

- Select chicken breast without skin to lower saturated fat in your diet.
- To boost calories, choose higher-fat yogurt and milk and regular peanut butter.
- Nut butters, such as peanut butter, are known to help thicken loose stool.
- Potatoes, together with milk, yogurt, chicken and peanut butter, pack a potassium punch.

IF FOLLOWING A LOW-FIBER DIET...

Finely chop the cilantro (do not include stems), peel the potatoes, use only a small amount of iceberg or Boston lettuce for the salad greens, and use smooth peanut butter.

Nutrients Per Serving	
Calories	399
Fat	11 g
Fiber	4 g
Protein	35 g
Carbohydrate	42 g

Warm Thai Chicken Salad

Marinade

1 cup	lower-fat plain yogurt	250 mL
1/4 cup	skim milk	60 mL
1 tbsp	chopped fresh cilantro	15 mL
1 tsp	curry powder	5 mL
1 tsp	ground ginger	5 mL
1 tsp	freshly squeezed lemon juice	5 mL
	Freshly ground black pepper	

Salad

6	boneless skinless chicken breasts (about 1 1/2 lbs/750 g)	6
6	medium red-skinned potatoes, cooked and quartered	6
6 cups	mixed torn salad greens	1.5 L

Peanut Dressing

1/3 cup	chicken broth	75 mL
1/4 cup	light peanut butter	60 mL
1/4 cup	sliced green onions	60 mL
3 tbsp	rice vinegar	45 mL
2 tbsp	sesame oil	30 mL
2 tbsp	grated gingerroot	30 mL
1 tbsp	sherry	15 mL
1 tbsp	soy sauce	15 mL
1 tbsp	granulated sugar	15 mL
1	clove garlic, minced	1
1/4 tsp	salt	1 mL

1. *Prepare the marinade:* In a shallow glass dish, combine ingredients. Add chicken and turn to coat. Cover and refrigerate overnight.
2. *Prepare the peanut dressing:* In a food processor or blender, process ingredients until smooth. Pour into jar; cover and refrigerate.
3. *Prepare the salad:* Remove chicken from marinade; grill or broil until no longer pink, adding potatoes for last 6 to 8 minutes.
4. Slice chicken crosswise into strips. Arrange greens on 6 plates; top with chicken and potatoes. Drizzle with dressing.

Smoked Turkey Toss

¼ cup	extra-virgin olive oil	60 mL
2 tbsp	balsamic vinegar	30 mL
1 tbsp	chopped fresh parsley	15 mL
1 tsp	dried basil	5 mL
1 tsp	liquid honey	5 mL
Pinch	salt	Pinch
Pinch	freshly ground black pepper	Pinch
8 cups	thinly sliced romaine lettuce	2 L
4 oz	thinly sliced smoked or cooked turkey breast, cut into strips	125 g
4 oz	part-skim mozzarella cheese, cut into cubes	125 g

1. In a small bowl or measuring cup, mix together oil, vinegar, parsley, basil, honey, salt and pepper. Chill.

2. In a large bowl, toss remaining ingredients. Cover and chill. Add dressing and toss.

IF FOLLOWING A LOW-FIBER DIET AND AVOIDING DIFFICULT-TO-DIGEST FOODS...

Use a small amount of iceberg lettuce instead of the romaine, finely chop the parsley (do not include stems), and remove casing from the turkey, if necessary. Dried flaked herbs and seasonings are okay on this diet.

Lower-fiber choice

Higher-protein choice

Source of sodium

MAKES 6 SERVINGS AS A SIDE SALAD

Tip

• This tasty salad is a good source of protein. To ensure that cheese is lower-fat, look for 20% or less milk fat (M.F.).

IBD Tips

• Compared to other meats, turkey has less calories and fat while still providing high-quality protein, vitamins and minerals. Many individuals with IBD report that poultry and fish are easier to digest than red meat.

• Choose smoked meat only occasionally, as it is considered a modifiable risk factor for cancer.

• Mozzarella contains relatively small amounts of lactose.

• Use regular mozzarella cheese if you are trying to gain weight.

• The cheese, deli meat and added salt provide the sodium in this recipe.

Nutrients Per Serving	
Calories	178
Fat	14 g
Fiber	1 g
Protein	10 g
Carbohydrate	4 g

Avocado Dressing

Here's a dressing with a light green color that's perfect for any salad or as a dip.

**MAKES ABOUT
2 CUPS (500 ML)
(2 TBSP/30 ML
PER SERVING)**

4 oz	cream cheese, cubed and softened	125 g
1/2 cup	buttermilk	125 mL
1/2 cup	mayonnaise	125 mL
1	ripe avocado	1
2 tsp	chopped fresh dill fronds	10 mL
1 tsp	freshly squeezed lemon juice	5 mL

Tip

• Cover the dressing tightly and refrigerate for up to 3 days.

IBD Tips

• This recipe is suitable for vegetarians who eat eggs. (Mayonnaise is usually made from egg, oil, and vinegar or lemon juice.)

• This recipe is high in calories thanks to the cream cheese, mayonnaise and avocado.

• Potassium is provided by the avocado, with a small contribution from the lemon juice.

1. In a food processor or blender, process cream cheese, buttermilk, mayonnaise, avocado, dill and lemon juice until smooth, about 2 minutes.

> **IF FOLLOWING A LOW-FIBER DIET AND AVOIDING DIFFICULT-TO-DIGEST FOODS...**
> Finely chop the dill fronds (do not include stems).

Nutrients Per Serving	
Calories	63
Fat	5 g
Fiber	1 g
Protein	2 g
Carbohydrate	3 g

Meat and Poultry

Meat and poultry provide many essential nutrients, such as protein, iron, zinc and B vitamins. These nutrients are important during times of disease activity and during remission, helping to maintain health. Good nutrition means eating a variety of healthful foods to maximize the nutrients delivered to your body, and including meat and poultry in your diet can be an important way to meet this goal.

Minimize Your Intake of Saturated Fat

Meat and poultry contain varying amounts of saturated fat, which is associated with health problems such as heart disease. To consume less saturated fat, choose lean cuts of beef and pork, usually called "round" or "loin," as these provide the least calories from fat. When preparing meats, trim visible fat before cooking, remove skin from poultry and drain fat after cooking. Lower-fat cooking methods include baking, roasting, broiling, grilling and braising.

IF YOU EXPERIENCE CRAMPING, CHOOSE GROUND MEATS

Some individuals with IBD report cramping after eating tougher cuts of red meat, likely because older animals have a lot of connective tissues and gristle (cartilage). To prevent unnecessary restrictions, choose ground meats. Because the connective tissue and fiber have been broken down mechanically, intolerance symptoms are minimized and less chewing is required. You can incorporate ground meat into your diet in sauces, soups, meatballs, meatloaf, or burgers.

Try Eating Your Largest Meal at Lunchtime

If you consume your largest meal for lunch rather than for dinner, you may find that you pass larger amounts of stool earlier in the evening. This allows you to empty your pelvic pouch or ileostomy or colostomy bag before bed, and you may not have to wake up at night (or not as often).

To reduce the amount of fat you're ingesting, place cooked ground beef in a colander and rinse under running water. If you're using it in a sauce, you won't taste the difference!

Eat Smaller Meals

Portion control and appetite are closely connected. If you're living with active disease, the effects of inflammatory cytokines can reduce appetite. During times of wellness, or while you're on high-dose steroids, however, you may struggle with hunger and have difficulty avoiding weight gain. Either way, "grazing" (eating frequent small meals throughout the day) is considered a healthy eating strategy. Remember, the key is five to six *small* meals. Prepare a meal as you normally would, then eat half the serving and put the rest aside for later (refrigerate and reheat, if necessary). If you don't feel like eating the remaining half later, choose a small snack.

Three ounces (90 g) of meat (a standard recommended serving size) is about the size of a deck of cards.

Make Sure You're Getting Enough Vitamin B_{12}

Vitamin B_{12} is plentiful in diets that contain meat, fish, dairy and eggs. This vitamin is important for your nervous system and helps prevent anemia. It takes just a small amount to meet the daily requirements, but if you have a disease that affects your terminal ileum, you could have difficulty absorbing this vitamin. If you experience chronic inflammation or have had surgical resections of your stomach or terminal ileum, ask your doctor about an injectable vitamin B_{12} replacement.

Four ounces (125 g) of raw meat is equal to about 3 ounces (90 g) of cooked meat.

THE FACTS ABOUT IRON

Meat contains both heme iron and non-heme iron. Iron is important for many functions in the body, including the transport and delivery of oxygen to the cells. Most of the body's iron is found in red blood cells (as hemoglobin) and in muscle cells (as myoglobin). About half the iron from meat, poultry and fish is heme iron, which is easily absorbed. Dairy foods, eggs and plant-based foods such as legumes, dark green leafy vegetables, nuts and fortified breads and cereals contain only non-heme iron, which is less easily absorbed. Vitamin C helps the body absorb non-heme iron, so include a source of vitamin C (from fruits and vegetables, or fruit juices such as orange juice) with meals. If you experience ongoing bleeding, especially small amounts of chronic blood loss, you may be at risk of iron deficiency, so be sure to discuss this with your doctor.

Avoid Scenarios That Promote Overeating

- Don't skip meals. Doing so can increase hunger, making it more likely that you will overeat at the next meal.
- Avoid foods that are high in fat or sugar; they are easy to overeat.
- Keep your portion size small. Some people rely on visual cues rather than hunger; if you're determined to clean your plate, you'll eat too much if your portion size is large.
- Minimize distractions. You are more likely to overeat (and also less likely to chew your food well) if you read or watch TV while eating.
- Pay attention to your moods. If you are bored, upset, stressed or lonely, you may try to make yourself feel better by overeating.

Higher-calorie choice

Lower-fat choice

Higher-protein choice

Source of sodium

MAKES 4 SERVINGS

IBD Tips

- Beef can be cooked to varying degrees of doneness. Tough or less tender cuts contain more connective tissue and should be cooked at low temperatures for longer periods of time. Choose lean cuts and remove any visible fat before cooking.

- Potassium is provided by steak, mushrooms, yogurt, peas and Worcestershire sauce. To increase the potassium content, serve over mashed potatoes instead of noodles.

- To increase the fat content, and thus the calories, use regular mushroom soup and full-fat sour cream or yogurt.

- To increase the sodium, use commercially prepared beef broth and mushroom soup that are not low-sodium.

Nutrients Per Serving	
Calories	447
Fat	8 g
Fiber	5 g
Protein	33 g
Carbohydrate	60 g

Beef Stroganoff

On a busy weeknight, it's always great to have a simple recipe, like this one, that requires little prep and only one pan to clean.

	Vegetable cooking spray	
12 oz	boneless sirloin grilling steak, cut into strips	375 g
1	large onion, sliced	1
¾ cup	sliced mushrooms	175 mL
3 cups	reduced-sodium beef broth	750 mL
1	can (10 oz/284 mL) condensed low-fat cream of mushroom soup, undiluted	1
2½ cups	fusilli pasta or spiral egg noodles	625 mL
1 cup	frozen peas	250 mL
1 tbsp	Worcestershire sauce	15 mL
¼ tsp	freshly ground black pepper	1 mL
¾ cup	light sour cream or plain yogurt	175 mL

1. Heat a large saucepan over medium-high heat. Spray with vegetable cooking spray. Working in batches, stir-fry beef for 3 to 4 minutes or until browned on all sides. Remove beef to a large bowl as each batch is completed.

2. Reduce heat to medium and add onion and mushrooms to saucepan; cook for 3 minutes or until lightly colored. Stir into beef.

3. In the same saucepan, combine broth and soup; bring to a boil. Add fusilli; bring back to a gentle boil and cook, stirring often, until fusilli is al dente (tender to the bite), about 12 minutes. Stir in peas, Worcestershire sauce and pepper; reduce heat and simmer for 3 minutes. Stir in beef mixture and sour cream; cook for about 5 minutes or until heated through.

IF FOLLOWING A LOW-FIBER DIET AND AVOIDING DIFFICULT-TO-DIGEST FOODS...

Finely chop onion and cook until soft, finely grind the black pepper (larger pieces can increase the risk of a food-related obstruction), use canned peas instead of frozen (the skin of frozen peas does not cook soft enough), and purée the mushrooms and the cream of mushroom soup, or use a soup without chunks of mushroom. Mushrooms are surprisingly hard to digest, and although those in canned soup are chopped into small pieces, they are a potential food obstruction.

Layered Beef and Noodle Bake

- *Preheat oven to 350°F (180°C)*
- *11- by 7-inch (28 by 18 cm) glass baking dish, greased*
- *Food processor*

8 oz	extra-lean ground beef	250 g
2	cloves garlic, minced	2
1 cup	chopped green onion tops, divided	250 mL
2	cans (each 8 oz/227 mL) tomato sauce	2
	Salt and freshly ground black pepper	
6 oz	whole wheat egg noodles	175 g
1 cup	low-fat cottage cheese	250 mL
1 cup	reduced-fat sour cream	250 mL
¼ cup	shredded reduced-fat Cheddar cheese	60 mL

1. In a large nonstick skillet, over medium-high heat, cook beef, garlic and half the green onions, breaking beef up with the back of a spoon, for 8 to 10 minutes or until beef is no longer pink. Drain off fat. Stir in tomato sauce, ½ cup (125 mL) water and a pinch each of salt and pepper; bring to a boil. Reduce heat to low, cover and simmer, stirring occasionally, for 10 minutes.

2. Meanwhile, in a large pot of boiling water, cook noodles according to package directions until just tender. Drain and set aside.

3. In a food processor, purée cottage cheese until smooth. Transfer to a medium bowl and stir in sour cream, the remaining green onions and a pinch each of salt and pepper.

4. Spread half the noodles in prepared baking dish. Top with half the cottage cheese mixture and half the meat sauce. Repeat layers with the remaining noodles, cottage cheese mixture and meat sauce. Sprinkle with Cheddar.

5. Bake in preheated oven for 30 to 40 minutes or until bubbling.

IF FOLLOWING A LOW-FIBER DIET AND AVOIDING DIFFICULT-TO-DIGEST FOODS…

Select regular egg noodles (not whole wheat) and tomato sauce without skins, seeds or difficult-to-digest vegetables. Finely grind the black pepper, and finely chop the green onions.

Lower-fiber choice

Higher-protein choice

Source of potassium

Source of sodium

MAKES 6 SERVINGS

Tip

- One bunch of green onions typically yields ½ cup (125 mL) chopped tops.

IBD Tips

- Boost calories in this recipe by choosing regular-fat ground beef, cottage cheese, sour cream and Cheddar.

- To reduce the amount of fat, place cooked ground beef in a colander and rinse under running water. If you're using it in a sauce or casserole, you won't taste the difference but your heart will thank you!

- Tomato sauce offers high potassium, and sodium is provided by the tomato sauce, cottage cheese and Cheddar cheese.

Nutrients Per Serving	
Calories	298
Fat	10 g
Fiber	4 g
Protein	23 g
Carbohydrate	30 g

MAKES 4 SERVINGS

IBD Tips

- To reduce the fat content, choose extra-lean ground beef and rinse in a colander after cooking, use an oil sprayer to minimize the amount of oil used, and make your own mashed potatoes for the topping instead of using hash browns.

- Potatoes are a source of potassium, and some is also provided by the beef and ketchup.

- Sodium sources include the hash browns, added salt, commercially prepared beef stock, ketchup and Worcestershire sauce.

Nutrients Per Serving	
Calories	424
Fat	21 g
Fiber	1 g
Protein	27 g
Carbohydrate	35 g

Crispy Shepherd's Pie

Shepherd's pie is traditionally made with a mashed potato crust, but this version takes advantage of frozen hash brown potatoes to produce a crispy and more convenient topping.

- *Preheat oven to 375°F (190°C)*
- *9-inch (23 cm) pie plate*

2 tbsp	vegetable oil, divided	30 mL
2 cups	frozen hash brown potatoes	500 mL
1 lb	lean ground beef, thawed if frozen	500 g
1 cup	diced onion	250 mL
1 tbsp	minced garlic	15 mL
1/4 tsp	salt	1 mL
	Freshly ground black pepper	
2 tbsp	all-purpose flour	30 mL
1 cup	beef stock	250 mL
1/2 cup	ketchup	125 mL
1 tbsp	Worcestershire sauce	15 mL

1. In a skillet, heat 1 tbsp (15 mL) of the oil over medium-high heat. Add potatoes and cook, stirring, until crisp, about 7 minutes. Using a slotted spoon, transfer to a paper towel–lined plate to drain.

2. Add remaining oil to pan. Add beef and onion and cook, breaking up meat, until beef is no longer pink inside, about 5 minutes. Drain off fat.

3. Return pan to element. Add garlic, salt and black pepper to taste. Cook, stirring, for 1 minute. Add flour and cook, stirring, for 1 minute. Add beef stock and bring to a boil. Cook, stirring, until mixture thickens, 3 minutes. Stir in ketchup and Worcestershire sauce and return to a boil.

4. Pour mixture into pie plate. Sprinkle potatoes over top. Bake in preheated oven until mixture is hot and bubbling, about 10 minutes.

IF YOU ARE WELL...

If there is no medical reason for you to avoid fiber or difficult-to-digest foods, consider adding corn along with the beef mixture in this pie. Just be sure to chew well!

IF FOLLOWING A LOW-FIBER DIET AND AVOIDING DIFFICULT-TO-DIGEST FOODS...

Finely grind the black pepper, as larger pieces can increase the risk of a food-related obstruction.

Meat Loaf "Muffins" with Barbecue Sauce

These meaty "muffins" are a favorite of kids and adults. Instead of making the sauce, substitute 1 cup (250 mL) of your favorite prepared barbecue sauce.

- *Preheat oven to 375°F (190°C)*
- *12-cup muffin tin, greased*

Meat Loaf "Muffins"

1½ lbs	lean ground beef	750 g
¾ cup	oatmeal or dry bread crumbs or cracker crumbs	175 mL
¼ cup	wheat bran	60 mL
1	can (5.4 oz/160 mL) 2% evaporated milk	1
1	egg	1
1 tsp	chili powder	5 mL
½ tsp	garlic powder	2 mL
¼ tsp	salt	1 mL
¼ tsp	freshly ground black pepper	1 mL

Barbecue Sauce

1 cup	ketchup	250 mL
¼ cup	finely chopped onion	60 mL
2 tbsp	brown sugar	30 mL
½ tsp	hot pepper sauce (optional)	2 mL

1. *Prepare the meat loaf "muffins":* In a large bowl, combine ground beef, oatmeal, bran, milk, egg, chili powder, garlic powder, salt and pepper. Divide mixture evenly among muffin cups, pressing down lightly.

2. *Prepare the barbecue sauce:* In another bowl, combine ketchup, onion, sugar and, if using, hot pepper sauce. Spoon about 1 tbsp (15 mL) sauce over each muffin.

3. Bake in preheated oven for 25 to 30 minutes or until meat is no longer pink in center.

IF FOLLOWING A LOW-FIBER DIET AND AVOIDING DIFFICULT-TO-DIGEST FOODS...

Use bread crumbs or cracker crumbs made from white flour, and substitute oat bran for the wheat bran.

Higher-calorie choice

Higher-protein choice

Source of soluble fiber

MAKES 6 SERVINGS

IBD Tips

- To increase the soluble fiber in this recipe, substitute oat bran for the wheat bran. Oat bran's "gelling" properties help to form loose stool. Because of this desirable effect, many low-fiber diets include oats and oat products despite the increased fiber content.

- Always use iodized salt — the added iodine is essential for your thyroid and for mental development.

- To reduce the fat in this recipe, choose extra-lean ground beef and evaporated skim milk, and substitute 2 egg whites for the egg (or use egg substitute).

Nutrients Per Serving	
Calories	396
Fat	19 g
Fiber	3 g
Protein	27 g
Carbohydrate	29 g

Lower-fiber choice

Higher-protein choice

Source of potassium

Source of sodium

MAKES 4 SERVINGS

Tips

- Feta cheese or shredded mozzarella can be substituted for the goat cheese in this interesting version of veal parmigiana.
- Boneless chicken or pork cutlets can replace the veal.

IBD Tips

- Use olive oil or canola oil for their heart-healthy fat profiles.
- Tomato sauce is rich in potassium; veal is also a source.
- Sodium is provided by the tomato sauce and cheese.
- Goat cheese does contain lactose, despite some claims that individuals with lactose intolerance can eat goat cheese but not cheese made from cow's milk. But it may not be an "all or nothing" situation — you may be able to tolerate some lactose, just not a lot.

Nutrients Per Serving	
Calories	253
Fat	11 g
Fiber	1 g
Protein	23 g
Carbohydrate	14 g

Veal Scaloppini with Goat Cheese and Tomato Sauce

- *Preheat oven to 450°F (230°C)*

1 lb	veal cutlets, pounded until thin	500 g
1	egg white	1
1/2 cup	dry bread crumbs	125 mL
1 tbsp	vegetable oil	15 mL
2 tsp	crushed garlic	10 mL
1 cup	tomato sauce	250 mL
2 oz	goat cheese, crumbled	50 g
	Chopped fresh parsley	

1. Dip veal in egg white, then in bread crumbs until coated.

2. In large nonstick skillet sprayed with nonstick vegetable spray, heat oil; sauté garlic for 1 minute. Add veal and cook just until tender and browned on both sides. Remove from heat.

3. Place tomato sauce in baking dish. Top with veal and sprinkle with goat cheese. Bake, uncovered, for 5 minutes or until heated through. Garnish with parsley.

> **IF FOLLOWING A LOW-FIBER DIET AND AVOIDING DIFFICULT-TO-DIGEST FOODS...**
>
> Choose bread crumbs made from white bread, tomato sauce without tomato skins or seeds or difficult-to-digest vegetables, and finely chopped parsley leaf (do not include stems).

Savory Lamb Chops

Tasty, elegant, simple and quick to make, this recipe is a keeper.

- *Preheat broiler or grill*

2 tbsp	bottled oil and vinegar dressing	30 mL
1 tbsp	Dijon mustard	15 mL
1½ lbs	lamb chops, thawed if frozen	750 g
2 tbsp	prepared sun-dried tomato pesto	30 mL

1. In a bowl, combine oil and vinegar dressing and mustard.
2. Pat lamb chops dry. Brush both sides with mixture.
3. Place on broiling pan about 6 inches (15 cm) from heat. Cook, turning once, until desired degree of doneness, 8 to 10 minutes. Serve topped with a dollop of pesto.

Pesto Sauce

"Pesto" simply means a sauce that is pounded in a mortar, but the name has become identified with Genovese pesto, which is made from a combination of basil, garlic, pine nuts, Parmesan cheese and olive oil. The popularity of this versatile and tasty sauce has encouraged manufacturers to introduce a prepared version of it and other varieties, such as red pepper and sun-dried tomato pesto. Although these sauces are traditionally served with pasta or fish, they are an excellent way of adding flavor to a broad range of dishes.

Higher-calorie choice

Lower-fiber choice

Higher-protein choice

Lactose-free choice

Source of sodium

MAKES 4 SERVINGS

IBD Tips

- Lamb usually comes from sheep less than a year old, whereas mutton is stronger-tasting meat from older sheep. Leg and loin lamb chops are considered lean cuts of meat. Be sure to serve lamb while it is hot, as its fat solidifies quickly.
- This recipe is appropriate for a low-fiber diet (no modifications are required).
- Lamb provides potassium. Seasonings that complement it include garlic, mustard, basil, mint, rosemary, sage, lemon zest, lime zest and orange zest.
- Sources of sodium in this recipe are the dressing, mustard and pesto.

Nutrients Per Serving	
Calories	590
Fat	43 g
Fiber	Trace
Protein	43 g
Carbohydrate	4 g

MAKES 4 SERVINGS

Tip

• Use 1 can (14 oz/398 mL) drained sliced peaches instead of fresh peaches for a year-round recipe. Or use fresh nectarines or mangos.

IBD Tips

• The most tender cuts of pork come from the loin. Pork must be cooked thoroughly to destroy parasitic worms that may be present in the flesh. Pork fat is visible and can easily be removed.

• Sources of potassium include orange juice, peaches, kiwi and pork.

• Commercially prepared chicken stock and added salt provide the sodium in this recipe.

• Mustard, onions, garlic, citrus juice, soy sauce and herbs complement the flavor of pork.

Nutrients Per Serving	
Calories	234
Fat	7 g
Fiber	2 g
Protein	23 g
Carbohydrate	19 g

Pork Chops with Peaches and Kiwi

Pork and fruit are a delicious combination usually reserved for special occasions. Here's an easy-to-make recipe that allows you to experience these great taste sensations on weeknights.

¾ cup	chicken stock	175 mL
½ cup	orange juice	125 mL
4 tsp	cornstarch	20 mL
2 tsp	granulated sugar	10 mL
1 tsp	minced garlic	5 mL
1 tsp	minced gingerroot (or ¼ tsp/1 mL ground ginger)	5 mL
½ tsp	grated lemon zest (optional)	2 mL
1 tsp	olive oil	5 mL
4	lean boneless or bone-in pork chops	4
1½ cups	sliced peaches	375 mL
½ cup	sliced (cut lengthwise) peeled kiwifruit	125 mL
	Salt and freshly ground black pepper	

1. In a medium bowl, combine stock, orange juice, cornstarch, sugar, garlic, ginger and, if using, lemon zest. Set aside.

2. In a large nonstick skillet, heat oil over medium-high heat. Add pork chops and sear for 1 to 2 minutes per side or until golden. Add stock mixture; bring to a boil. Reduce heat to medium-low and simmer for 5 to 6 minutes or until pork is cooked and just slightly pink at the center. Stir in peaches and kiwi. Season with salt and pepper to taste. Simmer for 1 to 2 minutes or until heated through.

> **IF FOLLOWING A LOW-FIBER DIET AND AVOIDING DIFFICULT-TO-DIGEST FOODS...**
>
> Finely mince the garlic and gingerroot, use peeled ripe peaches, and seed or omit the kiwi. It's okay to use orange juice with pulp, as this is soluble fiber.

Pizza with Red Peppers and Goat Cheese

- Preheat oven to 400°F (200°C)
- Baking sheet, lightly greased

1	10-inch (25 cm) pizza crust or prepared pizza dough (see tip, at left)	1
1 tbsp	olive oil	15 mL
1/4 cup	prepared sun-dried tomato pesto	60 mL
1 1/2 cups	finely shredded mozzarella cheese	375 mL
4 oz	prosciutto or thinly sliced smoked ham	125 g
2	roasted red bell peppers, chopped	2
4 oz	soft goat cheese, crumbled	125 g

1. Place crust on prepared baking sheet. Brush with oil and pesto.
2. Sprinkle mozzarella evenly over top. Tear prosciutto into thin strips and arrange evenly over cheese. Sprinkle red pepper then goat cheese evenly over prosciutto.
3. Bake in preheated oven until crust is golden and cheese is melted, 10 to 15 minutes.

Variation

Mini Pita Pizzas: If you don't have a pizza crust, try making mini pizzas with this recipe, using 4 to 6 pita breads. Follow the method above, leaving a 1/2-inch (1 cm) border around the edge of the pita and reduce the cooking time to about 6 minutes, just until the cheese melts.

IF YOU ARE WELL...

If there is no medical reason for you to avoid fiber or difficult-to-digest foods, consider adding sliced black olives or red onion to the toppings.

IF FOLLOWING A LOW-FIBER DIET AND AVOIDING DIFFICULT-TO-DIGEST FOODS...

Select pizza crust or dough made with white flour, remove any tough or chewy casing from the prosciutto or ham, and remove the skin of the roasted pepper.

Lower-calorie choice

Lower-fiber choice

Higher-protein choice

Source of sodium

MAKES 4 TO 6 SERVINGS

Tip

- When using prepared pizza dough, read the package instructions and adjust this method accordingly. I like to make a thin crust and bake the dough with nothing on it for about 7 minutes. Then I brush the warm crust with the olive oil and pesto and proceed as directed, reducing the remaining cooking time to 8 to 10 minutes. Watch carefully to ensure the edges of the crust don't burn.

IBD Tips

- Sources of sodium in this recipe include pesto, cheese and prosciutto or ham.
- Goat cheese does contain lactose, despite claims that individuals with lactose intolerance can eat goat cheese but not cheese made from cow's milk.

Nutrients Per Serving	
Calories	246
Fat	16 g
Fiber	Trace
Protein	18 g
Carbohydrate	9 g

Higher-calorie choice

Lower-fiber choice

Higher-protein choice

Source of potassium

Source of sodium

MAKES 2 SERVINGS

IBD Tips

- To make this recipe suitable for vegetarians who eat dairy, substitute soy-based deli meats, which are much lower in saturated fat and don't contain nitrites. They are still high in sodium.

- To add calories to this recipe, select regular-fat potato chips; to reduce fat, use baked chips.

- Substitute non-hydrogenated margarine for the butter if you are trying to reduce saturated fat.

- The sources of sodium are the deli meats, chips and cheese. Bread and salted butter also contribute.

Crazy Crunch Panini

A warm panini sandwich that is relatively easy to prepare is a helpful cooking solution during times of illness or low energy. Texture and crunch stimulate interest in food, especially if crunchy fresh vegetables and fruits are limited in your diet.

- *Preheat panini grill to high*

4	slices wheat bread (1/2-inch/1 cm thick slices)	4
1 tbsp	butter, melted	15 mL
2 oz	white American cheese, thinly sliced	60 g
1 oz	deli baked ham, thinly sliced	30 g
1 oz	deli smoked turkey breast, thinly sliced	30 g
1/4 cup	crushed potato or tortilla chips	60 mL

1. Brush one side of each bread slice with butter. Place two slices on a work surface, buttered side down, and evenly layer with cheese, ham, turkey and crushed chips. Cover with top halves, buttered side up, and press gently to pack.

2. Place sandwiches in grill, close the top plate and cook until golden brown, 3 to 4 minutes. Serve immediately.

IF FOLLOWING A LOW-FIBER DIET AND AVOIDING DIFFICULT-TO-DIGEST FOODS...

Choose bread made from refined flour, such as white or light rye. Use potato chips, as they are more refined than the corn flour used in tortilla chips. Remove any tough casing from the outside of the deli slices.

Deli Meats

Processed meats, such as deli ham and smoked turkey, should only be eaten occasionally. The preserving process — curing, smoking, salting and/or adding preservatives such as nitrites — in addition to a high sodium content and an often high saturated fat content, make them a less healthy choice. "Natural" versions still contain cultured celery extract, which is a source of naturally occurring nitrites.

Nutrients Per Serving	
Calories	456
Fat	24 g
Fiber	4 g
Protein	19 g
Carbohydrate	44 g

Crunchy Citrus Chicken

Serve these deliciously crunchy, tangy chicken breasts with roasted vegetables such as carrots, parsnips, garlic, rutabaga and butternut squash.

- *Preheat oven to 400°F (200°C)*
- *13- by 9-inch (33 by 23 cm) baking pan, lined with foil, lightly greased*

1	lemon	1
1	lime	1
1	orange	1
3 cups	GF corn flakes cereal, coarsely crushed	750 mL
3 tbsp	chopped fresh rosemary	45 mL
2 tbsp	minced fresh parsley	30 mL
2 tsp	paprika	10 mL
1/2 tsp	salt	2 mL
1/4 tsp	freshly ground black pepper	1 mL
4	skinless boneless chicken breasts	4

1. Zest the lemon, lime and orange. Juice half of each citrus fruit. Thinly slice the remaining half of each citrus fruit. Arrange fruit slices in bottom of prepared pan. Set aside.

2. On a pie plate, combine citrus juices. In a plastic bag, combine citrus zests, cereal, rosemary, parsley, paprika, salt and pepper. Roll chicken in citrus juice, then shake in seasoned crumbs. Place on citrus slices and sprinkle with leftover crumb mixture. Discard any excess juice.

3. Bake in preheated oven for 30 to 35 minutes, or until coating is golden brown and crispy, a meat thermometer inserted into the thickest part of a breast registers 170°F (75°C) and chicken is no longer pink inside.

IF FOLLOWING A LOW-FIBER DIET AND AVOIDING DIFFICULT-TO-DIGEST FOODS...

Finely chop the parsley leaves (do not include stems), finely grind the black pepper, and use 1 tbsp (15 mL) ground dried rosemary in place of fresh.

Lower-calorie choice

Lower-fat choice

Lower-fiber choice

Higher-protein choice

Lactose-free choice

Source of potassium

MAKES 4 SERVINGS

Tips

- Discard the plastic bag used for the coating mix — it is not safe to reuse anything when raw chicken is involved.

IBD Tips

- This recipe is gluten-free, which is important for individuals living with celiac disease or non-celiac gluten sensitivity.

- Rosemary is thought to play a role in reducing the formation of cancer-causing compounds during cooking.

- The juice of the citrus fruits supplies potassium, and its fresh fragrance stimulates interest in eating. The corn flakes supply some potassium as well.

Nutrients Per Serving	
Calories	317
Fat	5 g
Fiber	7 g
Protein	34 g
Carbohydrate	36 g

MAKES 6 SERVINGS

Tip

- Substitute Swiss cheese for the Cheddar if you prefer.

IBD Tips

- Many individuals with IBD report that they find poultry easier to digest than other types of meat.

- Don't skip this recipe just because it's made with broccoli! If you are well and there is no medical reason for you to avoid fiber or difficult-to-digest foods, try including broccoli in your diet. Broccoli is a source of beta carotene, vitamins C and E, folate, calcium and potassium. When selecting broccoli, choose firm, dark green, compact clusters of small buds, with none opened to show a yellow flower, and make sure the stem is not too thick or tough.

Chicken and Broccoli Bake

This tasty combination of noodles, cheese, chicken and vegetables in a creamy sauce is comfort food. Make this casserole the day before you intend to serve it and reheat for even better flavor.

- *Preheat oven to 350°F (180°C)*
- *Oblong baking dish, lightly greased*

6	chicken breast halves, skinned and boned	6
1	green onion, finely chopped	1
3 tbsp	butter or margarine	45 mL
2 tsp	freshly squeezed lemon juice	10 mL
3 tbsp	all-purpose flour	45 mL
2 cups	2% milk	500 mL
1 tbsp	chopped fresh parsley	15 mL
1/2 tsp	salt	2 mL
1/4 tsp	dried basil	1 mL
Pinch	freshly ground black pepper	Pinch
1 cup	shredded Cheddar cheese, divided	250 mL
1 cup	egg noodles	250 mL
2	medium tomatoes, sliced	2
2 cups	chopped broccoli, blanched	500 mL

1. In a large skillet over medium-high heat, cook chicken and onion in butter on 1 side until golden brown. Turn chicken to brown other side; sprinkle with lemon juice. Remove chicken. Whisk flour into pan juices; cook, stirring, for 2 minutes. Gradually whisk in milk, stirring constantly until smooth and thickened. Stir in seasonings and half of the cheese.

2. In a large pot of boiling water, cook noodles according to package directions or until tender but firm; drain well. Place cooked noodles in lightly greased oblong baking dish. Top with half of the sauce. Arrange tomato slices, broccoli and chicken on top of noodles. Cover with remaining sauce. Sprinkle with remaining cheese. Bake, uncovered, in preheated oven for about 30 minutes or until bubbling hot.

IF FOLLOWING A LOW-FIBER DIET AND AVOIDING DIFFICULT-TO-DIGEST FOODS...

Omit the broccoli. (When you decide to include broccoli in your diet again, start with the florets; the stems are higher in fiber and can be stringy.) Peel and seed the tomatoes (see page 169), and finely chop the parsley (do not include stems).

Nutrients Per Serving	
Calories	384
Fat	17 g
Fiber	2 g
Protein	38 g
Carbohydrate	20 g

Chicken and Eggplant Parmesan

- *Preheat oven to 425°F (220°C)*
- *Baking sheet, sprayed with vegetable spray*

4	crosswise slices of eggplant, skin on, approximately ½ inch (1 cm) thick	4
1	whole egg	1
1	egg white	1
1 tbsp	water or milk	15 mL
⅔ cup	seasoned bread crumbs	150 mL
3 tbsp	chopped fresh parsley (or 2 tsp/10 mL dried)	45 mL
1 tbsp	freshly grated Parmesan cheese	15 mL
1 lb	boneless skinless chicken breasts (about 4)	500 g
2 tsp	vegetable oil	10 mL
1 tsp	minced garlic	5 mL
½ cup	tomato pasta sauce	125 mL
½ cup	grated mozzarella cheese	125 mL

1. In small bowl, whisk together whole egg, egg white and water. On plate stir together bread crumbs, parsley and Parmesan. Dip eggplant slices in egg wash, then coat with bread-crumb mixture. Place on prepared pan and bake for 20 minutes, or until tender, turning once.

2. Meanwhile, pound chicken breasts between sheets of waxed paper to 1/4-inch (5 mm) thickness. Dip chicken in remaining egg wash, then coat with remaining bread-crumb mixture. Heat oil and garlic in nonstick skillet sprayed with vegetable spray and cook for 4 minutes, or until golden brown, turning once.

3. Spread 1 tbsp (15 mL) of tomato sauce on each eggplant slice. Place one chicken breast on top of each eggplant slice. Spread another 1 tbsp (15 mL) of tomato sauce on top of each chicken piece. Sprinkle with cheese and bake for 5 minutes or until cheese melts.

IF FOLLOWING A LOW-FIBER DIET AND AVOIDING DIFFICULT-TO-DIGEST FOODS...

Peel and seed the eggplant before cooking and bake until very soft, finely chop the parsley (do not include stems), use plain tomato sauce, and use seasoned bread crumbs made from white bread.

MAKES 4 SERVINGS

Tips

- Turkey, veal or pork scaloppini can replace chicken.
- A stronger cheese, such as Swiss, can replace mozzarella.
- A great dish to reheat the next day.

IBD Tips

- Eggplant is not typically found in a low-fiber diet; however, if it is peeled, seeded, cooked until soft, eaten in small amounts and chewed well, it can be included.
- If you are lactose intolerant, remember that aged hard cheeses have only a small amount of lactose and can often be tolerated. Parmesan is reportedly well tolerated by individuals who have trouble digesting larger amounts of lactose, such as the amount in a glass of milk.

Nutrients Per Serving	
Calories	317
Fat	10 g
Fiber	2 g
Protein	36 g
Carbohydrate	20 g

Lower-calorie choice

Lower-fiber choice

Higher-protein choice

MAKES 4 SERVINGS

IBD Tips

- No ingredient modifications are necessary, as this recipe is already low-fiber.

- Honey contains trace amounts of some vitamins, minerals and antioxidants, but because these amounts are so small they are not considered significant to our nutrition. The amount of antioxidants depends on the source of the pollen; in general, darker honey has a higher antioxidant content. But the bottom line is that, for the amount of honey we eat, it is really just a tasty form of sugar.

- Because this recipe calls for skinless chicken breasts and is flavored with honey and mustard, it is low in fat.

Nutrients Per Serving	
Calories	177
Fat	5 g
Fiber	Trace
Protein	21 g
Carbohydrate	12 g

Honey Dijon Chicken

You'd never guess by the taste just how quick and easy this recipe is to make!

- *Preheat oven to 350°F (180°C)*
- *Baking sheet, greased*

2 tbsp	all-purpose flour	30 mL
¼ tsp	salt	1 mL
¼ tsp	freshly ground black pepper	1 mL
4	boneless skinless chicken breasts (3 oz/90 g each)	4
2 tbsp	liquid honey	30 mL
2 tbsp	Dijon mustard	30 mL
1 tbsp	olive oil	15 mL

1. On a piece of waxed paper, combine flour, salt and pepper; coat chicken with mixture. In a small dish, combine honey and mustard; set aside.

2. In a skillet, heat oil over medium-high heat; quickly brown chicken on both sides. Place on greased baking sheet; spread with honey mixture. Bake in preheated oven for 10 to 15 minutes or until chicken is no longer pink inside.

Curried Chicken with Apples and Bananas

2 tbsp	vegetable oil	30 mL
1	3-lb (1.5 kg) chicken, skin removed and chicken cut into 6 to 8 pieces	1
1 cup	chopped onion	250 mL
1 tbsp	minced garlic	15 mL
2 tbsp	mild or medium curry powder	30 mL
2 tsp	ground turmeric	10 mL
1/2 tsp	ground cumin	2 mL
1/2 tsp	ground coriander	2 mL
1 cup	diced peeled tart apples	250 mL
1 1/2 cups	diced bananas	375 mL
1 1/2 cups	diced tomatoes	375 mL
1 cup	chicken stock	250 mL
1 cup	low-fat plain yogurt	250 mL
	Salt	

1. In a large saucepan or Dutch oven, heat 1 tbsp (15 mL) of the oil over medium-high heat. Add half of the chicken pieces and cook, turning once, until brown. Repeat with remaining oil and chicken. Transfer chicken to a plate and set aside.

2. Reduce heat to medium. Add onion and garlic; cook for 5 minutes or until soft. Stir in curry powder, turmeric, cumin and coriander; sauté for 1 minute.

3. Add apples, bananas, tomatoes and chicken stock; bring to a boil. Reduce heat and simmer, uncovered and stirring frequently, for 5 minutes or until liquid is reduced by half. Return chicken to pan; simmer, covered, for 30 minutes or until juices run clear when chicken is pierced with a fork.

4. Stir in yogurt; simmer for 15 minutes, stirring occasionally and watching for curdling. Season to taste with salt.

IF FOLLOWING A LOW-FIBER DIET AND AVOIDING DIFFICULT-TO-DIGEST FOODS...

Peel and seed the tomatoes (see page 169), and finely chop the onion.

MAKES 6 SERVINGS

IBD Tips

- Curry adds flavor, so don't hesitate to include it, as it can stimulate your taste buds during times of appetite loss. Ground spices are fine on a low-fiber diet and should be avoided only if necessary during times of illness, anal soreness or high ostomy outputs.

- Bananas are known for their stool-thickening effect.

- Peeling an apple helps reduce the insoluble fiber. Many individuals with IBD tolerate cooked apple better than raw.

- Bananas and tomatoes provide the potassium in this recipe.

- To boost sodium, use commercial chicken broth and add salt liberally.

- If you are trying to maintain or lose weight, use low-fat yogurt. If your goal is to gain weight, use full-fat yogurt.

Nutrients Per Serving	
Calories	273
Fat	9 g
Fiber	2 g
Protein	28 g
Carbohydrate	20 g

MAKES 4 SERVINGS

Tip

- If you prefer a spicier result, add 1 tsp (5 mL) Asian chili sauce along with the peanut butter.

IBD Tips

- Before you pass over this recipe because it has "spicy" in the title, remember that you can get all the taste while controlling the spice. Simply reduce the amount of curry powder and let everyone add their own chili sauce.

- Chicken thighs are tasty but are higher in fat than chicken breasts.

- Peanut butter is known to help thicken loose stool.

- Tomato juice, peanut butter and chicken provide potassium.

- Tomato juice, chili sauce, added salt and some peanut butters provide sodium.

Nutrients Per Serving	
Calories	467
Fat	25 g
Fiber	4 g
Protein	36 g
Carbohydrate	28 g

Spicy Peanut Chicken

Surprise your family with this exotic stew, which is easily made with pantry ingredients. If you're a heat seeker, add the Asian chili sauce.

1 tbsp	vegetable oil	15 mL
1 lb	boneless skinless chicken, cut into 1-inch (2.5 cm) cubes	500 g
1 cup	diced onion	250 mL
1 tbsp	minced garlic	15 mL
2 tsp	curry powder	10 mL
1 tsp	salt	5 mL
	Freshly ground black pepper	
1 cup	chopped red or green bell pepper or 1½ cups (375 mL) frozen mixed bell pepper strips	250 mL
1 tbsp	all-purpose flour	15 mL
2 cups	tomato juice	500 mL
¼ cup	peanut butter	60 mL
	Hot white rice	

1. In a skillet, heat oil over medium heat. Add chicken and onion and cook, stirring, until onions are softened and chicken is no longer pink inside, about 8 minutes.

2. Add garlic, curry powder, salt and black pepper to taste. Cook, stirring, for 1 minute. Add bell pepper and cook, stirring, for 1 minute. Add flour and cook, stirring, for 1 minute.

3. Add tomato juice. Bring to a boil. Cook, stirring, until thickened, about 5 minutes. Add peanut butter and stir until blended. Serve over hot white rice.

IF FOLLOWING A LOW-FIBER DIET AND AVOIDING DIFFICULT-TO-DIGEST FOODS...

Finely dice the onion, finely grind the black pepper, peel the bell pepper before chopping, and choose smooth peanut butter.

Slow-Cooked Creole Chicken

- *Electric slow cooker*

2 lbs	boneless skinless chicken thighs	1 kg
2 cups	diced green bell peppers	500 mL
1/2 cup	chopped green onions or cooking onions	125 mL
1	can (19 oz/540 mL) stewed tomatoes	1
1	can (5.5 oz/155 g) tomato paste	1
2 tsp	minced garlic	10 mL
1 tsp	hot pepper sauce	5 mL
1	bay leaf	1
2 tsp	dried thyme	10 mL
8 oz	spicy smoked Polish sausage, sliced	250 g

1. Place chicken thighs in bottom of slow cooker. Add peppers, onions, tomatoes, tomato paste, garlic, hot pepper sauce, bay leaf and dried thyme. Cook, covered, on Low heat setting for 4 to 5 hours. Increase heat setting to High; add sausage and cook for 20 to 30 minutes. Remove bay leaf.

IF FOLLOWING A LOW-FIBER DIET AND AVOIDING DIFFICULT-TO-DIGEST FOODS...

Peel the green peppers before dicing, finely chop the onions, use an equivalent amount of fresh tomatoes and peel and seed them (see page 169), and remove the casing from the sausage. Avoid the hot pepper sauce if you have high stoma outputs or are sore in the anal area from passing frequent liquidy stool.

Quick Microwave Rice

In a large microwave-safe bowl, combine 1 1/2 cups (375 mL) rice and 2 1/2 cups (625 mL) hot water. Cover completely and microwave on Medium-High for 20 minutes. Let stand for 2 to 3 minutes; fluff with a fork and serve. Rice freezes well, so save any leftovers in airtight containers and use as needed.

Lower-fiber choice

Higher-protein choice

Lactose-free choice

Source of potassium

Source of sodium

MAKES 8 SERVINGS

IBD Tips

- Sausage casings can be natural or synthetic. Natural casings are made from the cleaned intestinal membranes of animals such as cows and sheep. Some synthetic casings are edible. You'll know to remove it if it looks and feels like paper or thin plastic.

- If you have severe lactose intolerance, read the ingredient list on the sausage — hidden sources of lactose may have been added.

- If you don't like spicy smoked sausage, substitute turkey kielbasa; it is both milder and much lower in fat.

- Sources of potassium in this recipe are tomatoes, tomato paste and meat.

- Sources of sodium are canned tomatoes, tomato paste, sausage and possibly hot pepper sauce.

Nutrients Per Serving	
Calories	284
Fat	14 g
Fiber	2 g
Protein	27 g
Carbohydrate	12 g

MAKES 8 SERVINGS

Tips

• If your kids don't like rice, serve this dish over 1 lb (500 g) of spaghetti.

• Make up to 2 days ahead and reheat. Can be frozen for up to 6 weeks. Great for leftovers.

IBD Tips

• Pineapple juice contains potassium, as well as the digestive enzyme bromelain, which naturally digests protein and is the active ingredient in some meat tenderizers.

• Soft cooked white rice is known to help thicken loose stool.

• Tomato juice, ketchup and chili sauce provide sodium.

• Tomato juice is rich in potassium; chicken and pineapple juice are also sources.

Nutrients Per Serving	
Calories	351
Fat	6 g
Fiber	2 g
Protein	15 g
Carbohydrate	58 g

Sweet-and-Sour Chicken Meatballs over Rice

Meatballs

12 oz	ground chicken	375 g
¼ cup	finely chopped onions	60 mL
2 tbsp	ketchup	30 mL
2 tbsp	bread crumbs	30 mL
1	egg	1
2 tsp	olive oil	10 mL
2 tsp	minced garlic	10 mL
⅓ cup	chopped onions	75 mL
2 cups	tomato juice	500 mL
2 cups	pineapple juice	500 mL
½ cup	chili sauce	125 mL
2 cups	white rice	500 mL

1. *Prepare the meatballs:* In bowl, combine chicken, onions, ketchup, bread crumbs and egg; mix well. Form each 1 tbsp (15 mL) into a meatball and place on plate; set aside.

2. In large saucepan, heat oil over medium heat. Add garlic and onions and cook just until softened, approximately 3 minutes. Add tomato and pineapple juices, chili sauce and meatballs. Cover and simmer uncovered for 30 to 40 minutes just until meatballs are tender.

3. Meanwhile, bring 4 cups (1 L) of water to a boil. Stir in rice, reduce heat, cover and simmer for 20 minutes or until liquid is absorbed. Remove from heat and let stand for 5 minutes, covered. Serve meatballs and sauce over rice.

IF FOLLOWING A LOW-FIBER DIET AND AVOIDING DIFFICULT-TO-DIGEST FOODS...

Sauté onions until soft. If you are experiencing soreness in the anal area from passing frequent liquidy stool, omit the chili sauce. Some individuals report a burning sensation from foods containing tomato products; if this is a problem for you, limit your portion size.

Terrific Chicken Burgers

1	egg	1
½ cup	fine dry bread crumbs	125 mL
⅓ cup	finely chopped green onions	75 mL
1 tsp	ground coriander	5 mL
1 tsp	grated lemon zest	5 mL
½ tsp	salt	2 mL
¼ tsp	freshly ground black pepper	1 mL
1 lb	ground chicken or turkey	500 g
1 tbsp	vegetable oil	15 mL

1. In a bowl, beat egg; stir in bread crumbs, green onions, coriander, lemon zest, salt and pepper; mix in chicken. With wet hands, shape into four ¾-inch (2 cm) thick patties.

2. In a large nonstick skillet, heat oil over medium heat; cook patties for 5 to 6 minutes on each side or until golden brown on outside and no longer pink in center.

IF FOLLOWING A LOW-FIBER DIET AND AVOIDING DIFFICULT-TO-DIGEST FOODS…

Choose white bread crumbs and finely grind the black pepper.

Lower-fat choice

Lower-fiber choice

Higher-protein choice

Lactose-free choice

MAKES 4 BURGERS (1 PER SERVING)

Tip

- If burgers are starting to become mundane, put some excitement in the patties by adding shredded cheese right in the ground meat mixture for moist burgers with a twist.

IBD Tips

- If you are on a lactose-free diet, make sure the bread crumbs do not contain hidden sources of lactose (e.g., whey, curds, milk by-products, dry milk solids/powder) or consider making your own bread crumbs from lactose-free bread.

- Lean ground chicken and turkey are lower in fat than other types of meat.

- Many individuals with IBD report that they tolerate ground meat well.

Nutrients Per Serving	
Calories	227
Fat	14 g
Fiber	1 g
Protein	22 g
Carbohydrate	4 g

Turkey Cutlets in Savory Cranberry Gravy

Here's a great recipe for a holiday dinner if you don't feel like cooking an entire bird. It's absolutely delicious, attractive and will elicit compliments from the first bite. That said, it is also speedy enough for a quick weeknight meal served over fluffy white rice.

MAKES 4 SERVINGS

Tips

• Substitute chicken cutlets for the turkey if you prefer.

• If you prefer a bit of spice, add as much as 1/4 tsp (1 mL) cayenne pepper to the flour mixture.

IBD Tips

• Turkey is a great choice when you're trying to reduce your intake of saturated fat. Compared to other meats, turkey has fewer calories and less fat, but still provides high-quality protein, vitamins and minerals. Choose white meat and remove the skin *before* cooking.

• Sodium is provided by mustard and added salt, and can be boosted by using commercial chicken stock.

• Preheat oven to 250°F (120°C)

1/4 cup	all-purpose flour	60 mL
1/2 tsp	salt	2 mL
Pinch	freshly ground black pepper	Pinch
1 lb	turkey breast cutlets	500 g
2 tbsp	vegetable oil, divided	30 mL
1/2 cup	chicken stock or water	125 mL
1 tbsp	cider vinegar	15 mL
2 tbsp	packed brown sugar	30 mL
1 tbsp	Dijon mustard	15 mL
1	can (14 oz/398 mL) cranberry sauce, preferably whole berry	1

1. On a plate, combine flour, salt and black pepper. Dip turkey into flour mixture to coat evenly on both sides, shaking off excess.

2. In a skillet, heat 1 tbsp (15 mL) of the oil over medium-high heat. Sauté turkey, in batches, adding more oil as necessary, until golden outside and no longer pink inside, 2 to 3 minutes per side. Transfer to a deep platter and keep warm in preheated oven while making the sauce.

3. Add chicken stock and cider vinegar to pan. Cook, stirring and scraping pan to loosen any brown bits, until mixture is reduced by half, about 2 minutes. Add brown sugar and mustard and stir until blended. Stir in cranberry sauce and bring to a boil. Pour over cutlets and serve immediately.

> **IF FOLLOWING A LOW-FIBER DIET AND AVOIDING DIFFICULT-TO-DIGEST FOODS...**
>
> Choose a cranberry sauce without whole berries and finely grind the black pepper.

Nutrients Per Serving	
Calories	419
Fat	8 g
Fiber	1 g
Protein	30 g
Carbohydrate	59 g

Cajun-Style Turkey Cutlet with Citrus

Turkey cutlets are available fresh and frozen in most supermarkets and are a convenient way of enjoying turkey — without the leftovers!

2 tbsp	paprika	30 mL
1 tbsp	dried sage	15 mL
1 tsp	freshly ground black pepper	5 mL
½ tsp	salt	2 mL
½ tsp	garlic powder	2 mL
½ tsp	cayenne pepper	2 mL
6	turkey cutlets (3 oz/90 g each)	6
1 tbsp	vegetable oil	15 mL
1	large orange, peeled and sectioned	1
1	medium grapefruit, peeled and sectioned	1

1. Mix together paprika, sage, pepper, salt, garlic powder and cayenne; place on waxed paper. With meat mallet, pound turkey between 2 pieces of plastic wrap to ⅜-inch (9 mm) thickness. Coat cutlets well with seasoning mixture.

2. In a large skillet, heat oil over high heat; quickly brown turkey on both sides. Reduce heat and add orange and grapefruit; cook until turkey is no longer pink inside.

IF FOLLOWING A LOW-FIBER DIET AND AVOIDING DIFFICULT-TO-DIGEST FOODS...

Peel the orange and grapefruit and remove the membranes. (It may be easier to cut them in half and spoon out the pulpy part of the fruit, leaving the membranes behind). Citrus fruit can be included in a fiber-restricted diet, but some individuals with IBD report increased burning when passing stool after eating citrus fruit. If you are experiencing soreness in the anal area, you may wish to limit your portion size or avoid foods containing citrus.

Lower-calorie choice

Lower-fat choice

Lower-fiber choice

Higher-protein choice

Lactose-free choice

Source of potassium

MAKES 6 SERVINGS

IBD Tips

- Oranges are rich in potassium; grapefruit and turkey are also sources.

- Many individuals with IBD report that poultry and fish are easier to digest than other types of meat. In this recipe, turkey is combined with spices and citrus for a flavorful low-fat meal.

- Choose canola or olive oil for their favorable fatty acid profiles. Canola is a plant source of omega-3 fat, and olive oil is relatively high in monounsaturated fat.

Nutrients Per Serving	
Calories	153
Fat	4 g
Fiber	2 g
Protein	21 g
Carbohydrate	8 g

Turkey Apple Meatloaf

- *Preheat oven to 350°F (180°C)*
- *9- by 5-inch (23 by 12.5 cm) loaf pan, lightly greased*

2	cloves garlic, minced	2
1	egg	1
1	tart apple, such as Mutsu or Granny Smith, finely chopped	1
1 lb	lean ground turkey	500 g
½ cup	chopped onion	125 mL
⅓ cup	oat bran	75 mL
⅓ cup	ground flaxseed	75 mL
3 tbsp	prepared yellow mustard	45 mL
1 tbsp	ketchup	15 mL
1 tsp	salt	5 mL

1. In a large bowl, combine garlic, egg, apple, turkey, onion, oat bran, flaxseed, mustard, ketchup and salt. Pack into prepared loaf pan.

2. Bake in preheated oven for 45 to 60 minutes or until a meat thermometer inserted in the center registers an internal temperature of 175°F (80°C).

IF FOLLOWING A LOW-FIBER DIET AND AVOIDING DIFFICULT-TO-DIGEST FOODS...

Finely chop the onion and peel the apple.

MAKES 6 SERVINGS

Tip

- An extra meatloaf can be sliced to use in sandwiches or frozen for another day.

IBD Tips

- Oat bran and apple provide soluble fiber. Peeling an apple helps reduce the insoluble fiber. Many individuals with IBD tolerate cooked apple better than raw.

- Oat bran's "gelling" properties help to form loose stool. Because of this desirable effect, many low-fiber diets include oats and oat products despite the increased fiber content.

- Lean ground turkey is lower in fat than other varieties of meat.

- The added salt, ketchup and mustard supply sodium.

Nutrients Per Serving	
Calories	197
Fat	10 g
Fiber	3 g
Protein	17 g
Carbohydrate	11 g

Fish and Seafood

There are many benefits to eating fish on a regular basis. Fish is an excellent source of protein, vitamins and minerals, which are all important for achieving and maintaining good health. Many individuals with IBD report good tolerance to white fish, as the flavor is mild and the texture is relatively soft and easy to chew. There are many varieties of white fish, including snapper, tilapia, sole, cod and haddock. If you aren't as tolerant of other meats, it is important to include this source of high-quality protein and iron in your diet.

Shellfish can also contribute to a healthy, balanced diet. Mussels, clams, scallops, shrimp, oysters, lobster and abalone are low in calories and saturated fat, are excellent sources of protein and contain omega-3 fatty acids. Like fish, shellfish contribute to health by providing essential minerals and vitamins such as iron, zinc, copper and vitamin B_{12}. However, if you have a new ileostomy or your intestine is narrowed from inflammation or scar tissue, be careful with stringy, tough seafood such as shrimp, clams, octopus, squid, lobster and crab. Chew them very well or avoid them altogether.

The Facts About Mercury

Choose canned "light" tuna, as it contains other species of tuna, such as skipjack, yellowfin and tongol, which have lower mercury levels (and tend to cost less) than canned "white" albacore tuna.

Media articles about mercury levels in certain species of fish have caused many consumers to question the safety of these fish. Health experts advise limiting consumption of shark, swordfish and fresh and frozen tuna to one meal per week. Pregnant women, women of childbearing age and young children should eat no more than one meal per month of these fish. To minimize your exposure to mercury, vary the type of fish you choose and select smaller fish that are lower on the food chain and have had less time to accumulate contaminants. Good choices include char, herring, mackerel, salmon, sardines, trout, pollock and shrimp.

THE FACTS ABOUT OMEGA-3 FATS

Omega-3 fats help prevent heart disease, have been linked to better cognitive function in older adults, are necessary for brain development and may help treat disorders with an inflammatory component, such as rheumatoid arthritis. Because omega-3 fats have anti-inflammatory properties, it is worthwhile for individuals living with IBD to include them in their diet, although researchers have not yet determined a recommended amount.

Omega-3 fats have two dietary sources: seafood and plants. Marine sources such as fatty fish are best for providing eicosapentaenoic acid (EPA) and docosahexaenoic acid (DHA). Plant sources provide alpha-linolenic acid (ALA), which must be converted into EPA and DHA. Fish are able to convert ALA into EPA and DHA, but humans have a limited ability to do so. Plant-based sources of omega-3 fats include flax seeds, walnuts and canola oil. For full benefit, consume a variety of fish sources, plant sources and even omega-3-enriched foods such as eggs, dairy and juices.

The Facts About PCBs

Stock canned salmon in your pantry for times when you are busy or can't think of what to cook. For added calcium, crush and eat the bones, which are soft from the canning process. One can of salmon contains as much calcium as 1 cup (250 mL) of milk

Farmed salmon has received media attention due to concerns about PCBs (polychlorinated biphenyls), an environmental pollutant that accumulates in their fat stores. Studies have shown a possible link between consumption of PCBs and cancer. Farmed salmon are exposed to PCBs via their feed. While wild salmon also ingest some PCBs, their diet is more varied. To include this beneficial food in your diet while reducing the risk:

- Choose wild salmon (unfortunately, it is more expensive).
- Use canned salmon (almost all canned salmon is wild).
- Remove the skin and the fat under the skin before cooking salmon.
- Broil, bake, poach or grill instead of sautéing. This will allow some fat to drain off and still leave some omega-3 fats.

Fish Fillets with Basil Walnut Sauce

This easily prepared sauce, which is similar to pesto, is absolutely delicious.

- *Preheat broiler*
- *Broiler or roasting pan*

½ cup	fresh parsley, snipped and loosely packed	125 mL
½ cup	fresh basil, snipped and loosely packed	125 mL
3 tbsp	finely chopped walnuts	45 mL
2 tbsp	chicken broth	30 mL
2 tbsp	freshly grated Parmesan cheese	30 mL
1 tbsp	olive oil	15 mL
1 tbsp	balsamic vinegar or malt vinegar	15 mL
1 tsp	granulated sugar	5 mL
1	clove garlic, minced	1
½ tsp	freshly ground black pepper	2 mL
1½ lb	fish fillets (cod, haddock or halibut), 1 inch (2.5 cm) thick	750 g
¼ cup	dry white wine	60 mL
½	lemon	½
1 tbsp	butter or margarine	15 mL
	Salt and black pepper to taste	

1. In a food processor or blender, combine parsley, basil, walnuts, chicken broth, cheese, oil, vinegar, sugar, garlic and pepper. Process until smooth; add more broth if thinner sauce is desired.

2. Arrange fish in broiler or roasting pan. Pour wine into pan; squeeze lemon juice over fish. Dot with butter; sprinkle with salt and pepper. Broil for 5 minutes. Spoon sauce over top and broil for another 4 to 5 minutes, allowing total of 10 minutes per inch (2.5 cm) of thickness, or until fish flakes easily with fork.

IF FOLLOWING A LOW-FIBER DIET AND AVOIDING DIFFICULT-TO-DIGEST FOODS...

Use the leaves of the parsley and basil rather than the stems, and finely grind the black pepper (larger pieces can increase risk of a food-related obstruction).

Lower-calorie choice

Lower-fiber choice

Higher-protein choice

MAKES 6 SERVINGS

Tip

- This sauce, like pesto, is quite thick, but it can be thinned with chicken broth, if desired.

IBD Tips

- The alcohol content of wine evaporates with cooking.

- Walnuts are a good source of omega-3 fats. In this recipe, they are puréed to a smooth consistency, making them easier to tolerate for individuals with active disease. Although marine sources of omega-3 fat are the best sources, plant-based sources are still worth including in your diet.

- Commercial chicken broth, cheese, butter or margarine, and added salt all contribute to the overall sodium content of this recipe.

Nutrients Per Serving	
Calories	200
Fat	9 g
Fiber	Trace
Protein	25 g
Carbohydrate	3 g

Vegetarian choice

Lower-fiber choice

Higher-protein choice

Source of sodium

MAKES 4 SERVINGS

Tips

- Try to make the relish as close to the time of serving as possible; otherwise, the cucumber will make the sauce too watery.
- Use cod, snapper or haddock.
- Use 1½ tsp (7 mL) dried dillweed if fresh dill is unavailable.
- The flatter the fish, the faster it cooks.
- Prepare fish early in the day and keep refrigerated until ready to bake.

IBD Tips

- This recipe is suitable for vegetarians who eat fish, dairy and eggs.
- Choose a non-hydrogenated margarine to limit saturated and trans fats.
- To boost calories, use full-fat yogurt, mayonnaise and milk.

Nutrients Per Serving	
Calories	274
Fat	9 g
Fiber	1 g
Protein	27 g
Carbohydrates	20 g

Crunchy Fish with Cucumber Dill Relish

Relish

2 cups	finely chopped cucumbers	500 mL
⅓ cup	chopped fresh dill	75 mL
⅓ cup	2% yogurt	75 mL
¼ cup	finely diced green onions (about 2 medium)	60 mL
¼ cup	finely diced green bell pepper	60 mL
3 tbsp	light mayonnaise	45 mL
1 tsp	minced garlic	5 mL

Crunchy Fish

2 cups	corn flakes cereal	500 mL
1 tbsp	freshly grated Parmesan cheese	15 mL
1 tsp	minced garlic	5 mL
½ tsp	dried basil	2 mL
1	egg	1
3 tbsp	2% milk	45 mL
3 tbsp	all-purpose flour	45 mL
1 lb	firm white fish fillets	500 g
1 tbsp	margarine or butter	15 mL

1. *Prepare the relish:* In bowl, combine cucumbers, dill, yogurt, green onions, green peppers, mayonnaise and garlic; mix to combine and set aside.

2. *Prepare the fish:* Put corn flakes, Parmesan, garlic and basil in food processor; process until fine and put on a plate. In shallow bowl, whisk together egg and milk. Dust fish with flour.

3. Dip fish fillets in egg wash, then coat with crumb mixture. In large nonstick skillet sprayed with vegetable spray, melt margarine over medium heat. Add fillets and cook for 5 minutes or until browned, turn and cook for 2 minutes longer, or until fish is browned and flakes easily when pierced with a fork. Serve topped with cucumber dill relish.

IF FOLLOWING A LOW-FIBER DIET AND AVOIDING DIFFICULT-TO-DIGEST FOODS...

Peel and seed the cucumbers, finely chop the dill (do not include stems) or use dried dillweed, sauté the green onions until soft, and peel the green pepper before dicing.

Tandoori Haddock

Purchased tandoori paste makes an easy marinade for white fish. This Indian-inspired dish can be made quickly for a great weeknight meal.

- *Rimmed baking sheet, lightly greased*

¼ cup	tandoori paste (see tip, at right)	60 mL
¼ cup	low-fat yogurt	60 mL
1 tbsp	freshly squeezed lemon juice	15 mL
4	haddock fillets (about 14 oz/420 g total)	4

1. In a shallow dish, combine tandoori paste, yogurt and lemon juice. Add fish, turning to coat evenly. Cover and refrigerate for 20 to 30 minutes. Meanwhile, preheat broiler, with rack set 4 inches (10 cm) from the top.
2. Place fish on baking sheet and broil for 10 minutes or until fish is opaque and flakes easily with a fork and the top is lightly browned.

Variation

This works well with most firm white fish fillets or steaks, such as halibut or orange roughy. We have even tested it with salmon, and it works great! Adjust the broiling time depending on the thickness of the fish.

Vegetarian choice

Lower-calorie choice

Lower-fat choice

Lower-fiber choice

Higher-protein choice

Source of sodium

MAKES 4 SERVINGS

Tip

- Most supermarkets now carry tandoori paste. You can usually find it in the ethnic food aisle where Indian and Asian sauces are displayed.

IBD Tips

- This recipe is suitable for vegetarians who eat fish and dairy, and is appropriate for a low-fiber diet.
- Keep the fish fillets in your freezer and the tandoori paste in your pantry for days when you want to prepare something quick without going to the grocery store.
- Prepared sauces and pastes are usually high in sodium.
- To boost calories, use full-fat yogurt.
- For a lactose-free version, use soy yogurt.

Nutrients Per Serving	
Calories	113
Fat	1 g
Fiber	Trace
Protein	20 g
Carbohydrate	4 g

Vegetarian choice

Lower-calorie choice

Higher-calorie choice

Higher-protein choice

Lactose-free choice

Source of sodium

MAKES 2 SERVINGS

Tips

- This recipe can be doubled or tripled.
- Canned or frozen peas work well in this curry. If using canned peas, be sure to drain them before adding to the recipe. Cook frozen peas according to package instructions.

IBD Tips

- This recipe is appropriate for vegetarians who eat fish.
- Canned salmon provides potassium, and you can crush the bones for added calcium. It's also a great way to get vitamin D and omega-3 fats!
- Coconut milk is high in saturated fat and calories.
- Sodium is provided by the canned salmon and fish sauce.

Nutrients Per Serving	
Calories	619
Fat	50 g
Fiber	7 g
Protein	27 g
Carbohydrate	25 g

Thai-Style Salmon Curry

If you're fond of Thai food, here's an easy way to taste its unique flavors. Look for fish sauce in the Asian foods section of well-stocked supermarkets.

1	can (14 oz/398 mL) coconut milk	1
1 to 2	fresh chili peppers, minced, or 3 whole dried red chili peppers	1 to 2
1	can (7$\frac{1}{2}$ oz/213 g) salmon, drained	1
1 cup	cooked green peas (see tip, at left)	250 mL
2 tbsp	fish sauce	30 mL
2 tbsp	freshly squeezed lemon juice	30 mL
1 tbsp	freshly squeezed lime juice	15 mL
1 tsp	packed brown sugar	5 mL
	Finely chopped cilantro (optional)	
	Hot white rice or noodles	

1. In a saucepan over medium heat, combine coconut milk and chili peppers. Bring to a simmer.

2. Add salmon and peas and cook, stirring, being careful not to let the mixture boil, about 3 minutes. Add fish sauce, lemon juice, lime juice and brown sugar and cook, stirring, for 1 minute. Taste for seasoning, adding more fish sauce, lemon or lime juice, or brown sugar, if desired.

3. Remove dried peppers, if using. Pour over rice or noodles. Garnish with cilantro, if using. Serve immediately.

IF FOLLOWING A LOW-FIBER DIET AND AVOIDING DIFFICULT-TO-DIGEST FOODS...

Use ground chili peppers and reduce the amount, use canned green peas (the skin of fresh or frozen green peas does not cook soft enough), and finely chop the cilantro (do not include stems).

Orange Hoisin Salmon

A quick and easy fish dish with Asian flair.

- *Preheat broiler, with rack set 4 inches (10 cm) from the top*
- *Rimmed baking sheet, lightly greased*

2 tbsp	hoisin sauce	30 mL
1 tbsp	frozen orange juice concentrate	15 mL
2 tsp	grated orange zest	10 mL
2 tsp	liquid honey	10 mL
Pinch	salt	Pinch
Pinch	freshly ground black pepper	Pinch
4	salmon fillets (about 1½ lbs/750 g total)	4
	Vegetable cooking spray	

1. In a small bowl, combine hoisin sauce, orange juice concentrate, orange zest and honey.
2. Place salmon on baking sheet and baste both sides with hoisin mixture. Season with salt and pepper.
3. Broil for 7 to 10 minutes or until fish is opaque and flakes easily with a fork.

> **IF FOLLOWING A LOW-FIBER DIET AND AVOIDING DIFFICULT-TO-DIGEST FOODS...**
>
> Finely grind the black pepper (larger pieces can increase the risk of a food-related obstruction).

Vegetarian choice

Lower-fiber choice

Higher-protein choice

Lactose-free choice

MAKES 4 SERVINGS

IBD Tips

- This recipe is appropriate for vegetarians who eat fish.
- While this recipe contains frozen orange juice concentrate, not enough of it is used for the recipe to be considered rich in potassium.
- Zest is the outer skin of a citrus fruit such as an orange or lemon. The oils it contains add a strong flavor to foods. However, the white membrane under the zest is usually bitter, so don't scrape too deep with your grater or peeler.
- Honey contains trace amounts of some vitamins, minerals and antioxidants, but these amounts are too small to be considered significant to our nutrition.

Nutrients Per Serving	
Calories	314
Fat	17 g
Fiber	Trace
Protein	30 g
Carbohydrate	8 g

Vegetarian choice

Lower-calorie choice

Lower-fiber choice

Higher-protein choice

Lactose-free choice

Baked Salmon with Ginger and Lemon

Fresh ginger gives such a sparkling flavor to salmon — or any fish, for that matter. Dried ground ginger just doesn't impart the same crisp taste.

MAKES 4 SERVINGS

Tips

- Buy gingerroot that is firm and unwrinkled, with a gingery aroma. Mature, thick-skinned ginger has a more intense flavor than tender, thin-skinned roots. Store it in a sealable plastic bag in the refrigerator. It will keep for several weeks. Or peel it and freeze in a freezer bag. Grate what you need for a recipe while it's still frozen and return the rest to the freezer.

IBD Tips

- This recipe is suitable for vegetarians who eat fish.
- Sodium is provided by soy sauce and can be boosted by selecting regular-sodium soy sauce.

- *Preheat oven to 375°F (190°C)*
- *Shallow baking dish*

4	skinless salmon fillets (each 4 oz/125 g)	4
2	green onions	2
1	clove garlic, minced	1
1½ tsp	minced gingerroot	7 mL
1 tsp	granulated sugar	5 mL
2 tbsp	reduced-sodium soy sauce	30 mL
1 tsp	grated lemon zest	5 mL
1 tbsp	freshly squeezed lemon juice	15 mL
1 tsp	sesame oil	5 mL

1. Arrange salmon in a single layer in baking dish.

2. Thinly slice green onions and set aside green parts for garnish. In a bowl, combine white part of green onions, garlic, ginger, sugar, soy sauce, lemon zest, lemon juice and oil. Pour marinade over salmon. Let stand at room temperature for 15 minutes, or cover and refrigerate for up to 1 hour.

3. Bake, uncovered, in preheated oven for 17 to 20 minutes or until fish is opaque and flakes easily when tested with a fork.

4. Arrange salmon on serving plates and spoon sauce from dish over top. Sprinkle with reserved green onions.

> **IF FOLLOWING A LOW-FIBER DIET AND AVOIDING DIFFICULT-TO-DIGEST FOODS...**
> Finely chop the green onions.

Nutrients Per Serving	
Calories	181
Fat	7 g
Fiber	0 g
Protein	26 g
Carbohydrate	3 g

Salmon Pizza Pinwheels

Add these pinwheels to lunchbags or serve them as easy after-school snacks.

* *Preheat oven to 400°F (200°C)*
* *Baking sheet, lined with parchment paper*

1	can (7½ oz/213 g) salmon, drained, deboned and broken into chunks	1
2 tbsp	soft cream cheese	30 mL
	Flour for dusting	
1	tube (14 oz/391 g) refrigerated pizza dough	1
1 cup	shredded Italian cheese blend (about 4 oz/125 g)	250 mL
4	green onions, thinly sliced	4

1. In a bowl, using a fork, mix salmon and cream cheese.

2. On a lightly floured surface, roll dough into a rectangle about 14 by 10 inches (36 by 25 cm). Spread salmon mixture right to the edges on three sides and about 1 inch (2.5 cm) from the short edge farthest from you (the filling will be pushed to this edge when the dough is rolled up).

3. Scatter cheese, then green onions over the salmon. Beginning with the short end closest to you, roll up the dough as tightly as possible, jelly-roll fashion, to form a log.

4. Pat the ends to flatten slightly and, using a serrated knife, cut the cylinder into 10 slices. Lay, cut side up, on prepared pan.

5. Bake in preheated oven for about 20 minutes, until crust is golden and cheese is molten. Let pinwheels rest for 5 minutes before serving.

Omega-3 Fats

Marine sources of anti-inflammatory omega-3 fats — which include cold-water fatty fish, such as salmon, mackerel, sardines, anchovies, and tuna — provide omega-3s in the forms most easily used by the body.

Vegetarian choice

Lower-calorie choice

Higher-protein choice

Source of sodium

MAKES 10 PINWHEELS (1 PER SERVING)

IBD Tips

* This recipe is suitable for vegetarians who eat seafood, dairy and eggs.

* Recipes using canned ingredients may be easier to prepare during times of illness.

* For a low-fiber version of this recipe, finely mince the green onion or omit it.

* Boost calories by selecting canned salmon packed in oil and full-fat cream cheese.

* Crush the bones of the canned salmon for added calcium and vitamin D.

* Sodium is provided by canned salmon and cheese.

* Cheese is known to help thicken loose stool.

Nutrients Per Serving	
Calories	160
Fat	6 g
Fiber	1 g
Protein	12 g
Carbohydrate	17 g

Vegetarian choice

Higher-calorie choice

Lower-fiber choice

Higher-protein choice

Source of potassium

Source of sodium

**MAKES 4 BURGERS
(1 PER SERVING)**

Tips

- Panko is Japanese-style bread crumbs.

IBD Tips

- This recipe is suitable for vegetarians who eat seafood, dairy and eggs.

- This recipe may be lactose-free, depending on the ingredients used to make the panko.

- Consider crushing the bones of the canned salmon for added calcium. It's also a great way to get vitamin D.

- Sodium is provided by the canned salmon and soy sauce.

- Potassium is provided by the soy sauce and tomato.

Nutrients Per Serving	
Calories	405
Fat	14 g
Fiber	2 g
Protein	31 g
Carbohydrate	42 g

Open Sesame Salmon Burgers

Sesame lovers can get their fix with this Asian-inspired fish burger.

- *Preheat broiler, placing oven rack one level down from top position*
- *Broiling pan, covered with generously greased foil*

1	egg	1
2 tbsp	mayonnaise	30 mL
1 tbsp	toasted sesame oil	15 mL
2 tsp	soy sauce	10 mL
2	cans (each 6 oz/170 g) boneless, skinless salmon, drained and broken into chunks	2
½ cup	panko bread crumbs (see tip, at left)	125 mL
4	leaves leaf lettuce	4
4	sesame seed buns	4
	Sesame Mayo (see recipe, opposite)	
4	slices tomato	4
¼ cup	thinly sliced red onion	60 mL

1. In a bowl, using a fork, mix egg, mayonnaise, sesame oil and soy sauce. Gently squeeze salmon to remove excess moisture and add to the bowl. Add panko crumbs and mix well.

2. Divide salmon mixture into 4 portions and shape each into a patty approximately $4\frac{1}{2}$ inches (11 cm) in diameter. Place each on prepared pan as completed.

3. Place patties under preheated broiler for about 5 minutes, until tops are golden brown. Carefully turn over and broil for about 4 minutes, until flipside is golden brown. Remove from oven and set aside for 2 minutes to firm up.

4. Place lettuce on bottoms of buns and place patties on top. Slather patties with sesame mayo and top with tomato and onion. Replace tops of buns and serve immediately.

> **IF FOLLOWING A LOW-FIBER DIET AND AVOIDING DIFFICULT-TO-DIGEST FOODS...**
>
> Avoid whole wheat varieties of panko and choose buns made with all-purpose or white flour. Remove the sesame seeds from the buns, peel and seed the tomatoes (see page 169), use only a small amount of iceberg or Boston lettuce (and chew it well), and finely mince the red onion.

Making Fish Burgers

- To counteract dryness, add a bit of mayonnaise, oil or butter to the mix. Salmon needs less than tuna. Full-fat mayo is preferable, but the lower-fat kind will work. Another potential moistener is sour cream.
- Squeeze excess moisture from the fish to ensure that the mixture won't be too wet to handle. You should be able to gently pat the mixture into patties.
- Cook fish burgers under the broiler or on the grill, as cooking them in a skillet increases the chances that they will crumble. If using the barbecue, place the burgers on greased foil rather than directly on the grate (a recipe for disaster).
- Be gentle with the patties. Use a spatula to lift them from your work surface or plate to the pan, and turn them carefully with two short-handled spatulas as they cook.

IBD Tips

- Recipes using canned ingredients may be easier to prepare during times of illness.
- Boost calories by selecting canned salmon packed in oil.

Sesame Mayo

¼ cup	mayonnaise	60 mL
2 tsp	toasted sesame oil	10 mL
2 tsp	toasted sesame seeds (see tip, at right)	10 mL
½ tsp	finely grated lime zest	2 mL
½ tsp	freshly squeezed lime juice	2 mL
¼ tsp	soy sauce	1 mL
¼ tsp	Asian chili sauce (such as sambal oelek or Sriracha)	1 mL

1. In a measuring cup, stir together mayonnaise, sesame oil, sesame seeds, lime zest, lime juice, soy sauce and chili sauce.

MAKES ABOUT ⅓ CUP (75 ML) (1 TBSP/15 ML PER SERVING)

Tip

- Toast sesame seeds in a dry skillet over medium heat, shaking the pan often, for 2 to 3 minutes, until seeds start to clump and turn golden and fragrant. Immediately transfer to a bowl. Even easier, buy toasted sesame seeds, which are available in many supermarkets. For an attractive presentation, use toasted mixed white and black sesame seeds.

IF FOLLOWING A LOW-FIBER DIET AND AVOIDING DIFFICULT-TO-DIGEST FOODS...

Purée the sesame seeds and sambal oelek (Sriracha is already ground). Spice adds great flavor, and should only be avoided if necessary during illness or anal soreness from frequent loose stool.

Nutrients Per Serving	
Calories	64
Fat	6 g
Fiber	0 g
Protein	0 g
Carbohydrate	1 g

MAKES 2 SERVINGS

Tip

- Give the batter a stir before cooking each batch.

IBD Tips

- This recipe is appropriate for vegetarians who eat dairy, eggs and fish.
- This recipe is suitable for a low-fiber diet.
- Eat smoked fish only occasionally; it is considered a modifiable risk factor for cancer.
- Potatoes are a rich source of potassium; salmon is also a source.
- If you are trying to minimize calories, chose a fat-free sour cream. If you are maintaining your weight, look for sour cream with less than 2% milk fat. If you are trying to gain weight, go for full-fat sour cream.
- If you omit the sour cream, this recipe is a lactose-free choice.

Nutrients Per Serving	
Calories	407
Fat	19 g
Fiber	7 g
Protein	15 g
Carbohydrate	45 g

Potato Pancakes with Smoked Salmon

Potato pancakes, also known as latkes, are one of the world's great comfort foods.

- *Preheat oven to 250°F (120°C)*

1	can (19 oz/540 mL) whole white potatoes, drained, or 2 medium potatoes, cooked and peeled	1
½ cup	diced onion	125 mL
1	egg, beaten	1
1 tbsp	all-purpose flour	15 mL
½ tsp	salt	2 mL
	Freshly ground black pepper	
2 tbsp	vegetable oil (approx.)	30 mL
4	slices smoked salmon, thawed if frozen	4
	Sour cream	

1. Shred potatoes on coarse grater and finely chop any leftover bits.
2. In a bowl, combine potatoes, onion, egg, flour, salt and black pepper to taste. Mix well. Shape into 4 small, thin pancakes.
3. In a nonstick skillet, heat oil over medium heat. Fry pancakes, in batches, turning once, until golden, about 3 minutes per side. Add more oil as required. Keep cooked pancakes warm in preheated oven.
4. To serve, place 2 pancakes on each plate. Top each with a piece of salmon and a dollop of sour cream.

Parmesan-Crusted Snapper with Tomato Olive Sauce

Here's a quick and easy dish that takes advantage of the rich Mediterranean flavors of bottled antipasto sauce.

1 cup	coarse dry bread crumbs, such as panko	250 mL
½ cup	freshly grated Parmesan cheese	125 mL
½ tsp	salt	2 mL
	Freshly ground black pepper	
1 lb	snapper or other firm white fish fillets, patted dry, cut into 4 pieces	500 g
2 tbsp	mayonnaise	30 mL
1 tbsp	vegetable oil	15 mL
½ cup	bottled antipasto sauce (see tip, at left)	125 mL

1. In a bowl, combine bread crumbs, Parmesan, salt and black pepper to taste. Spread mixture on a plate.

2. Brush fish evenly with mayonnaise, then dip in crumb mixture.

3. In a skillet, heat oil over medium heat. Add fish and cook, turning once, until it flakes easily when tested with a knife and outside is crisp and golden, about 3 minutes per side. Serve immediately topped with antipasto sauce.

IF FOLLOWING A LOW-FIBER DIET AND AVOIDING DIFFICULT-TO-DIGEST FOODS...

Skip the antipasto sauce (especially if it contains olives). Instead, use a plain tomato sauce made from tomatoes with the skins and seeds removed.

MAKES 4 SERVINGS

Tips

- There are many kinds of antipasto sauce on the market. When making this recipe, check the label to ensure that it contains tomato and black olives.

- For a hint of spice, add a pinch of cayenne pepper to the bread crumb mixture.

IBD Tips

- This recipe is appropriate for vegetarians who eat fish, dairy and eggs.

- White fish is light and may be easier to eat if you are not feeling well.

- Hard aged cheeses are often tolerated by individuals with lactose intolerance. They contain very small amounts of lactose, especially when compared to milk.

- Cheese, salt, mayonnaise and antipasto provide sodium.

Nutrients Per Serving	
Calories	344
Fat	15 g
Fiber	1 g
Protein	20 g
Carbohydrate	30 g

Vegetarian choice

Higher-calorie choice

Lower-fiber choice

Higher-protein choice

Source of potassium

Source of sodium

Old-Fashioned Tuna Noodle Casserole

Tuna casserole is certainly easy to prepare and evokes a warm sense of nostalgia.

MAKES 4 SERVINGS

IBD Tips

- This recipe is suitable for vegetarians who eat seafood, dairy and eggs.

- Recipes using canned ingredients may be easier to prepare during times of illness. You can also shred cheese in advance and store it in the freezer for when you need it.

- To maximize calories, use regular soup (not lower-fat), whole milk, full-fat cheese, tuna packed in oil and regular (not baked) potato chips.

- Canned soup, tuna, cheese and potato chips provide sodium. Potato chips also provide potassium.

- Potato chips and cheese help thicken loose stool.

- Preheat oven to 350°F (180°C)
- 8-inch (20 cm) square baking dish

6 oz	broad egg noodles	175 g
1	can (10 oz/284 mL) condensed reduced-sodium cream of mushroom soup	1
1/2 cup	whole milk	125 mL
1 cup	shredded Cheddar cheese (4 oz/125 g)	250 mL
1	can (6 oz/170 g) tuna in water, drained and broken into chunks	1
1 cup	green peas, thawed if frozen	250 mL
2 tbsp	chopped pimiento	30 mL
	Salt	
1 cup	crushed potato chips	250 mL

1. In a large pot of boiling salted water over medium heat, cook noodles for 10 to 12 minutes, until tender. Drain and set aside.

2. Meanwhile, in a saucepan over medium-low heat, cook soup, milk and Cheddar for about 5 minutes, until mixture is hot and cheese has melted. Add tuna, peas, pimiento and cooked noodles. Stir to combine and season to taste with salt.

3. Scrape mixture into baking dish and sprinkle chips overtop. Bake in preheated oven for 30 minutes, until sauce is bubbly and topping is golden. Remove from heat and set aside for 10 minutes before serving.

IF FOLLOWING A LOW-FIBER DIET AND AVOIDING DIFFICULT-TO-DIGEST FOODS...

Choose regular egg noodles rather than whole-grain or whole wheat pasta, purée the cream of mushroom soup (or choose a soup without chunks of mushroom), use canned peas (the skin of fresh or frozen green peas does not cook soft enough), and finely chop or purée the pimiento. Mushrooms are surprisingly hard to digest, and although those in canned soup are chopped into small pieces, they can potentially contribute to a food obstruction. Pimiento (or pimento) is a pepper available in sweet and hot varieties. Spice adds great flavor, and should only be avoided if necessary during illness or anal soreness from frequent loose stool.

Nutrients Per Serving	
Calories	627
Fat	26 g
Fiber	8 g
Protein	33 g
Carbohydrate	68 g

Tuna and Olive Rotini

A bit of tuna can go a long way in pasta. This rotini is both visually appealing and tasty.

12 oz	rotini	375 g
2	cans (each 3 oz/85 g) tuna in olive oil, with oil	2
1 cup	sliced pitted green olives (20 large)	250 mL
1	small red bell pepper, slivered	1
1	large clove garlic, minced	1
2 tbsp	extra virgin olive oil	30 mL
½ tsp	salt (approx.)	2 mL
¼ tsp	freshly ground black pepper	1 mL
½ cup	fresh parsley leaves, coarsely chopped	125 mL

1. In a large pot of boiling salted water, cook rotini over medium heat for about 12 minutes, until tender to the bite (al dente). Scoop out about ½ cup (125 mL) cooking water and set aside. Drain pasta.

2. Meanwhile, in a large warmed serving bowl, stir together tuna with oil, olives, red pepper, garlic, extra virgin olive oil, salt and pepper. Add rotini. If the pasta seems dry or clumpy, add enough reserved cooking water to moisten and loosen it. Add salt to taste, if necessary.

3. Scatter parsley overtop and serve immediately.

Variations

Substitute an equal quantity of salmon or sardines for the tuna.

If the seafood you are using is not packed in olive oil, add an extra 2 tbsp (30 mL) extra virgin olive oil to this dish.

IF FOLLOWING A LOW-FIBER DIET AND AVOIDING DIFFICULT-TO-DIGEST FOODS...

Choose regular rotini rather than whole-grain or whole wheat pasta, purée the olives, mince and sauté the red bell pepper, finely grind the black pepper, and finely chop the parsley leaves (do not include stems).

Vegetarian choice

Higher-calorie choice

Higher-protein choice

Lactose-free choice

Source of sodium

MAKES 4 SERVINGS

IBD Tips

- This recipe is suitable for vegetarians who eat seafood.

- Recipes using canned ingredients may be easier to prepare during times of illness.

- Calories are boosted in this recipe by tuna packed in oil, the high amount of monounsaturated fat found naturally in olives, and additional olive oil.

- Sodium is provided by canned tuna and olives.

Nutrients Per Serving	
Calories	300
Fat	13 g
Fiber	2 g
Protein	17 g
Carbohydrate	28 g

**MAKES 32 PIECES
(8 PER SERVING)**

Tips

- To prepare the cucumber for this recipe, peel it, cut it lengthwise into ½-inch (1 cm) strips, then cut each strip lengthwise into ¼-inch (0.5 cm) strips.

- Nori sheets are almost square. Luckily, you can use the perforations on them as a placement guide. They should be perpendicular to the slats of the sushi mat.

- When spreading the rice over the nori, be aware that it will be very sticky, so moisten your fingers as needed. Don't compact the rice onto the nori too enthusiastically. You should still be able to see the individual grains of rice.

- For neater cuts, let the rolls sit briefly before slicing. It also helps to wipe the knife on a wet towel before each cut.

Nutrients Per Serving	
Calories	53
Fat	2 g
Fiber	1 g
Protein	4 g
Carbohydrate	4 g

Tuna and Cucumber Sushi Rolls

4	sheets nori	4
4 cups	Sushi Rice (see recipe, page 240)	1 L
4 tsp	toasted sesame seeds	20 mL
1	can (6 oz/170 g) tuna in water, drained and broken into flakes	1
4	strips cucumber (each 8 by ½ by ¼ inch/ 20 by 1 by 0.5 cm)	4
⅓ cup	carrot, cut into matchsticks	75 mL
¼ cup	Wasabi Mayonnaise (see recipe, opposite)	60 mL
1 tbsp	tobiko roe (optional)	15 mL

1. Place sushi mat on top of a large cutting board with bamboo strips running crosswise. Place a bowl of cold water next to the board.

2. Lay 1 sheet of nori, shiny side down, with the longer side facing you and the perforations perpendicular to the bamboo strips on the mat (see tip, at left). Place about 1 cup (250 mL) rice on top. Using the tip of a fork, break up large clumps and push rice loosely across nori. With moistened fingers, spread rice evenly over nori, gently patting it down (see tip, at left). Spread right to the edges but leave a ½- to 1-inch (1 to 2.5 cm) border at the top.

3. Sprinkle 1 tsp (5 mL) sesame seeds evenly over rice. Lay one-quarter of the tuna, 1 strip cucumber and one-quarter of the carrot matchsticks horizontally and evenly across the rice, almost at the center (about 3 inches/7.5 cm from the bottom).

4. Lift mat and bottom edge of nori and fold it over filling. Pulling back on the mat, run your fingers from the center to the ends to tuck in nori and create an even cylinder. Roll nori up to border at top (you can either let go of the mat and finish rolling by hand or push the mat over the cylinder). When you get to the border, use the mat to pull back on the roll to tighten it a bit, then roll to the end. From the top, roll the sushi mat completely around the cylinder and press and squeeze along its length to create a firm, even roll. Pat the ends of the cylinder to push in any protruding rice or fillings. Set the roll aside, seam side down. Repeat with remaining ingredients. Let rolls rest for 5 minutes before slicing.

5. Place a roll on cutting board. If ends are ragged, slice them off neatly, using a small, sharp knife. Cut roll in half, then cut each half into 4 pieces. Repeat with remaining rolls.

6. Place sushi slices, rice side up, on a serving platter. Garnish each with a dab of Wasabi Mayonnaise and a sprinkling of tobiko, if using, dividing equally. Serve immediately.

Variation

Substitute an equal quantity of salmon or mackerel for the tuna.

IF YOU ARE WELL...

If there is no medical reason for you to avoid fiber or difficult-to-digest foods, use the nori, whole sesame seeds, raw carrot and wasabi mayonnaise. During times of better health, enjoy foods such as sushi and the great flavor provided by spices (they should only be avoided if necessary during illness or anal soreness from frequent loose stool).

IF FOLLOWING A LOW-FIBER DIET AND AVOIDING DIFFICULT-TO-DIGEST FOODS...

Use ground sesame seeds or tahini, peeled seeded cucumber, soft cooked carrot sticks, white (not brown) sushi rice and plain mayonnaise. Include the roe, if desired.

Wasabi Mayonnaise

**MAKES ABOUT
²⁄₃ CUP (150 ML)
(1 TBSP/15 ML PER
SERVING)**

Wasabi mayonnaise is trendy, tasty and versatile. It is a great finishing touch for sushi and so much more. You can spread it on wraps, party sandwiches or lobster rolls; use it to give tuna salad a contemporary twist; add it to deviled egg filling; smear it on fish burgers or croquettes; or simply dollop it alongside fresh sliced tomatoes and canned seafood, such as crab, tuna and salmon.

½ cup	mayonnaise	125 mL
1 tsp	wasabi powder	5 mL
1	green onion, finely chopped	1
1 tbsp	finely chopped fresh parsley	15 mL

1. In a small measuring cup, stir together mayonnaise and wasabi powder. Stir in green onion and parsley.

2. Serve immediately or transfer to a small airtight storage tub and refrigerate for up to 3 days.

IBD Tips

- This recipe is suitable for vegetarians who eat seafood and eggs.
- White rice, including sticky varieties like white sushi rice, is helpful for thickening stool.
- Boost calories by selecting tuna packed in oil and using full-fat mayonnaise.
- Canned tuna provides sodium, and some nori sheets may contain additional sodium.

Nutrients Per Serving	
Calories	42
Fat	4 g
Fiber	0 g
Protein	0 g
Carbohydrate	1 g

Sushi Rice

The Japanese say rice is the heart of sushi. Leftover sushi rice is delicious. Enjoy it as a side dish, use it to experiment with other types of sushi rolls or make informal hand rolls or sushi salad.

Tips

• Sushi rice is sold in supermarkets and Asian grocery stores. It is sticky but not mushy and may be short- or medium-grain. White sushi rice is most commonly used, but brown sushi rice is also available. Sushi rice may be labeled "Japanese rice" or "sticky rice." A popular type of sushi rice developed in California is Calrose.

• You need plenty of cold water to efficiently rinse the starchy sushi rice. It helps to tilt the handle of the pan against the rim of the sink, then let water run into the pan in a slow stream on one side and spill out the other.

• Fanning dissipates steam and helps the individual rice grains maintain their shape. You can grab a magazine to fan the rice, use a bamboo fan or even set up an electric fan to blow on the rice. After mixing and fanning, the rice should be moist and shiny, not mushy or broken.

• *Rimmed baking sheet*

2 cups	white sushi rice (see tip, at left)	500 mL
2½ cups	cold water, plus more for rinsing rice	625 mL
1 tbsp	salt, divided	15 mL
⅓ cup	unseasoned rice vinegar	75 mL
3 tbsp	granulated sugar	45 mL

1. Place rice in a saucepan (preferably nonstick). Rinse and swish with cold running water until the water runs clear (see tip, at left). Drain rice in a sieve and return to saucepan. Add 2½ cups (625 mL) cold water. Set aside for 1 hour.

2. Add 1 tsp (5 mL) salt to saucepan and bring to a boil over high heat. Stir well, reduce heat to low and cover. Simmer for about 15 minutes, until rice is tender and water has been absorbed. Remove from heat. Lift off lid and place a clean tea towel over top of saucepan. Replace lid and set aside for 10 minutes.

3. Meanwhile, in a very small saucepan, combine vinegar, sugar and remaining 2 tsp (10 mL) salt. Cook, stirring, over medium heat for 1 to 2 minutes, until sugar dissolves and mixture is warm (be careful not to boil). Remove from heat and set aside.

4. Transfer rice to baking sheet and, using the tip of a fork, quickly spread it across the sheet (it doesn't have to be tidy). Drizzle vinegar mixture evenly over top. With one hand, use a short-handled spatula to gently mix, using scooping and flipping motions. With the other hand, fan the rice (see tip, at left). (Better still, enlist a helper to fan.) Mix the rice gently; do not mash. Mix and fan for 5 minutes, until vinegar is absorbed and rice has cooled.

Uses for Sushi Rice

For a quick hand roll, spread a handful of rice at one end of a sheet of nori (it doesn't have to be tidy), lay any filling you like diagonally across the rice, then roll up the nori in a cone shape.

To make simple sushi salad, put sushi rice in a bowl, top with cut vegetables such as cucumber, carrot or avocado and drizzle with a bit of soy sauce.

Nutrients Per Serving	
Calories	263
Fat	0 g
Fiber	2 g
Protein	4 g
Carbohydrate	59 g

Tuna and Rice Casserole

Here's a delicious change from the usual tuna noodle casserole — and it takes less than 10 minutes to prepare! It's easy enough for older children and teens to make on their own; younger children can help by shredding the cheese.

* *Preheat oven to 350°F (180°C)*
* *8-inch (20 cm) square baking dish, greased*

1	can (10 oz/284 mL) condensed cream of mushroom soup	1
1¼ cups	instant rice	300 mL
1 cup	milk	250 mL
½ cup	water	125 mL
1	can (6 oz/170g) water-packed tuna, drained	1
1 cup	frozen peas	250 mL
¼ cup	finely chopped onion	60 mL
1 tsp	freshly squeezed lemon juice	5 mL
	Freshly ground black pepper to taste	
½ cup	shredded Cheddar cheese	125 mL
	Paprika to taste	

1. In a large bowl, stir together soup, rice, milk, water, tuna, peas, onion, lemon juice and pepper. Pour into a greased 8-inch (2 L) square baking dish. Sprinkle with cheese and paprika. Bake in preheated oven for 30 to 35 minutes or until bubbling and rice is tender.

IF FOLLOWING A LOW-FIBER DIET AND AVOIDING DIFFICULT-TO-DIGEST FOODS...

Use canned peas instead of frozen (the skin of frozen peas does not cook soft enough), use white rice, and purée the cream of mushroom soup, or use a soup without chunks of mushroom. Mushrooms are surprisingly hard to digest, and although those in canned soup are chopped into small pieces, they are a potential food obstruction.

Vegetarian choice

Lower-fiber choice

Higher-protein choice

Source of potassium

Source of sodium

MAKES 4 SERVINGS

IBD Tips

* This recipe is suitable for vegetarians who eat fish and dairy.
* Canned soup, canned tuna, and cheese all provide sodium.
* To boost calories in this recipe, choose regular canned soup instead of low-fat, full-fat milk and Cheddar cheese, and tuna packed in oil rather than water. This increases the fat content, but for short-term weight gain goals is considered an acceptable way to boost calories.
* White rice is known to help thicken stool.

Nutrients Per Serving	
Calories	330
Fat	12 g
Fiber	2 g
Protein	19 g
Carbohydrate	35 g

Vegetarian choice

Higher-calorie choice

Lower-fiber choice

Higher-protein choice

Lactose-free choice

Source of sodium

MAKES 4 SERVINGS

Tips

- For a spicier version, increase the amount of curry paste. But be careful — a little goes a long way.
- Garnish with cilantro sprigs and/or red bell pepper strips, if desired.

IBD Tips

- This recipe is appropriate for vegetarians who eat seafood.
- Coconut milk is fine to use; it is dried shredded coconut that is an obstruction risk. Coconut milk is surprisingly high in saturated fat, and thus calories, but reduced-fat versions are available.
- To minimize food obstruction after surgery, avoid this recipe for 6 weeks.
- Sodium is provided by the curry paste and fish sauce.

Nutrients Per Serving	
Calories	379
Fat	19 g
Fiber	2 g
Protein	27 g
Carbohydrate	26 g

Coconut Shrimp Curry

Many Thai cooks make their own curry paste, but bottled versions are now available in supermarkets with a well-stocked Asian foods section. This quick and easy recipe is delicious over hot white rice.

1 tbsp	vegetable oil	15 mL
1 lb	peeled and deveined shrimp, thawed if frozen	500 g
	Freshly ground black pepper	
1 tbsp	red curry paste	15 mL
1 cup	coconut milk	250 mL
2 tbsp	fish sauce	30 mL
2 tbsp	lime juice	30 mL
1 tbsp	granulated sugar	15 mL
	Hot white rice	

1. In a skillet, heat oil over medium-high heat. Add shrimp and cook, stirring, until they firm up and turn pink, 3 to 5 minutes. Season with black pepper to taste. Using a slotted spoon, transfer to a deep platter and keep warm. Return pan to element.

2. Add red curry paste and cook, stirring, until it releases its aroma, 1 to 2 minutes. Stir in coconut milk, fish sauce, lime juice and sugar. Bring to a boil. Simmer for 1 to 2 minutes to combine flavors. Pour over shrimp.

3. Serve immediately over hot white rice.

> **IF FOLLOWING A LOW-FIBER DIET AND AVOIDING DIFFICULT-TO-DIGEST FOODS...**
>
> Finely grind the black pepper (larger pieces can increase the risk of a food-related obstruction). If you are experiencing disease activity or are sore in the anal area from passing frequent liquidy stool, reduce the amount of curry paste rather than exclude it from this tasty recipe.

Shrimp in Tomato Sauce with Feta

This Greek specialty has a bold combination of flavors. Serve over hot white rice.

- *Preheat broiler*
- *6-cup (1.5 L) shallow baking or gratin dish*

2 tbsp	vegetable oil	30 mL
1 lb	peeled and deveined shrimp, thawed if frozen	500 g
2 tbsp	minced garlic	30 mL
	Freshly ground black pepper	
¼ cup	freshly squeezed lemon juice	60 mL
1 cup	tomato sauce	250 mL
4 oz	crumbled feta cheese (about 1 cup/250 mL)	125 g

1. In a skillet, heat oil over medium-high heat. Add shrimp and cook, stirring, until they firm up and turn pink, 3 to 5 minutes. Using a slotted spoon, transfer to baking dish. Reduce heat to medium-low and return pan to element.

2. Add garlic and black pepper to taste. Cook, stirring, for 1 minute. Add lemon juice and stir. Add tomato sauce and bring to a simmer.

3. Pour mixture over shrimp. Sprinkle with cheese. Place under preheated broiler until cheese begins to melt and turn brown, about 3 minutes.

IF FOLLOWING A LOW-FIBER DIET AND AVOIDING DIFFICULT-TO-DIGEST FOODS...

Finely grind the black pepper (larger pieces can increase the risk of a food-related obstruction) and choose a plain tomato sauce that does not contain difficult-to-digest vegetables.

Vegetarian choice

Higher-protein choice

Source of potassium

Source of sodium

MAKES 4 SERVINGS

IBD Tips

- This recipe is appropriate for vegetarians who eat seafood and dairy.

- To minimize food obstruction after surgery, avoid this recipe for 6 weeks.

- Choose canola or olive oil for their favorable fatty acid profiles.

- To boost sodium, choose commercial tomato sauce or add salt liberally to homemade tomato sauce.

- Tomato sauce is a rich source of potassium and sodium.

- If you want to decrease calories from fat, choose light feta cheese (about 17% M.F.). Read the label carefully, as the word "light" or "lite" can refer to color, flavor or texture, not necessarily calories or fat.

Nutrients Per Serving

Calories	317
Fat	16 g
Fiber	3 g
Protein	31 g
Carbohydrate	13 g

Vegetarian choice

Higher-calorie choice

Lower-fat choice

Lower-fiber choice

Higher-protein choice

Source of potassium

Source of sodium

MAKES 6 SERVINGS

IBD Tips

- This recipe is suitable for vegetarians who eat seafood, dairy and eggs.

- Crabmeat is low in fat, as is surimi (imitation crab). Surimi is made from mild-flavored white fish such as pollock. Surimi was developed in Japan; the name means "minced fish."

- To boost calories in this recipe, use full-fat ricotta cheese, mozzarella and milk. This increases the fat content, but for short-term weight gain goals this is considered an acceptable way to boost calories.

- Commercial tomato pasta sauce provides potassium and sodium. The cheese also provides sodium.

Nutrients Per Serving	
Calories	392
Fat	10 g
Fiber	2 g
Protein	25 g
Carbohydrate	53 g

Jumbo Shells Stuffed with Crabmeat, Cheese and Dill

- *Preheat oven to 350°F (180°C)*
- *13- by 9-inch (33 by 23 cm) baking dish*

18	jumbo pasta shells	18
6 oz	crabmeat or surimi (imitation crab)	175 g
1¾ cups	5% ricotta cheese	425 mL
⅔ cup	shredded low-fat mozzarella cheese	150 mL
2	green onions, sliced	2
3 tbsp	low-fat milk	45 mL
1	large egg	1
¼ cup	chopped fresh dill (or 1 tsp/5 mL dried)	60 mL
¼ tsp	freshly ground black pepper	1 mL
1 cup	tomato pasta sauce	250 mL
3 tbsp	low-fat milk	45 mL

1. In a large pot of boiling water, cook shells for 14 minutes or until tender; drain. Rinse under cold running water; drain. Set aside.

2. In a bowl combine crabmeat, ricotta cheese, mozzarella cheese, green onions, milk, egg, dill and pepper. Stuff approximately 2½ tbsp (35 mL) mixture into each pasta shell.

3. In a bowl combine tomato sauce and milk; spread half over bottom of baking dish. Add stuffed shells; pour remaining sauce over top. Bake, covered with foil, for 20 minutes or until heated through.

IF FOLLOWING A LOW-FIBER DIET AND AVOIDING DIFFICULT-TO-DIGEST FOODS...

Use semolina pasta shells, finely slice the green onions and sauté until soft, finely chop the dill (do not include stems), and finely grind the black pepper.

Vegetarian and Vegan Entrées

Vegetarian and vegan cuisines have gained much publicity in recent years due to the established health benefits. There are different types of vegetarianism, but all vegetarians eat plant products. An ovo-vegetarian will also eat eggs, and an ovo-lacto-vegetarian will eat eggs and dairy, while a pesco-vegetarian will eat fish. A strict vegetarian, or vegan, will eat no animal products of any type. A semi-vegetarian is more liberal and will eat fish, poultry and, less frequently, a little red meat, but still relies mostly on plant foods. This chapter provides recipes that contain eggs, dairy or only plant-based ingredients to meet the needs of different vegetarians. Pesco-vegetarians will also want to refer to the Fish and Seafood chapter, as many of the recipes there are suitable for them.

The health-promoting benefits of a plant-based diet are thought to derive from the fact that this diet contains complex carbohydrates, vitamins and minerals, is low in saturated fat and is usually high in fiber. This last attribute, high fiber, is a potential challenge for individuals living with symptomatic IBD. For that reason, certain recipes are accompanied by modifications that will help keep your meals safe, tasty and nutritious.

Look for Plant-Based Meat and Dairy Substitutes

To meet the needs of vegetarians and vegans looking for meat substitutes, the food industry produces a number of products made of high-quality plant-based protein. Most are made from wheat, soy, soy milk or cereal products free of animal fats. Textured vegetable protein (soy protein) is formulated to look and taste like meat, fish or poultry.

For vegans and some vegetarians, most supermarkets carry plant-based beverages as dairy alternatives. Replacements for egg can include banana, corn or potato starch, arrowroot flour, soy milk powder with water, silken tofu or a specific egg replacer. Soy margarine can be used in place of butter or regular margarine, as it does not contain whey, a dairy product. Soy yogurt, cheese and frozen desserts are also widely available.

The challenge from a nutritional perspective is to make sure the same quality and quantity of nutrients are available from the alternative ingredient as from its animal counterpart. For vegans and some vegetarians, a multivitamin with minerals will help ensure that they are getting adequate daily nutrients.

Make Sure You're Getting Enough Vitamin B_{12}

It is of paramount importance that vegans find an adequate source of vitamin B_{12}, as the only reliable sources are animal products. Some fermented soy products contain vitamin B_{12}, but not in its active form. Alternative sources of vitamin B_{12} include fortified soy milk and cereals, supplements and nutritional yeasts. If you have experienced chronic inflammation in your terminal ileum or have had surgical resections in your stomach or terminal ileum, speak with your doctor about the possible need for vitamin B_{12} injections.

Some commercial enzyme products, such as Beano or Phazyme, may not be appropriate for vegans; be sure to check with the manufacturer.

EAT GAS-PRODUCING FOODS CAUTIOUSLY

Including legumes in the diet can make you gassy. Be sure to soak dry beans and discard the water before cooking, and rinse canned beans well. Regularly eating legumes will help your body get used to them. Fermented soy products such as tempeh and miso are not as gas-forming as their unfermented counterparts. Other gas-producing foods can include vegetables from the cabbage family, grapes and melons. Ginger, cumin and fennel are considered helpful for digestion, so experiment with adding them to recipes.

THE FACTS ABOUT COMPLEMENTARY PROTEINS

A complete protein is one that contains all the essential amino acids your body requires (amino acids are the building blocks that make up a protein; "essential" means that our bodies cannot synthesize them and we rely on an external source to get them). While proteins from meat, fish, poultry, cheese, eggs and milk are complete, proteins from plant-based foods tend to be lacking in one or more essential amino acids (one exception is soy protein).

The solution is to choose plant proteins that provide complementary amino acids. Complementary proteins could include black beans and rice, peanut butter on wheat bread, or tofu and stir-fried vegetables. Research has shown that complementary plant proteins do not need to be eaten at the same meal — or even over the course of the same day — to prevent protein deficiency. If you are getting enough energy from a plant-based diet (that is, enough to maintain your weight) and you vary the protein source (legumes, grains, vegetables, seeds, nuts) you will consume high-quality complete protein. (Of course, if you consume dairy, eggs or fish, this is much easier to achieve.)

Remember that there may be times when you have higher protein requirements, for example, when you are taking high-dose steroids, have significant weight loss and malnutrition, or are experiencing ongoing blood loss in stool. These can be very frustrating times, as previously tolerated foods may now be difficult to digest. At these times, you might want to consider nutritional supplements. Speak with your doctor or registered dietitian for advice.

Reduce Fiber by Juicing Your Fruits and Vegetables

Plant-based diets are more challenging when you are asked to follow a fiber-restricted diet. Many individuals compromise by juicing their fruits and vegetables, thus preserving the vitamins, minerals, phytonutrients and calories while eliminating much of the fiber. Be sure to add water if using fruits in your juice, as fruits with the fiber removed are an even more concentrated source of natural sugar and can contribute to osmotic diarrhea.

If you are experiencing frequent liquidy stools, you will need to replace fluid and electrolytes. If your diet contains few commercially prepared foods and beverages, be sure to add salt to replace the sodium you are losing through your gastrointestinal tract. It is also important to replace potassium, which is abundant in fruits and vegetables.

> Other nutrients of concern for the vegetarian include vitamins A, B_2 (riboflavin) and D_3, calcium, iron, zinc and selenium. For those living with IBD *and* following vegetarian diets, alternative food sources may not always be tolerated; during times of symptomatic disease, it may be worthwhile to consider supplements of these nutrients.

Vegetarian choice

Higher-calorie choice

Higher-protein choice

Source of potassium

Source of sodium

MAKES 2 SERVINGS

Tip

- If the handle of your skillet is not ovenproof, wrap it in aluminum foil.

IBD Tips

- This recipe is appropriate for vegetarians who eat eggs and dairy.

- Spinach is not typically found in a low-fiber diet, so avoid this recipe unless you are well.

- Aged hard cheeses have only small amounts of lactose. Small amounts of Parmesan are often well tolerated by individuals who have trouble digesting lactose.

- Cooked spinach is rich in potassium.

- The cheese, pesto and added salt provide sodium.

Nutrients Per Serving	
Calories	423
Fat	26 g
Fiber	6 g
Protein	28 g
Carbohydrate	20 g

Spinach Frittata

A frittata is an Italian omelet in which the ingredients are cooked with the eggs rather than being folded into them, French style. There are several methods for making this versatile dish. I prefer this one — which partially cooks the eggs on top of the stove, then finishes them in the oven — as it is essentially foolproof.

- *Preheat oven to 425°F (220°C)*
- *Ovenproof skillet with heatproof handle and lid (see tip, at left)*

6	eggs, beaten	6
1 tbsp	vegetable oil	15 mL
½ cup	diced onion	125 mL
1 tsp	dried Italian seasoning	5 mL
½ tsp	salt	2 mL
	Freshly ground black pepper	
1	package (10 oz/300 g) frozen chopped spinach, thawed and squeezed dry, or 1 package (10 oz/300 g) spinach, washed, stems removed and chopped	1
¼ cup	freshly grated Parmesan cheese	60 mL
2 tbsp	prepared sun-dried tomato pesto	30 mL

1. In a bowl, lightly beat eggs. Set aside.

2. In an ovenproof skillet, heat oil over medium heat. Add onion and cook, stirring, until softened, about 3 minutes. Stir in Italian seasoning, salt and black pepper to taste. Add spinach and stir well.

3. Reduce heat to low. Cover and cook until spinach is wilted, about 5 minutes. Slowly pour eggs over spinach. Increase heat to medium. Cover and cook until mixture begins to form a crust on the bottom, 2 to 3 minutes.

4. Sprinkle with Parmesan cheese and transfer pan to preheated oven. Bake, uncovered, until eggs are set but frittata is still soft in the center, about 3 minutes. Cut into wedges and serve topped with a dollop of pesto.

IF YOU ARE WELL...

If there is no medical reason for you to avoid fiber or difficult-to-digest foods, include spinach in your diet. Spinach is packed with nutrients, especially folate and carotenoids, which act as antioxidants in the body. Spinach is also a source of calcium and iron; however, these are not well absorbed. I often recommend starting with chopped cooked spinach, as this recipe calls for, and with small amounts.

Eggplant Pilaf

4 cups	unpeeled diced eggplant (about 1 medium)	1 L
1 tbsp	salt	15 mL
2 tbsp	olive oil	30 mL
1 tsp	salt	5 mL
1/2 tsp	freshly ground black pepper	2 mL
1/2 tsp	turmeric	2 mL
2	cloves	2
Pinch	ground cumin	Pinch
1	onion, finely diced	1
1 cup	finely chopped leek (1 medium)	250 mL
4	cloves garlic, minced	4
2 cups	rice (preferably basmati)	500 mL
3 cups	boiling water	750 mL
1/4 cup	olive oil	60 mL

1. Place the cubed eggplant and salt in bowl; add cold water to cover. Mix well and set aside.

2. In a heavy-bottomed pot with a tight-fitting lid, heat 2 tbsp (30 mL) oil over high heat for 30 seconds. Add salt, black pepper, turmeric, cloves and cumin; stir for 30 seconds. Add onions and stir-fry for 1 minute. Add chopped leek and continue stir-frying for 1 minute. Add garlic and stir-fry for 30 seconds.

3. Add rice and stir-fry until grains are shiny, about 1 to 2 minutes. (Don't worry if the spices start to scorch on the bottom of the pan; the next addition will cure that.)

4. Add boiling water, and pull pot off heat as it sizzles and splutters for 30 seconds. Reduce heat to low; return pot to heat, cover tightly and let it simmer for 20 minutes. Then remove from heat but do not uncover. Let rice mixture rest for 10 minutes to temper.

5. Meanwhile, in a large frying pan, heat 1/4 cup (60 mL) oil over high heat for 1 minute. Drain eggplant cubes and add to oil (carefully: there will be spluttering). Fry for 6 to 7 minutes, stirring and tossing actively, until all the cubes have softened and have started to brown. Remove from heat and set aside.

6. Fluff rice and add fried eggplant, folding from the bottom up to distribute the eggplant, as well as the onions and leeks that will have risen to the top of the rice. Transfer to a presentation dish and serve immediately.

Vegan choice

Lower-calorie choice

Lactose-free choice

MAKES 8 SERVINGS

IBD Tips

- Eggplant adds a hearty, satisfying quality to a meal. It is not typically found in low-fiber diets, but if the skin and seeds are removed and it is cooked very soft, eaten in small amounts and chewed well, it can be included. The bitterness is concentrated just below the peel, so larger varieties should be peeled. Eggplant also provides potassium.

- Soft cooked white rice is known to help thicken loose stool.

IF FOLLOWING A LOW-FIBER DIET AND AVOIDING DIFFICULT-TO-DIGEST FOODS...

Peel and seed the eggplant and stir-fry until very soft, omit the leek, and remove cloves before eating.

Nutrients Per Serving	
Calories	151
Fat	11 g
Fiber	3 g
Protein	2 g
Carbohydrate	13 g

MAKES 10 SERVINGS

IBD Tips

- This recipe is suitable for vegetarian diets. If following a vegan diet, use soy margarine in place of regular margarine and replace the granulated sugar with a vegan substitute, such as unbleached cane sugar.

- Chickpeas and squash provide the potassium in this recipe.

IF FOLLOWING A LOW-FIBER DIET...

Pinch the skin from the chickpeas, peel and seed the summer squash or zucchini, finely mince the onion, omit the raisins, finely grind the black pepper, select white couscous, and finely chop the parsley leaves (do not include stems).

Nutrients Per Serving

Calories	229
Fat	3 g
Fiber	6 g
Protein	7 g
Carbohydrate	44 g

Slow Cooker Squash Couscous

Preparing one-pot meals using a slow cooker may be a helpful cooking solution during times of illness. This delicious meal simmers away while you go on with your day.

- *Minimum 5-quart slow cooker*

1	butternut squash (about 1$\frac{1}{2}$ lbs/750 g)	1
3 cups	cooked or rinsed drained canned chickpeas	750 mL
2 cups	chopped yellow summer squash or zucchini	500 mL
$\frac{1}{2}$ cup	thinly sliced onion	125 mL
$\frac{1}{2}$ cup	raisins	125 mL
2 tbsp	granulated sugar	30 mL
2 tsp	ground ginger	10 mL
$\frac{1}{2}$ tsp	ground turmeric	2 mL
$\frac{1}{2}$ tsp	freshly ground black pepper	2 mL
4 cups	vegetable stock	1 L
2 tbsp	non-hydrogenated margarine	30 mL
1 cup	couscous	250 mL
$\frac{1}{4}$ cup	coarsely chopped fresh parsley	60 mL

1. Peel butternut squash and cut the flesh into 1-inch (2.5 cm) cubes; you should have 4 to 5 cups (1 to 1.25 L) cubed squash.

2. In slow cooker stoneware, combine butternut squash, chickpeas, summer squash, onion, raisins, sugar, ginger, turmeric, pepper, stock and margarine. Cover and cook on Low for 4 to 5 hours or until vegetables are tender.

3. Uncover, increase heat to High and cook for 15 minutes or until liquid is reduced slightly. Using a slotted spoon, remove vegetable mixture to a large bowl. Cover and keep warm.

4. Place couscous in a large bowl and pour in 1 cup (250 mL) of the hot broth from the slow cooker. Cover with plastic wrap and let stand for 5 to 10 minutes or until couscous is plumped. Fluff with a fork.

5. Spoon vegetable mixture over couscous and ladle the remaining broth over top. Sprinkle with parsley.

Baked Orzo and Beans

Orzo — a jumbo rice look-alike — may be the most versatile of all pastas. This recipe comes from a long line of similarly baked Greek dishes, but borrows from Italian cuisine in its cheese topping.

- *Preheat oven to 350°F (180°C)*
- *10-cup (2.5 L) casserole with lid*

2½ cups	orzo	625 mL
1 tbsp	olive oil	15 mL
½ cup	sliced red onion	125 mL
2	tomatoes, roughly chopped	2
2 cups	Tomato Sauce (see recipe, page 267)	500 mL
2 cups	cooked red kidney beans	500 mL
1 cup	tomato juice	250 mL
1 cup	shaved Parmesan cheese	250 mL
1 tbsp	extra-virgin olive oil	15 mL
	Few sprigs fresh parsley, chopped	
	Grated Romano cheese (optional)	

1. In a large pot of boiling salted water, cook orzo until al dente, about 10 minutes.

2. Meanwhile, in a skillet, heat oil over high heat for 30 seconds; add onions and cook, stirring, for 1 or 2 minutes, until slightly charred. Remove from heat and set aside.

3. When orzo is cooked, drain well and transfer to casserole. Add sautéed onions to orzo and stir to combine. Add tomatoes and tomato sauce; mix thoroughly. Add cooked beans; fold until evenly distributed.

4. Cover orzo mixture and bake in preheated oven, covered, for 30 minutes. Remove from oven and mix in tomato juice. Top with Parmesan shavings and return to the oven, uncovered, for another 10 to 12 minutes, until the cheese is melted. Serve on pasta plates, making sure each portion is topped with some of the melted cheese. Drizzle a few drops of extra-virgin olive oil on each portion and garnish with chopped parsley. Serve immediately, with Romano, if using, as an accompaniment.

IF FOLLOWING A LOW-FIBER DIET AND AVOIDING DIFFICULT-TO-DIGEST FOODS...

Finely chop the red onion, peel and seed the tomatoes (see page 145), pinch the skin from the kidney beans, and finely chop the parsley (do not include stems).

Vegetarian choice

Higher-calorie choice

Lower-fat choice

Higher-protein choice

Source of soluble fiber

Source of potassium

MAKES 4 TO 6 SERVINGS

IBD Tips

- This recipe is appropriate for vegetarians who eat dairy.

- Tomatoes, tomato sauce, tomato juice and beans provide potassium.

- Boost sodium by choosing canned kidney beans and commercial tomato sauce and tomato juice. The cheese also provides sodium.

- While kidney beans provide a good dose of soluble fiber, they are still a higher-fiber food and may cause gas; if you are not used to eating them, start with a small amount.

Nutrients Per Serving	
Calories	398
Fat	11 g
Fiber	7 g
Protein	21 g
Carbohydrate	56 g

Vegan choice

Lower-calorie choice

Lower-fat choice

Lactose-free choice

Source of soluble fiber

Source of potassium

Source of sodium

MAKES 8 SERVINGS

Tips

• Nothing can really substitute for the flavor of saffron, but the pretty yellow-orange color it creates can be mimicked with 1/2 tsp (2 mL) ground turmeric.

IBD Tips

• Potatoes, tomatoes, chickpeas and sweet potato are all sources of potassium.

• Canned tomatoes and chickpeas and commercial vegetable broth boost the sodium in this recipe.

• Chickpeas provide soluble fiber, but remember that they may make you gassy; if you are not used to eating them, start with a small amount.

Nutrients Per Serving	
Calories	175
Fat	3 g
Fiber	5 g
Protein	5 g
Carbohydrate	34 g

Moroccan Vegetable Tagine

This colorful and healthy blend of vegetables scented with saffron, lemon and parsley works beautifully served with steamed whole wheat couscous or brown rice.

1 tbsp	olive oil	15 mL
2	onions, chopped	2
2	cloves garlic, finely chopped	2
2	Yukon gold potatoes, peeled and cubed	2
2	large carrots, cut into short sticks	2
1/2	large sweet potato, peeled and cut into short sticks	1/2
1 tbsp	grated gingerroot	15 mL
1 tsp	ground cumin	5 mL
1 tsp	ground cinnamon	5 mL
1	can (19 oz/540 mL) diced tomatoes	1
1	can (19 oz/540 mL) chickpeas, drained and rinsed	1
4 cups	vegetable broth	1 L
Pinch	saffron strands (optional)	Pinch
1/4 cup	chopped fresh parsley	60 mL
	Juice of 1 lemon	
	Salt and freshly ground black pepper	
2 tbsp	hot pepper sauce (optional)	30 mL

1. In a large saucepan, heat oil over medium-high heat. Add onions, garlic, potatoes, carrots, sweet potato, ginger, cumin and cinnamon; cook, stirring often, for 10 minutes. Stir in tomatoes; cook for 2 minutes. Stir in chickpeas, broth and saffron (if using); bring to a boil. Reduce heat, cover and simmer for 30 minutes, until vegetables are just tender. Stir in parsley and lemon juice. Season to taste with salt and pepper. Stir in hot sauce (if using).

> **IF FOLLOWING A LOW-FIBER DIET AND AVOIDING DIFFICULT-TO-DIGEST FOODS...**
>
> Finely chop the onions, peel and seed an equivalent amount of fresh tomatoes (see page 169), pinch the skin from the chickpeas, and finely chop the parsley (do not include stems). If you are sore in the anal area from frequent loose stools, omit the black pepper and hot pepper sauce. Small amounts of soft cooked carrots are okay. Choose white couscous or white rice as your side dish.

Vegetable Moussaka

This is a great lower-fat vegetarian version of a Greek classic. The rich cream sauce normally used in moussaka has been replaced with a tofu mixture that gives all the taste with a fraction of the fat!

- *Preheat oven to 350°F (180°C)*
- *Baking sheets, greased*
- *13- by 9-inch (33 by 23 cm) baking pan, greased*

2	medium eggplants	2
1 tsp	salt	5 mL
1	medium onion, chopped	1
1	clove garlic, minced	1
1	can (19 oz/540 mL) chickpeas, drained and rinsed	1
1	can (28 oz/796 mL) tomatoes	1
1 tbsp	dried oregano	15 mL
1 tbsp	dried basil	15 mL
½ tsp	ground cinnamon	2 mL
½ tsp	freshly ground black pepper	2 mL
¼ cup	freshly grated Parmesan cheese	60 mL
Topping		
1 lb	tofu	500 g
1	medium onion, quartered	1
2	egg whites	2
Pinch	ground nutmeg	Pinch

1. Slice eggplants lengthwise into ¼-inch (5 mm) thick slices; sprinkle with salt. Drain in colander for 30 minutes. Bake in preheated oven for 15 minutes. Turn and bake for 15 minutes longer.

2. In a nonstick skillet sprayed with nonstick cooking spray, cook onion and garlic, stirring, for 2 minutes. Add chickpeas, mashing slightly. Stir in tomatoes, oregano, basil, cinnamon, pepper and ½ tsp (2 mL) salt; bring to a boil. Reduce heat and simmer, uncovered, for 20 minutes, stirring occasionally. Process in food processor until mixture resembles coarse meal.

3. In greased baking pan, layer half of the eggplant, then all of the chickpea mixture, half of the Parmesan, then remaining eggplant.

4. *Prepare the topping:* Purée ingredients for topping; spread over moussaka. Sprinkle with remaining cheese. Bake in preheated oven for 30 minutes.

Vegetarian choice

Lower-calorie choice

Lower-fat choice

Higher-protein choice

Source of soluble fiber

Source of potassium

Source of sodium

MAKES 8 SERVINGS

IBD Tips

- This recipe is appropriate for vegetarians who eat eggs and dairy.

- Eggplant is not typically found in low-fiber diets, but if the skin and seeds are removed and it is cooked very soft, eaten in small amounts and chewed well, it can be included.

IF FOLLOWING A LOW-FIBER DIET...

Peel and seed the eggplant and bake until very soft, pinch skin from the chickpeas, and peel and seed an equivalent amount of fresh tomatoes (see page 169).

Nutrients Per Serving	
Calories	187
Fat	5 g
Fiber	6 g
Protein	12 g
Carbohydrate	26 g

MAKES 8 SERVINGS

IBD Tips

- This recipe is suitable for vegetarians who eat dairy and eggs.
- Boost calories by selecting higher-fat sour cream, ricotta and mozzarella. For short-term weight gain goals, an increased fat content is considered an acceptable way to boost calories.
- Ground meat replacements are often soy-based, a good-quality protein. They may also contain varying amounts of wheat, legumes and vegetables.
- Pasta sauce provides potassium in this recipe.
- Cheese, pasta sauce and vegetarian ground beef replacement provide sodium.

Nutrients Per Serving	
Calories	376
Fat	14 g
Fiber	8 g
Protein	27 g
Carbohydrate	35 g

Tangy Meatless Lasagna

An Italian-flavored ground meat alternative gives delicious texture and flavor to this lasagna. It's a delicious way to introduce your family to meat alternatives.

- *13- by 9-inch (33 by 23 cm) glass baking dish*

12	whole wheat lasagna noodles	12
2 tbsp	canola or olive oil	30 mL
1 cup	finely chopped onion	250 mL
1	clove garlic, minced	1
1½ cups	reduced-sodium tomato pasta sauce	375 mL
1	package (12 oz/340 g) Italian-seasoned vegetarian ground beef replacement	1
1	egg	1
1 cup	light sour cream	250 mL
1 cup	light ricotta cheese	250 mL
2 cups	shredded part-skim mozzarella cheese	500 mL

1. In a large pot of boiling salted water, cook lasagna noodles according to package directions until almost tender but still firm (they will finish cooking in the oven). Drain and rinse under cold running water. Drain and lay flat on a plate; set aside.

2. In a large saucepan, heat oil over medium heat. Sauté onion for 3 to 4 minutes or until softened. Add garlic and sauté for 30 seconds. Stir in pasta sauce and bring to a boil. Reduce heat and simmer, stirring occasionally, for 10 minutes. Remove from heat and stir in ground beef replacement. Set aside.

3. In a small bowl, whisk egg until blended. Stir in sour cream, ricotta and ½ cup (125 mL) of the mozzarella.

4. Spread about 2 tbsp (30 mL) sauce over bottom of baking dish. Arrange 3 lasagna noodles on top and spread with half the remaining sauce. Top with 3 noodles and spread with sour cream mixture. Top with 3 noodles and spread with the remaining sauce. Arrange the remaining 3 noodles on top and sprinkle with the remaining mozzarella.

5. Bake in preheated oven for 30 minutes or until bubbling and golden. Let stand for 15 minutes before serving.

IF FOLLOWING A LOW-FIBER DIET AND AVOIDING DIFFICULT-TO-DIGEST FOODS...

Use semolina noodles in place of whole wheat noodles and choose a plain tomato sauce that does not contain difficult-to-digest vegetables, tomato skins or seeds.

Caribbean Rice and Beans

2 tbsp	olive oil	30 mL
1	onion, finely chopped	1
2	cloves garlic, minced (about 2 tsp/10 mL)	2
1½ cups	long-grain white rice	375 mL
1	bay leaf	1
6	whole cloves (or ¼ tsp/1 mL ground cloves)	6
1½ tbsp	tomato paste	22 mL
½ tsp	ground allspice	2 mL
½ tsp	salt (optional)	2 mL
¼ tsp	hot pepper flakes	1 mL
1	can (14 oz/398 mL) coconut milk	1
1¼ cups	water	300 mL
1	can (14 to 19 oz/398 to 540 mL) red kidney beans, drained and rinsed, or 1 cup (250 mL) dried kidney beans, soaked, cooked and rinsed	1

1. In a heavy pot, heat oil over medium heat for 30 seconds. Add onion and cook, stirring, for 3 minutes or until softened. Add garlic and cook, stirring, for 30 seconds. Add rice and cook, stirring, for 4 minutes or until coated and hot. Remove from heat.

2. Add bay leaf, cloves, tomato paste, allspice, salt, if using, and hot pepper flakes and stir well. Stir in coconut milk and water. Increase heat to medium-high and bring to a boil, stirring often to prevent sticking. Reduce heat to low, cover and simmer for 18 minutes or until rice is tender and liquid is absorbed.

3. Add kidney beans and stir well. Cover and cook for 2 minutes. Remove from heat. Discard bay leaf and cloves. Serve piping hot.

IF FOLLOWING A LOW-FIBER DIET AND AVOIDING DIFFICULT-TO-DIGEST FOODS...

Use ground hot pepper flakes and pinch the skin from the kidney beans to reduce the insoluble fiber. If you are sore in the anal area from frequent loose stools, reduce the amount of tomato paste and omit the hot pepper flakes.

Vegan choice

Lactose-free choice

Source of soluble fiber

Source of potassium

Source of sodium

MAKES 6 TO 8 SERVINGS

IBD Tips

- White rice is known to help thicken loose stool. Be sure to cook it soft if you have any concerns about obstruction.

- Coconut milk is surprisingly high in saturated fat, and thus calories, but reduced-fat versions are available.

- Because legumes are economical, low-fat and full of nutrients, they are worth adding to the diet. If you don't normally eat them, start slowly.

- There are many beans and peas in the legume family, including chickpeas (garbanzo beans), black beans, kidney beans, navy beans, pinto beans, split peas, lima beans, black-eyed peas, great northern beans, lentils, peanuts and soy beans. They are available dried, canned, fresh or frozen.

Nutrients Per Serving	
Calories	313
Fat	15 g
Fiber	3 g
Protein	7 g
Carbohydrate	40 g

Vegan choice

Higher-protein choice

Lactose-free choice

Source of potassium

MAKES 4 TO 6 SERVINGS

IBD Tip

- To help prevent onions from making you cry when you're slicing them, try using a sharp knife, setting up a fan to blow the fumes away, placing the onion in the freezer for 10 minutes beforehand or even wearing goggles!

- Olive oil is not only flavorful, but contains a high proportion of monounsaturated fat and is considered a heart-healthy choice.

- Potatoes provide the potassium punch in this recipe.

Shepherd's Pie

Here's a new version of an old standby that everyone will enjoy. Delicious when hot out of the oven, it also makes a great leftover.

- *Preheat oven to 375°F (190°C)*
- *8-cup (2 L) casserole dish, greased*

1 tbsp	olive oil	15 mL
1	onion, finely chopped	1
1 cup	vegetable stock	250 mL
12 oz	soy ground meat alternative	375 g
10 oz	frozen mixed vegetables (about 1½ cups/375 mL), thawed and drained	300 g
2 cups	Garlic Mashed Potatoes (see recipe, page 295)	500 mL
1½ cups	shredded vegan Cheddar cheese alternative	375 mL
	Salt and freshly ground black pepper	

1. In a large skillet, heat oil over medium heat for 30 seconds. Add onion and cook, stirring, for 3 minutes or until softened. Add vegetable stock and cook for 3 minutes. Add soy ground meat alternative. Reduce heat to low, cover and cook for 10 minutes or until heated through.

2. Add vegetables and stir well. Cook for 5 minutes or until heated through. Transfer to prepared casserole dish. Top with mashed potatoes, spreading evenly. Sprinkle vegan Cheddar cheese alternative over top.

3. Bake in preheated oven for 25 minutes or until potatoes and cheese form a soft crust on top.

IF YOU ARE WELL...

If there is no medical reason for you to avoid fiber or difficult-to-digest foods, choose a package of frozen vegetables that includes corn and peas.

IF FOLLOWING A LOW-FIBER DIET AND AVOIDING DIFFICULT-TO-DIGEST FOODS...

Choose frozen cauliflower, carrots and green beans and cook until soft. You can also substitute with canned vegetables, as these are softer. Canned vegetables will increase the sodium content of this recipe.

Nutrients Per Serving	
Calories	253
Fat	12 g
Fiber	6 g
Protein	21 g
Carbohydrate	18 g

Falafel in Pita

These tasty treats are a gift from the Middle East, where they are eaten the way hamburgers are in North America. Liberally garnished, they make a great lunch or light dinner.

1	can (19 oz/540 mL) chickpeas, drained and rinsed	1
½ cup	sliced green onion	125 mL
2 tbsp	freshly squeezed lemon juice	30 mL
1 tbsp	minced garlic	15 mL
1 to 2 tsp	curry powder	5 to 10 mL
1	egg	1
2 tbsp	vegetable oil	30 mL
½ cup	all-purpose flour	125 mL
4	pita breads	4
	Chopped peeled cucumber	
	Chopped tomato	
	Shredded lettuce	
	Plain yogurt	

1. In a food processor, combine chickpeas, onion, lemon juice, garlic, and curry powder to taste. Process until blended but chickpeas retain their texture. Using your hands, shape into 4 large patties.

2. In a shallow bowl, lightly beat egg. In a skillet, heat oil over medium heat. Dip each patty into the egg, then into the flour, coating both sides well. Fry until golden and heated through, about 2 minutes per side.

3. Fill each pita bread with a falafel and garnish with cucumber, tomato, lettuce and yogurt, as desired.

IF FOLLOWING A LOW-FIBER DIET AND AVOIDING DIFFICULT-TO-DIGEST FOODS...

Pinch the skin from the chickpeas, choose pita bread made with white flour, seed the cucumber, peel and seed the tomato (see page 169), and use only a small amount of iceberg (head) lettuce and chew well.

Vegetarian choice

Higher-calorie choice

Lower-fat choice

Source of soluble fiber

Source of potassium

Source of sodium

MAKES 4 SERVINGS

IBD Tips

- This recipe is appropriate for vegetarians who eat eggs and dairy.

- Chickpeas provide soluble fiber, but remember that legumes may make you gassy; if you are not used to eating them, start with a small amount.

- Curry powder adds flavor — don't be afraid to include this wonderful spice!

- To boost calories, garnish with full-fat yogurt or sour cream.

Nutrients Per Serving	
Calories	474
Fat	12 g
Fiber	12 g
Protein	16 g
Carbohydrate	80 g

MAKES 5 SERVINGS

Tips

- In some locations, chickpeas are known as garbanzo beans.
- If you prefer, use 2 tbsp (30 mL) chopped fresh mint leaves in place of the dried.

IBD Tips

- Oats are the best source of a soluble fiber called beta glucan.
- Chickpeas and oats provide the soluble fiber in this recipe.
- Always use iodized salt — the added iodine is essential for your thyroid and for mental development.
- Use olive oil or canola oil in this recipe for their heart-healthy fat profiles.
- Canned chickpeas provide potassium and sodium.

Nutrients Per Serving	
Calories	273
Fat	13 g
Fiber	6 g
Protein	7 g
Carbohydrate	32 g

Tasty Chickpea Cakes

We love this version of the Middle Eastern specialty, falafel. The combination of seasoning and oatmeal, which can't be detected in the final result, make this a satisfying main dish.

½ cup	rolled oats (quick-cooking or old-fashioned)	125 mL
1 tbsp	freshly squeezed lemon juice	15 mL
1	can (14 to 19 oz/398 to 540 mL) chickpeas, drained and rinsed, or 1 cup (250 mL) dried chickpeas, soaked, cooked and drained	1
2 tbsp	coarsely chopped Italian parsley	30 mL
1	small onion, coarsely chopped	1
3	cloves garlic, minced (1 tbsp/15 mL)	3
2 tsp	cumin seeds	10 mL
2 tsp	dried mint (see tip, at left)	10 mL
1 tsp	chili powder	5 mL
½ tsp	salt	2 mL
¼ tsp	freshly ground black pepper	1 mL
¼ cup	olive or vegetable oil	60 mL
3 tbsp	cornmeal or bread crumbs	45 mL

1. In food processor, combine oats with lemon juice and pulse 3 or 4 times or until blended. Add chickpeas and parsley and pulse 10 times or until chickpeas are ground and mixture is blended but not puréed.

2. Add onion, garlic, cumin seeds, mint, chili powder, salt and pepper. Pulse 5 times or until mixed. (The large pieces of onion and the chickpeas should be broken down, but the mixture should have a coarse texture.)

3. With moistened hands, shape mixture into 5 cakes, each about 2½ inches (6.25 cm) in diameter and ¾ inch (2 cm) thick. Sprinkle cornmeal on both sides.

4. In a large skillet, heat oil over high heat until hot but not smoking. Add cakes and fry for 1 minute. Reduce heat to medium and fry for 1 to 2 minutes longer or until browned. Flip cakes and fry for 2 to 3 minutes longer or until browned on both sides and hot in the center. Serve immediately.

IF FOLLOWING A LOW-FIBER DIET AND AVOIDING DIFFICULT-TO-DIGEST FOODS...

Pinch the skin from the chickpeas, finely chop the parsley (do not include stems), finely chop the onion, use ground cumin instead of seeds, and use white bread crumbs instead of cornmeal.

Tofu Patties

This is a great way to prepare tofu. For children, make mini patties.

- *Preheat oven to 325°F (160°C)*
- *9-inch (23 cm) square baking pan, lightly greased*

10 oz	firm tofu, mashed	300 g
¾ cup	quick-cooking rolled oats	175 mL
2 tbsp	soy sauce	30 mL
½ tsp	dried basil	2 mL
½ tsp	dried oregano	2 mL
½ tsp	garlic powder	2 mL
½ tsp	onion powder	2 mL
	Salt and freshly ground black pepper	

1. In a medium bowl, combine tofu, oats, soy sauce, basil, oregano, garlic powder, onion powder, and salt and pepper to taste. Knead for a few minutes. Shape into 1-inch (2.5 cm) thick patties and place in prepared pan.

2. Bake in preheated oven for 20 to 25 minutes or until lightly browned.

IF YOU ARE WELL...

If there is no medical reason for you to avoid fiber or difficult-to-digest foods, experiment with fixings such as relish, pickled peppers, sauerkraut, raw onions, chutney or salsa, tomato and lettuce.

IF FOLLOWING A LOW-FIBER DIET AND AVOIDING DIFFICULT-TO-DIGEST FOODS...

Stick with mayonnaise, ketchup and mustard (there are many flavor varieties) and a small amount of iceberg (head) lettuce for your toppings. If you eat dairy, add a slice of melted cheese.

Vegan choice

Lower-calorie choice

Lower-fiber choice

Higher-protein choice

Lactose-free choice

Source of sodium

MAKES 6 SERVINGS

Tip

- Look for tofu made with calcium. Look for "calcium sulfate" or "calcium chloride" in the ingredients list to make sure the tofu you are buying is a source of calcium.

IBD Tips

- Consider serving on a bun with hummus. Spreads made from roasted peppers or eggplant will also add great flavor!
- Despite the increased fiber, many low-fiber diets include oats and oat products because they thicken loose stool.
- Soy sauce is rich in sodium.

Nutrients Per Serving	
Calories	83
Fat	3 g
Fiber	2 g
Protein	6 g
Carbohydrate	10 g

MAKES 2 TO 4 SERVINGS

Tip

• You can find smoked barbecued tofu in most major supermarkets or natural foods stores. If you can't find it, use the same amount of extra-firm tofu, cubed. Place the cubes on a double layer of paper towels. Let drain for 20 minutes. Pour off water and set tofu aside.

IBD Tip

• Potato chips supply potassium, sodium and lots of calories! Potato chips may slow stool outputs, but be careful how often you consume them. They don't provide a lot of nutrition, and they will contribute to weight gain.

Nutrients Per Serving	
Calories	120
Fat	6 g
Fiber	1 g
Protein	6 g
Carbohydrate	10 g

Barbecued Tofu Nuggets

• *Preheat oven to 375°F (190°C)*
• *Rimmed baking sheet, greased*

6 oz	smoked barbecued tofu, cut into 12 cubes (see tip, at right)	175 g
1/3 cup	barbecue sauce	75 mL
1 1/2 cups	finely crushed plain potato chips or barbecue-flavor potato chips	375 mL

1. Pat tofu dry with paper towels and brush all over with barbecue sauce. Place potato chips in a bowl. One at a time, drop cubes into potato chips, lightly tossing to ensure all sides are coated.

2. Place nuggets on prepared pan, 2 to 3 inches (5 to 7.5 cm) apart. Bake in preheated oven for 12 minutes or until hot and crispy. Let cool on pan for 1 minute. Using a metal spatula, transfer to a serving platter.

Variation

Substitute 1/3 cup (75 mL) soy mayonnaise for the barbecue sauce.

IF FOLLOWING A LOW-FIBER DIET AND AVOIDING DIFFICULT-TO-DIGEST FOODS...

Serve this recipe with a white rice or noodle dish. For a tasty meal, add sliced seeded peeled cucumber on the side.

Asian-Style Baked Tofu

This tasty tofu can be eaten as a snack, as an appetizer or in an Asian stir-fry. It can be served hot or cold.

- *Preheat oven to 350°F (180°C)*
- *8-inch (20 cm) square glass baking dish*

¼ cup	reduced-sodium soy sauce	60 mL
¼ cup	vegan teriyaki sauce	60 mL
2 tbsp	freshly squeezed lime juice	30 mL
1 tbsp	finely grated gingerroot	15 mL
2	cloves garlic, minced (about 2 tsp/10 mL)	2
1 lb	firm or extra-firm tofu, cut in 1-inch (2.5 cm) cubes and drained (see tip, at right)	500 g

1. In a small bowl, whisk together soy sauce, teriyaki sauce, lime juice, ginger and garlic.

2. Arrange tofu evenly over the bottom of baking dish. Add sauce and stir until cubes are completely covered with sauce. Marinate for 1 hour at room temperature or in the refrigerator for at least 2 hours or for up to 8 hours.

3. Bake, uncovered, in preheated oven for 35 to 40 minutes, stirring and turning pieces over after 20 minutes, or until tofu is firm and liquid is absorbed.

MAKES 4 TO 6 SERVINGS

Tips

- To drain tofu, place the cubes on a plate lined with a double layer of paper towels. Cover with another paper towel and another plate and place a weight on top of the plate to press the water from the tofu. Let stand for 30 minutes. Drain off water.

- Although tofu is a staple in the vegan diet, it can be high in fat. If you're concerned about fat intake, look for lower-fat versions, which work well in both this dish and Italian-Style Baked Tofu (see recipe, page 262).

IBD Tips

- This recipe is appropriate for a low-fiber diet.

- If you need to boost your sodium intake, use regular soy sauce.

Nutrients Per Serving	
Calories	71
Fat	2 g
Fiber	Trace
Protein	6 g
Carbohydrate	7 g

Vegan choice

Lower-calorie choice

Lower-fiber choice

Higher-protein choice

Lactose-free choice

Source of sodium

MAKES 4 TO 6 SERVINGS

Tip

• To drain tofu, place the cubes on a plate lined with a double layer of paper towels. Cover with another paper towel, then another plate. Place a weight on top of the plate to press the water out of the tofu. Let stand for 30 minutes. Drain off water.

IBD Tips

• Tofu provides good-quality protein and is high in polyunsaturated fat. Read the label to choose a tofu set with calcium.

• The salad dressing and added salt provide sodium.

Nutrients Per Serving	
Calories	73
Fat	5 g
Fiber	Trace
Protein	5 g
Carbohydrate	2 g

Italian-Style Baked Tofu

Like Asian-Style Baked Tofu (see recipe, page 261), this recipe is versatile. Serve it as an appetizer, in salads, or crumbled and used as a cheese substitute in Italian dishes. You can also use this to make a sauce (see variation, below) for pasta or potatoes.

* *Preheat oven to 350°F (180°C)*
* *8-inch (20 cm) square glass baking dish*

1 lb	firm or extra-firm tofu, cut in 1-inch (2.5 cm) cubes and drained (see tip, at left)	500 g
2	cloves garlic, minced (about 2 tsp/10 mL)	2
1 tsp	dried oregano	5 mL
1 tsp	dried basil	5 mL
¼ tsp	salt, or to taste	1 mL
	Freshly ground black pepper	
¼ cup	prepared Italian salad dressing	60 mL

1. In baking dish, combine tofu, garlic, oregano, basil and salt and pepper to taste. Drizzle with dressing, then stir until tofu is evenly coated. Marinate for 1 hour at room temperature or in the refrigerator for at least 2 hours or for up to 8 hours.

2. Bake, uncovered, in preheated oven, for 35 to 40 minutes, stirring and turning pieces over after 20 minutes, or until tofu is firm and liquid is absorbed.

Variation

Before baking, add 1 can (14 oz/398 mL) seasoned diced tomatoes to tofu and mix well. Serve over pasta.

IF FOLLOWING A LOW-FIBER DIET AND AVOIDING DIFFICULT-TO-DIGEST FOODS...

Choose flaked dried spices and finely grind the black pepper. If making the variation with tomatoes, peel and seed and equivalent amount of fresh tomatoes (see page 169).

Sesame Noodles with Tofu

This dish, without tofu, is often offered as an appetizer in Chinese restaurants. We've added tofu to make it a meal. Serve it warm or let cool to room temperature.

10 oz	rice noodles	300 g
6 cups	hot water	1.5 L
½ cup	coarsely chopped green onions (white and green parts), divided	125 mL
⅓ cup	natural non-homogenized peanut butter	75 mL
¼ cup	sesame oil	60 mL
3 tbsp	reduced-sodium soy sauce	45 mL
1½ tbsp	tahini	22 mL
1 tbsp	granulated natural cane sugar, or to taste	15 mL
Dash	hot sesame oil, or to taste (see tip, at right)	Dash
8 oz	Asian-Style Baked Tofu (see recipe, page 261)	250 g
1	cucumber, peeled and sliced into 2½- by ½-inch (6 by 1 cm) strips	1

1. In a bowl, soak noodles in hot water for 20 minutes or until soft (or prepare according to package directions). Drain and transfer to a large serving bowl.

2. In a small bowl, combine all but 2 tbsp (30 mL) of the green onions, peanut butter, sesame oil, soy sauce, tahini, sugar and hot sesame oil. (This should become a thick, light brown sauce. If your mixture is too thick, stir in up to 1 tbsp/15 mL water.) Pour about two-thirds of the sauce over noodles. Add tofu and gently toss to coat evenly.

3. Place the cucumber slices around the perimeter of the noodles. Pour the remaining sauce over top and sprinkle with remaining green onions.

Variation

Garnish with 2 tbsp (30 mL) chopped peanuts and a sprig of parsley.

IF FOLLOWING A LOW-FIBER DIET AND AVOIDING DIFFICULT-TO-DIGEST FOODS...

Omit the green onions, use smooth peanut butter, use only regular sesame oil, and seed the cucumber.

Vegan choice

Higher-calorie choice

Lactose-free choice

MAKES 4 TO 6 SERVINGS

Tips

- Use all-natural, non-homogenized peanut butter for best results.

- Make sure to taste the sauce when mixing, as the amount of sugar may need to be adjusted based on the brand of peanut butter you use. Some are saltier than others.

- You can find hot sesame oil in Asian markets or well-stocked supermarkets. If you can't find it, use regular sesame oil.

IBD Tips

- If you need to boost your sodium intake, use regular soy sauce.

- Tahini contains polyunsaturated and monounsaturated fats, calcium, vitamin E and antioxidants.

Nutrients Per Serving	
Calories	461
Fat	23 g
Fiber	3 g
Protein	15 g
Carbohydrate	49 g

MAKES 4 SERVINGS

Tips

- Freeze the tofu cubes prior to preparation; this enhances the texture of the tofu so it's more poultry-like.
- This dish goes well with jasmine rice or noodles.

IBD Tips

- Tomatoes are rich in potassium; tofu is also a source.
- Tofu provides high-quality protein and is high in polyunsaturated fat. Read the label to choose a tofu set with calcium.
- Almonds are a good source of calcium.
- Use heart-healthy olive oil or canola oil in this recipe.

Nutrients Per Serving	
Calories	149
Fat	9 g
Fiber	4 g
Protein	7 g
Carbohydrate	14 g

Nutty Tofu and Green Vegetable Stir-Fry

This spicy, nutty tofu recipe has the flavor of an Asian satay dish and is guaranteed to please both vegetarians and non-vegetarians!

1 tbsp	vegetable oil	15 mL
8 oz	firm tofu, cubed	250 g
1	green bell pepper, thinly sliced	1
1½ cups	green beans, trimmed	375 mL
½ tsp	salt	2 mL
4	cloves garlic, minced	4
1	onion, chopped	1
1	tomato, chopped	1
¼ cup	coarsely ground almonds	60 mL
½ cup	water (approx.), divided	125 mL
½ tsp	granulated sugar	2 mL
½ tsp	ground turmeric	2 mL
½ tsp	ground cumin	2 mL
½ tsp	ground coriander	2 mL

1. In a large skillet, heat oil over medium heat. Lightly brown tofu on all sides, then remove from pan and set aside.

2. Add green pepper, green beans and salt to skillet; stir-fry until tender-crisp, about 5 minutes. Add garlic, onion and tomato; stir-fry for 5 minutes. Stir in tofu pieces. Stir in almonds, ¼ cup (60 mL) of the water and sugar. Reduce heat to low and cook for 5 minutes. Stir in turmeric, cumin and coriander, then the remaining ¼ cup (60 mL) water (add more if the mixture becomes too dry and sticks to the pan).

> **IF FOLLOWING A LOW-FIBER DIET AND AVOIDING DIFFICULT-TO-DIGEST FOODS...**
>
> Peel and finely chop the green pepper, peel away the stringy vein along the length of the green beans and cook until soft (or use canned green beans), peel and seed the tomato (see page 169), and use almond butter or finely ground almonds.

Pasta

Pasta can be used in soups, salads, appetizers, as a meat accompaniment and in main dishes. Most of the recipes in this chapter are intended to be served as side dishes.

Pasta is usually made from a coarsely ground durum wheat called semolina. Durum wheat is a high-protein grain and has a higher concentration of carotenoid pigments than bread wheats, giving pasta its characteristic yellow color. It also produces firm pasta that maintains its form when cooked and is less likely to stick. In North America, pasta is enriched with the B vitamins thiamin, riboflavin and niacin, and sometimes with iron.

In addition to providing some protein, pasta is a source of complex carbohydrate. People trying to lose weight on low-carbohydrate diets sometimes avoid it; however, it is usually the additions to pasta — the butter and cream sauces and cheese — that are high in calories and should be limited.

There are over 150 different shapes and sizes of pasta, including fettuccine, linguine, spaghetti, spaghettini, ziti, rigatoni, farfalle, penne, fusilli, rotini, macaroni, cannelloni, ravioli, tortellini, gnocchi, ditali, lasagna and conchiglie (shells), to name just a few.

Tips for Cooking Pasta

- Cook pasta in a large pot with enough rapidly boiling water to avoid sticking. It is ready when it is tender yet still firm to the bite, also known as "al dente."
- Adding a small amount of oil to the cooking water will help to keep pasta pieces separate.
- Fresh pasta cooks much faster than dried pasta, so adjust your cooking times if using fresh.
- Pasta can increase to anywhere from two to four times its original volume when cooked!
- Rinsing enriched pasta with water once it's cooked will increase the loss of vitamins and minerals.
- When reheating pasta, pour boiling water over it just before serving, then combine it with sauce. This helps you avoid soft and sticky pasta and sauce combinations.

Be sure to read the labels of "whole grain," "whole wheat" or "multigrain" pastas, as they vary in fiber content. If you are following a low-fiber diet, avoid these selections.

Take the Time to Chew Well

If you are concerned about your tolerance to the food you're eating or a food-related obstruction, be sure to eat in a relaxed environment and take your time. Distractions like eating in front of the TV, enjoying good conversation or paying attention to small children will take your attention away from chewing well.

THE FACTS ABOUT CHEESE

Many pasta dishes call for cheese, which can be a problem for the lactose intolerant. But remember that the amount of lactose you can tolerate may fall along a "spectrum" (you can tolerate some, just not a lot). Parmesan cheese, like other hard cheeses, contains relatively small amounts of lactose and is often tolerated by individuals with mild to moderate lactose intolerance.

Choose the fat content of cheese according to your personal goals. If you are trying to gain weight, select full-fat versions for the short term. If you are trying to eat healthy and minimize calories, chose a reduced-fat version. Regular Cheddar cheese, for example, is over 30% milk fat; if you can find cheese that contains less than 15% milk fat, you are making great strides toward reducing saturated fat in your diet. When choosing a "light" version, always read the label carefully, as the word "light" or "lite" can refer to color, flavor or texture, not necessarily calories or fat.

To save money, buy blocks of cheese on sale, shred the cheese in advance and store it in your freezer.

Tomatoes are rich in lycopene, which is thought to reduce the risk of prostate cancer.

Tomato Sauce

This is a generic tomato-basil-garlic sauce that works not only with spaghetti, but with whatever recipe calls for a tomato enhancement. It freezes well, and is easy to make in large batches. It is very useful to have on hand.

3 lbs	ripe tomatoes (see tip, at right)	1.5 kg
1/3 cup	olive oil	75 mL
Pinch	salt	Pinch
8	cloves garlic, roughly chopped	8
1/2 tsp	hot pepper flakes	2 mL
1 1/2 tbsp	dried basil or 1/4 to 1/2 cup (50 to 125 mL) chopped fresh basil, packed down	22 mL
1 tbsp	balsamic vinegar	15 mL
6	sun-dried tomatoes, finely chopped	6

1. Blanch tomatoes in boiling water for 30 seconds. Over a bowl, peel, core and seed them. Chop tomatoes roughly and set aside. Strain any accumulated tomato juices from bowl; add half of the juices to the chopped tomatoes. Save or freeze the other half for recipes that call for tomato juice.

2. In a large, deep frying pan or pot, heat oil over high heat for 30 seconds. Add salt and stir. Add chopped garlic and stir-fry for 30 seconds. Add the hot pepper flakes and stir-fry for 30 seconds.

3. Add chopped tomatoes and juices. Stir-cook until boiling. Add basil (if using dried), the vinegar and sun-dried tomatoes. Mix well, and reduce heat to medium-low. Cook for 20 to 25 minutes, maintaining a steady bubbling, stirring occasionally.

4. If using fresh basil, add it now to taste (no amount is too much). Stir in, and continue cooking for 5 minutes. Remove from heat and cover. Let rest for 5 to 10 minutes to develop flavor. Stir to redistribute the oil that has risen to the top, and serve immediately.

IF FOLLOWING A LOW-FIBER DIET AND AVOIDING DIFFICULT-TO-DIGEST FOODS...

Finely chop the garlic and use sun-dried tomato paste instead of chopped sun-dried tomatoes. If using fresh basil, finely chop the leaves and do not include stems. You might also want to consider using hot pepper sauce or ground dried hot pepper instead of flakes.

Vegan choice

Higher-calorie choice

Lactose-free choice

Source of potassium

MAKES 4 CUPS (1 L) OR 8 SERVINGS

Tip

• Canned, whole plum tomatoes can replace fresh. Use 2 cans (each 28 oz/796 mL), reserving 2 cups (500 mL) of the juice for use if the sauce needs thinning.

IBD Tips

• If you use canned tomatoes, the sauce will contain tomato seeds, so be sure use this substitution only when you are feeling well.

• Adjust the amount of added salt to boost sodium, if needed.

• Tomatoes provide the potassium in this recipe.

Nutrients Per Serving	
Calories	205
Fat	11 g
Fiber	5 g
Protein	6 g
Carbohydrate	25 g

MAKES 4 TO 6 SERVINGS

Tips

- Substitute 14 oz (420 g) soy ground meat alternative for the meatless meatballs. Pinch off small pieces and roll into balls approximately 1 inch (2.5 cm) in diameter.

- Soy meat alternatives come in a variety of textures. Those found in the refrigerated section of your supermarket tend to be moister than those found in the frozen section. The moist versions are easiest to work with when forming soyballs.

IBD Tips

- Boost sodium by using commercial tomato sauce.

- Tomatoes are rich in potassium.

Nutrients Per Serving	
Calories	332
Fat	14 g
Fiber	7 g
Protein	19 g
Carbohydrate	34 g

Spaghetti and Soyballs

Here's an old standard with a contemporary vegan twist. You get the health benefits of soy, the great taste of tomato sauce and the satisfaction of comfort food.

8 oz	spaghetti	250 g
¼ cup	dry bread crumbs	60 mL
2 tbsp	coarsely chopped fresh oregano (or 2 tsp/10 mL dried)	30 mL
1 tbsp	coarsely chopped fresh parsley (or 1 tsp/5 mL dried)	15 mL
1 tbsp	whole wheat or unbleached all-purpose flour	15 mL
1	package (14 oz/420 g) meatless meatballs (see tips, at left)	1
4 cups	tomato sauce	1 L
3 tbsp	olive oil	45 mL
	Grated vegan Parmesan cheese alternative (optional)	

1. In a pot of boiling salted water, cook spaghetti for 8 minutes or until tender to the bite. Drain.

2. Meanwhile, in a bowl, combine bread crumbs, oregano, parsley and flour. Add meatballs and toss until evenly coated. Transfer to a plate, shaking off excess crumb mixture. Set aside.

3. In a pot, heat tomato sauce over low heat until heated through.

4. Meanwhile, in a large nonstick skillet, heat oil over medium-high heat for 30 seconds. Add meatballs and cook, turning, until lightly browned and crispy. Using a slotted spoon, transfer to tomato sauce. Simmer, uncovered, for 5 minutes or until heated through.

5. Divide hot spaghetti among plates. Spoon soyballs and sauce over top.

IF FOLLOWING A LOW-FIBER DIET AND AVOIDING DIFFICULT-TO-DIGEST FOODS...

Choose white bread crumbs, use all-purpose flour, finely chop oregano and parsley (do not include stems) or use dried, and select a plain tomato sauce that does not contain difficult-to-digest vegetables.

Italian-Style Macaroni

This macaroni dish provides fewer calories and less fat than conventional macaroni and cheese.

- *Preheat oven to 375°F (190°C)*
- *6-cup (1.5 L) baking dish*

2 cups	tomato juice	500 mL
1 cup	chicken broth	250 mL
2 tbsp	finely chopped onion	30 mL
1	clove garlic, minced	1
1 tsp	dried Italian seasoning	5 mL
Pinch	salt	Pinch
Pinch	freshly ground black pepper	Pinch
2 cups	cooked elbow macaroni	500 mL
1 cup	shredded old Cheddar cheese	250 mL

1. In a medium saucepan, combine tomato juice, broth, onion, garlic and seasonings. Cook over low heat, uncovered, for about 25 minutes or until reduced by half.

2. Stir tomato sauce into cooked macaroni. Spoon into 6-cup (1.5 L) baking dish. Sprinkle with cheese. Bake in preheated oven for about 25 minutes.

Higher-calorie choice

Lower-fiber choice

Higher-protein choice

Source of potassium

Source of sodium

MAKES 4 SERVINGS

Tip

- The sauce will be thin when added to the macaroni but will thicken during the oven baking. If desired, replace Cheddar cheese with Parmesan.

IBD Tips

- This recipe is appropriate for a low-fiber diet if the black pepper is finely ground.

- The sources of sodium in this recipe are tomato juice, commercial chicken broth, added salt and cheese.

- Tomato juice is rich in potassium.

Nutrients Per Serving	
Calories	240
Fat	10 g
Fiber	1 g
Protein	12 g
Carbohydrate	25 g

Vegetarian choice

Higher-calorie choice

Higher-protein choice

Source of potassium

Source of sodium

MAKES 6 SERVINGS

IBD Tips

- Canned soup, canned tomatoes, cheese and added salt provide the sodium in this recipe.

- Tomatoes and tomato juice are rich in potassium.

- You can substitute non-hydrogenated margarine for the butter if you are trying to reduce saturated fat.

Mac and Cheese with Tomatoes

- *Preheat oven to 350°F (180°C)*
- *8-cup (2 L) baking dish, lightly greased*

12 oz	elbow macaroni	375 g
½ cup	dry bread crumbs	125 mL
2 tbsp	melted butter	30 mL
1	can (28 oz/796 mL) tomatoes, coarsely chopped, including juice	1
1	can (10 oz/284 mL) condensed Cheddar cheese soup	1
2 cups	shredded Cheddar cheese	500 mL
1 tsp	salt	5 mL
	Freshly ground black pepper	

1. Cook macaroni in a pot of boiling salted water until tender to the bite, about 8 minutes. Drain.

2. In a bowl, combine bread crumbs and melted butter. Set aside.

3. In a large bowl, combine tomatoes, Cheddar cheese soup, Cheddar cheese, salt and black pepper to taste. Add hot macaroni and stir well.

4. Transfer mixture to prepared baking dish. Spread bread crumb mixture evenly over top. Bake in preheated oven until crumbs are golden and mixture is bubbling, about 25 minutes.

Variation

Mac and Cheese with Cauliflower: Add 3 cups (750 mL) cauliflower florets to macaroni cooking water after it has been boiling for 2 minutes. (Break up larger florets to ensure size uniformity.) Return to a boil and cook until both cauliflower and macaroni are firm to the bite, about 5 minutes. Add 1 tbsp (15 mL) basil pesto to the tomato mixture before stirring in the cauliflower mixture.

IF FOLLOWING A LOW-FIBER DIET AND AVOIDING DIFFICULT-TO-DIGEST FOODS...

Avoid whole wheat bread crumbs, peel and seed an equivalent amount of fresh tomatoes (see page 169), and finely grind the black pepper. If making the variation, cook the cauliflower until soft. Cauliflower is a gas-producing food, so eat only a small portion at first.

Nutrients Per Serving	
Calories	383
Fat	19 g
Fiber	4 g
Protein	17 g
Carbohydrate	38 g

Linguine Alfredo

12 oz	linguine noodles	375 g
4 tsp	margarine	20 mL
2 tbsp	all-purpose flour	30 mL
2 cups	2% milk	500 mL
¼ cup	freshly grated Parmesan cheese	60 mL
¼ tsp	ground nutmeg	1 mL
	Freshly ground black pepper	

1. Cook linguine according to package directions or until firm to the bite. Drain and place in serving bowl.

2. Meanwhile, in small saucepan, melt margarine; add flour and cook, stirring, for 30 seconds. Add milk and cook on medium heat, stirring constantly, just until thickened, approximately 3 minutes. Add cheese, nutmeg and pepper to taste; stir until combined. Pour over pasta and toss well.

Vegetarian choice

Higher-calorie choice

Lower-fat choice

Higher-protein choice

Source of sodium

MAKES 4 SERVINGS

Tip

- Sauce can be made ahead and refrigerated for up to 2 days. Reheat gently, adding more milk to thin.

IBD Tips

- This recipe is appropriate for a low-fiber diet if the black pepper is finely ground.

- Boost calories by using homogenized milk or cream.

- Margarine, like cow's milk, is fortified with vitamin D, and non-hydrogenated margarine contains much less saturated fat than butter.

- Margarine and cheese provide sodium.

Nutrients Per Serving	
Calories	470
Fat	9 g
Fiber	3 g
Protein	18 g
Carbohydrate	77 g

Pasta with Broccoli Herb Sauce

MAKES 5 SERVINGS

Tip

• As this sauce is thick, like pesto, it is best served with a long pasta such as spaghetti, spaghettini or fettuccine because it will cling to the pasta.

IBD Tips

• When selecting broccoli, choose firm, dark green compact clusters of small flower buds. Broccoli is a gas-producing food, so start with small portions.

• Olive oil is not only flavorful, but contains a high proportion of monounsaturated fat and is considered a heart-healthy choice.

This broccoli sauce is similar to a basil pesto sauce and is intended to be thick. If you prefer a thinner sauce, add chicken or vegetable stock while processing. Serve over fettuccine, fusilli or linguine. What a great way to encourage kids to eat their broccoli!

2³⁄₄ cups	chopped broccoli	675 mL
¹⁄₃ cup	olive or vegetable oil	75 mL
¹⁄₃ cup	freshly grated Parmesan cheese	75 mL
¹⁄₄ cup	chopped fresh parsley	60 mL
1 tbsp	chopped fresh basil	15 mL
12 oz	pasta	375 g

1. Place broccoli and 2 tbsp (30 mL) water in a 4-cup (1 L) microwave-safe bowl. Microwave, covered, on High for about 5 minutes; drain.

2. In a food processor, purée broccoli, oil, cheese, parsley and basil until broccoli is finely chopped.

3. Cook pasta in boiling water according to package directions or until tender but firm. Drain well and toss with vegetable mixture. Serve immediately.

IF YOU ARE WELL...

If there is no medical reason for you to avoid fiber or difficult-to-digest foods, include broccoli in your diet. Broccoli provides beta carotene, vitamins C and E, folate, calcium and potassium. And, as a member of the cabbage family, it is considered anticarcinogenic.

IF FOLLOWING A LOW-FIBER DIET AND AVOIDING DIFFICULT-TO-DIGEST FOODS...

Finely chop the parsley and basil (do not include stems). While broccoli is not normally part of a low-fiber diet, you can reduce fiber by using a smaller amount of only broccoli florets and omitting the stems. Because the broccoli is puréed, the risk of food obstruction is minimized.

Nutrients Per Serving	
Calories	422
Fat	16 g
Fiber	4 g
Protein	13 g
Carbohydrate	56 g

Pasta with Spinach Pesto

12 oz	pasta (any variety)	375 g
1½ cups	fresh spinach, washed and well packed down	375 mL
¼ cup	water or chicken stock	60 mL
3 tbsp	olive oil	45 mL
2 tbsp	toasted pine nuts	30 mL
3 tbsp	freshly grated Parmesan cheese	45 mL
1½ tsp	crushed garlic	7 mL
	Freshly ground black pepper	

1. Cook pasta in boiling water according to package instructions or until firm to the bite. Drain and place in serving bowl.
2. Meanwhile, in food processor, purée spinach, water, oil, nuts, cheese, garlic and pepper until smooth. Pour over pasta.

Vegetarian choice

Higher-calorie choice

Lower-fiber choice

Source of potassium

MAKES 4 TO 6 SERVINGS

Tips

- For variety, add to pasta 8 to 12 oz (250 to 375 g) of cooked meat, chicken or fish.
- Toast pine nuts on top of stove in skillet for 2 to 3 minutes, until brown.
- Dry spinach well after washing.
- Refrigerate sauce up to 3 days ahead or freeze for up to 6 weeks.

IBD Tips

- Spinach is packed with nutrients, especially folate and carotenoids, which act as antioxidants in the body. The calcium and iron in spinach are not well absorbed due to binding compounds called oxalates, but spinach does provide potassium and magnesium.
- Because the spinach and pine nuts are puréed, the risk of food obstruction is minimized.

Nutrients Per Serving	
Calories	325
Fat	10 g
Fiber	2 g
Protein	10 g
Carbohydrate	48 g

MAKES 2 TO 4 SERVINGS

Tip

- Approximately 2 cups (500 mL) small-shell pasta yields 3 cups (750 mL) cooked pasta.

IBD Tips

- If you are trying to gain weight, it's okay to increase your fat intake for the short term. Use homogenized milk or cream and full-fat yogurt.

- Add more color to this recipe by choosing red- or green-colored pasta (sold, for example, as vegetable bow ties or tricolor fusilli). The pasta is usually colored by tomato or spinach powder.

- Milk, yogurt, zucchini and tomatoes together provide some potassium.

Aphrodite's Pasta

Aphrodite was the Greek goddess of love, and this recipe, which makes 2 main-course servings, is perfect for a romantic dinner! If you wish, you can also make this as a side dish to serve 4.

½ cup	2% milk	125 mL
4 tsp	cornstarch	20 mL
1 tsp	finely minced gingerroot	5 mL
1 tsp	finely minced garlic	5 mL
½ cup	lower-fat plain yogurt	125 mL
1	small zucchini, cut into strips	1
3 cups	drained cooked pasta (bow ties, shells or fusilli)	750 mL
	Freshly ground black pepper	
2 tbsp	coarsely chopped fresh parsley	30 mL
½ cup	diced seeded tomatoes	125 mL

1. In a medium saucepan, mix milk and cornstarch until smooth. Add ginger and garlic; bring to a boil, stirring constantly, and cook until thickened.

2. Stir in yogurt and zucchini; simmer for 2 to 3 minutes. Stir in pasta; simmer for 1 to 2 minutes or until hot. Season with pepper to taste. Garnish with parsley and tomatoes.

IF YOU ARE WELL...

If there is no medical reason for you to avoid fiber or difficult-to-digest foods, substitute other vegetables in this recipe to increase variety, and thus nutrients, in your diet.

IF FOLLOWING A LOW-FIBER DIET AND AVOIDING DIFFICULT-TO-DIGEST FOODS...

Peel and seed the zucchini and cook until soft, finely grind the black pepper, finely chop the parsley (do not include stems), and peel the tomatoes (see page 169).

Nutrients Per Serving	
Calories	242
Fat	2 g
Fiber	3 g
Protein	9 g
Carbohydrate	46 g

Pasta with Roasted Vegetables and Goat Cheese

This dish is a great way to increase your vegetable intake. Prepare the recipe with the ingredients here or with any favorite vegetables. Leftovers are delicious served cold or reheated for lunch the next day.

- *Preheat oven to 425°F (220°C)*
- *Large rimmed baking sheet, greased*

4 cups	cubed zucchini	1 L
2 cups	cubed eggplant	500 mL
2 cups	coarsely chopped red bell peppers	500 mL
1 cup	coarsely chopped sweet white or red onions	250 mL
2 tbsp	olive oil	30 mL
1½ tsp	dried Italian seasoning or French herbs	7 mL
8 oz	rotini, penne or other pasta	250 g
3½ to 4 oz	soft crumbled goat cheese	100 to 125 g
	Freshly grated Parmesan cheese (optional)	

1. Combine zucchini, eggplant, peppers and onions in a large bowl. Add oil and Italian seasoning; toss to coat. Place vegetables in a single layer on prepared baking sheet; roast in preheated oven, stirring occasionally, for 30 to 40 minutes or until vegetables are golden and slightly softened.

2. Meanwhile, in a pot of boiling water, cook pasta according to package directions or until tender but firm; drain.

3. Toss vegetables with pasta. Sprinkle goat cheese over top; toss to combine or leave as is and sprinkle with Parmesan cheese, if desired.

IF FOLLOWING A LOW-FIBER DIET AND AVOIDING DIFFICULT-TO-DIGEST FOODS...

Peel and seed zucchini and eggplant, peel and finely chop red peppers, finely chop onions, and roast vegetables until soft. If using fresh herbs, finely chop leaves and do not include stems.

MAKES 4 SERVINGS

Tip

- Vegetables can be roasted up to 1 day in advance. Reheat in a hot oven for 5 to 10 minutes or until piping hot.

IBD Tip

- Goat cheese does contain lactose, despite some claims that individuals with lactose intolerance can eat goat cheese but not cheese made from cow's milk. But it may not be an "all or nothing" situation — you may be able to tolerate some lactose, just not a lot.

Nutrients Per Serving	
Calories	395
Fat	13 g
Fiber	6 g
Protein	14 g
Carbohydrate	56 g

Vegetarian choice

Higher-calorie choice

Lower-fat choice

Higher-protein choice

Source of potassium

MAKES 6 SERVINGS

Tip

- In the refrigerator, basil only keeps for a day or two. So try to buy basil no earlier than a day before you need it. Don't wash the leaves; just put the basil in a paper bag (or perforated plastic bag). Basil also bruises easily — quickly turning from a beautiful green to an ugly brown-black color — so don't chop it until just before you're ready to add it to the recipe.

IBD Tips

- This recipe is appropriate for vegetarians who eat dairy.

- Tomatoes provide the potassium in this recipe.

- Feta cheese is high in salt. To further increase sodium, boil pasta in salted water and use commercial roasted tomato sauce in place of the plum tomatoes.

Nutrients Per Serving	
Calories	310
Fat	7 g
Fiber	3 g
Protein	12 g
Carbohydrate	49 g

Roasted Garlic and Tomatoes with Ricotta Cheese over Rotini

- *Preheat oven to 450°F (230°C)*
- *Baking sheet, lined with foil*

1	head garlic, top ½ inch (1 cm) cut off, loosely wrapped in foil	1
5	large ripe plum tomatoes, cut in half crosswise	5
½ cup	5% ricotta cheese	125 mL
2 oz	feta cheese, crumbled	60 g
½ cup	chopped fresh basil (or 1 tsp/5 mL dried)	125 mL
1 tbsp	olive oil	15 mL
½ tsp	freshly ground black pepper	2 mL
12 oz	rotini	375 g

1. Place garlic and tomatoes on prepared baking sheet. Roast in preheated oven for 30 minutes or until tomatoes are charred; let cool. Squeeze garlic out of skins.

2. In a food processor or blender, combine roasted tomatoes (with their juices) and garlic; pulse on and off several times until combined but still chunky. Transfer mixture to a bowl; add ricotta cheese, feta cheese, basil, olive oil and pepper. Set aside.

3. In a large pot of boiling water, cook rotini for 8 to 10 minutes or until tender but firm; drain. In a serving bowl, combine pasta and sauce; toss well. Serve immediately.

IF FOLLOWING A LOW-FIBER DIET AND AVOIDING DIFFICULT-TO-DIGEST FOODS...

Peel and seed tomatoes (see page 169), finely chop basil (do not include stems) or use dried, and finely grind the black pepper.

Roasted Red Pepper and Ricotta Purée over Rotini

Higher-calorie choice

Lower-fat choice

Lower-fiber choice

Higher-protein choice

• *Preheat oven to broil*

12 oz	rotini	375 g
1	medium sweet red bell pepper	1
1²/₃ cups	ricotta cheese	400 mL
2 tbsp	vegetable oil	30 mL
½ cup	chicken stock	125 mL
2 tbsp	freshly grated Parmesan cheese	30 mL
1½ tsp	crushed garlic	7 mL
½ cup	chopped basil (or 2 tsp/10 mL dried)	125 mL
	Parsley	

MAKES 6 SERVINGS

Tips

• The skin of sweet peppers will come off easily if, after broiling, you place the peppers in a plastic or paper bag for 10 minutes, then peel.

• Prepare sauce early in day. Pasta must be hot before adding sauce.

IBD Tips

• Canned chicken stock provides more sodium than homemade.

• Choose heart-healthy canola oil or olive oil in this recipe.

1. Broil pepper until charred on all sides, approximately 15 minutes. Let cool; remove top, then skin, seed and cut into quarters. Set aside.

2. Cook pasta in boiling water according to package instructions or until firm to the bite. Drain and place in serving bowl.

3. In food processor, purée ricotta cheese, red pepper, oil, stock, Parmesan cheese, garlic and basil until well combined. Pour over pasta. Toss and garnish with parsley.

IF FOLLOWING A LOW-FIBER DIET AND AVOIDING DIFFICULT-TO-DIGEST FOODS...

Finely chop the basil and parsley (do not include stems) or use dried.

Nutrients Per Serving	
Calories	368
Fat	10 g
Fiber	2 g
Protein	18 g
Carbohydrate	51 g

MAKES 6 SERVINGS

Tip

• Prepare sauce early in day. Reheat gently, adding more stock if sauce becomes too dense.

IBD Tips

• Carrots and sweet potatoes provide beta carotene, a powerful antioxidant.

• Rainbow tortellini filled with cheese also works well in this recipe. The pasta is usually colored by tomato or spinach powder and is filled with ricotta, Romano and Parmesan cheeses.

• To reduce saturated fat, choose non-hydrogenated margarine instead of butter.

• Commercial chicken or vegetable stock provides more sodium than homemade.

Nutrients Per Serving	
Calories	296
Fat	9 g
Fiber	3 g
Protein	12 g
Carbohydrate	42 g

Spinach Cheese Tortellini in Puréed Vegetable Sauce

1 lb	cheese and/or spinach tortellini	500 g
1 tbsp	margarine or butter	15 mL
1 tsp	crushed garlic	5 mL
1 cup	finely diced carrots	250 mL
1 cup	finely diced zucchini	250 mL
1½ cups	chicken or vegetable stock	375 mL
⅓ cup	chopped fresh basil (or 1½ tsp/ 7 mL dried)	75 mL
2 tbsp	freshly grated Parmesan cheese	30 mL

1. Cook pasta in boiling water according to package instructions or until firm to the bite. Drain and place in serving bowl.

2. In a small nonstick skillet, melt margarine; add garlic, carrots and zucchini. Cook until tender, approximately 8 minutes. Add stock and basil; simmer on medium heat for 5 minutes. Purée in food processor on and off for 30 seconds. Pour over pasta. Add cheese, and toss.

Variation

You can substitute sweet potatoes for carrots.

IF FOLLOWING A LOW-FIBER DIET AND AVOIDING DIFFICULT-TO-DIGEST FOODS...

Choose spinach-*flavored* pasta rather than spinach-*filled* tortellini, peel and seed the zucchini, and finely chop the basil (do not include stems) or use dried. Because the carrots and zucchini in the sauce are puréed, it is not as important to cook them until soft.

Stuffed Pasta Shells

In this dish, which is perfect for entertaining, jumbo pasta shells are stuffed with ricotta, Cheddar-style and Parmesan cheeses, sun-dried tomatoes and herbs, then baked in a creamy sauce. Make it the centerpiece of a delicious meal.

- *Preheat oven to 350°F (180°C)*
- *13- by 9-inch (33 by 23 cm) baking dish*

2	cloves garlic	2
1/4 cup	chopped onion	60 mL
1 tbsp	olive oil	15 mL
1	can (14 oz/398 mL) tomato sauce	1
2 cups	5% ricotta cheese	500 mL
3/4 cup	shredded lower-fat medium Cheddar-style cheese, divided	175 mL
1/2 cup	freshly grated Parmesan cheese, divided	125 mL
1/4 cup	diced sun-dried tomatoes	60 mL
2 tbsp	chopped fresh basil	30 mL
3 tbsp	chopped fresh parsley	45 mL
1 tbsp	finely chopped green onions	15 mL
1 tsp	coarsely ground black pepper	5 mL
1	egg, lightly beaten	1
24	jumbo pasta shells, cooked and drained	24
1 2/3 cups	2% milk, divided	400 mL
5 tsp	cornstarch	30 mL
1/2 tsp	salt	2 mL

1. In a saucepan, sauté garlic and onion in oil until tender. Add tomato sauce; simmer over low heat for 8 to 10 minutes or until reduced slightly. Pour into 13- by 9-inch (3 L) baking dish.

2. Combine ricotta, 1/2 cup (125 mL) of the Cheddar, 1/4 cup (60 mL) of the Parmesan, tomatoes, basil, 2 tbsp (30 mL) of the parsley, onions, 1/2 tsp (2 mL) of the pepper and egg. Spoon into pasta shells and arrange in single layer over sauce.

3. In a saucepan, heat 1 1/2 cups (375 mL) of the milk. Whisk cornstarch into remaining milk; whisk into hot milk and cook, stirring, until sauce thickens and boils. Stir in salt and remaining Parmesan, parsley and pepper; cool for 5 minutes. Pour over prepared shells. Cover with foil.

4. Bake in preheated oven for 40 to 45 minutes or until hot and bubbly. Remove foil and sprinkle with remaining Cheddar; bake just until cheese melts.

Vegetarian choice

Higher-calorie choice

Lower-fiber choice

Higher-protein choice

Source of potassium

Source of sodium

MAKES 8 SERVINGS

IBD Tips

- Tomato sauce is rich in potassium.
- Cheese, canned tomato sauce and added salt boost sodium in this recipe.

IF YOU ARE WELL...

Add drained thawed chopped spinach to the ricotta cheese mixture as a variation.

IF FOLLOWING A LOW-FIBER DIET...

Finely chop the onion, choose plain tomato sauce, use sun-dried tomato paste or omit the sun-dried tomatoes, finely chop the basil and parsley (do not include stems), and finely grind the black pepper.

Nutrients Per Serving	
Calories	309
Fat	11 g
Fiber	2 g
Protein	19 g
Carbohydrate	32 g

Vegetarian choice

Lower-fat choice

Lower-fiber choice

Higher-protein choice

Source of potassium

Source of sodium

MAKES 6 SERVINGS

Tips

• Once unpackaged, tofu should be stored in the refrigerator in water to cover. To keep tofu fresh for as long as a week, change the water daily.

IBD Tips

• This recipe is appropriate for vegetarians who eat dairy.

• Part-skim mozzarella cheese has less saturated fat and calories than regular mozzarella.

• Tomatoes are rich in potassium; tofu also contributes some.

• To boost sodium, use commercial tomato sauce and canned mushrooms and boil the pasta in salted water.

Nutrients Per Serving	
Calories	117
Fat	2 g
Fiber	2 g
Protein	11 g
Carbohydrate	16 g

Lasagna Roll-Ups

Here's a great lasagna recipe for any vegetarians in your family or circle of friends.

• *Preheat oven to 350°F (180°C)*
• *8-inch (20 cm) square baking pan*

2	large cloves garlic, minced	2
1 tsp	olive oil	5 mL
2 cups	chopped mushrooms	500 mL
½ cup	diced red bell pepper	125 mL
1 tsp	dried thyme	5 mL
1 tsp	fennel seed	5 mL
¼ tsp	salt	1 mL
Pinch	freshly ground black pepper	Pinch
4 oz	firm tofu, drained and crumbled	125 g
2 cups	tomato sauce	500 mL
6	cooked lasagna noodles	6
1 cup	shredded part-skim mozzarella cheese	250 mL

1. In a large skillet over medium-high heat, cook garlic in hot oil for about 2 minutes. Add mushrooms, red pepper and seasonings; cook over high heat, stirring constantly, for about 5 minutes or until liquid evaporates and vegetables are tender. Add tofu.

2. Spoon half of the tomato sauce into bottom of 8-inch (2 L) square baking pan. Spread about ⅓ cup (75 mL) mushroom mixture over each cooked noodle. Divide cheese evenly over filling on each noodle. Roll up, jelly roll–style. Arrange rolls seam side down in baking dish. Spoon remaining tomato sauce over rolls.

3. Cover and bake in preheated oven for 15 minutes; remove cover and bake for about 10 minutes.

> **IF FOLLOWING A LOW-FIBER DIET AND AVOIDING DIFFICULT-TO-DIGEST FOODS...**
>
> Finely chop, purée or omit the mushrooms, peel the red pepper before dicing, use ground fennel seed, and finely grind the black pepper.

Side Dishes

When we think of side dishes, we usually think of recipes based on vegetables or grains, both of which are powerhouses of nutrition. Vegetables provide carbohydrate, fiber, B vitamins such as folate, vitamins A and C, potassium, magnesium and antioxidants. Most are low in calories and fat. Rice, barley and couscous provide complex carbohydrate, protein, fiber, riboflavin, thiamin, niacin, iron and magnesium. They are low in fat (and the little they do have is mostly polyunsaturated) and have no cholesterol.

The variety of vegetables available in the marketplace makes it easy to incorporate color, flavor and texture into meals, thereby making them more appetizing. However, most people consume far less than the recommended amount of vegetables on a daily basis. Individuals living with IBD often want to eat vegetables, but are apprehensive based on past experiences. The recipes in this chapter have been carefully chosen because they are easy to prepare, contain desirable ingredients that are generally tolerated, and convert easily to a low-fiber version.

Maximize the Nutritional Value of Vegetables

The nutritional value of a vegetable is affected by how it is stored and prepared, and how long it is exposed to air, heat or water. Flavor, texture and appearance are also affected. Most vegetables can be eaten raw, and if they are fresh their nutritional value is maximal. Some vegetables are more tasty and easily digested when cooked, but cooking decreases water-soluble vitamin content, so it is important to cook vegetables for as short a time as possible. Nutrient losses can be limited by cooking vegetables at a high temperature for a short time (e.g., in a pressure cooker) or steaming using the microwave.

Frozen and canned vegetables still provide good-quality nutrients and are considered an acceptable healthy and convenient option. Canned vegetables are softer because they are cooked during processing, so a relatively short reheating time is needed. Frozen vegetables, when properly blanched and frozen, are comparable in nutritional value to fresh.

Canned vegetables are easy to store and add to meals quickly. Most brands are also high in salt, so they can help replenish sodium losses from loose stool or an ileostomy.

To preserve vitamin content when boiling vegetables, add them to the water after it is boiling.

Go for Green and Orange!

Try to eat at least one dark green and one orange vegetable each day. Choose vegetables prepared with little or no added fat, sugar or salt, unless you are specifically targeting these additives for health reasons. Select fresh, frozen, canned, juiced or dried vegetables, depending on your disease status. If you are following a low-fiber diet, try green vegetables such as canned asparagus tips or canned green peas for folate. Choose orange vegetables such as soft cooked carrots, squash or sweet potato or canned pumpkin purée for carotenoids, which your body converts to vitamin A.

HOW TO TRANSITION FROM A FIBER-RESTRICTED DIET TO YOUR REGULAR DIET

Begin by choosing the fruits and vegetables you have missed eating the most. Start with one at a time and eat small portions, then slowly increase the amount back to your usual portion size. Begin with fully cooked vegetables, then try tender-crisp vegetables, and finally move on to raw vegetables. Concentrate on chewing your food well and take the time to discover what foods are more difficult for you to digest. Gradually, you'll become more confident about what foods you can safely incorporate into your diet.

Keep vegetables in the vegetable crisper of your fridge. The crisper is less cold and more humid than upper shelves, which helps prevent vegetables from drying out.

Tangy Green Beans

A robust citrus vinaigrette combined with subtle-tasting green beans makes for a great combination of flavors.

1 tbsp	sesame oil	15 mL
3 cups	chopped trimmed green beans (1-inch/2.5 cm pieces)	750 mL

Citrus Vinaigrette

1 tbsp	grated orange zest	15 mL
⅓ cup	freshly squeezed orange juice	75 mL
⅓ cup	rice vinegar	75 mL
¼ cup	vegetable oil	60 mL
¼ tsp	Dijon mustard	1 mL
2	cloves garlic, minced (about 2 tsp/10 mL)	2
¼ tsp	grated gingerroot	1 mL

1. *Prepare the vinaigrette:* In a serving bowl, whisk together orange zest and juice, rice vinegar, oil, mustard, garlic and ginger. Set aside.
2. In a nonstick skillet, heat sesame oil over medium heat for 1 minute. Add green beans, reduce heat to low and cook, stirring, for 3 to 4 minutes or until coated and bright green. Add vinaigrette and toss well. Let stand for 5 minutes or until flavors are blended. Serve immediately.

Variation

If you're trying to reduce your dietary fat intake, steam the beans for 3 to 4 minutes instead of frying them and omit the sesame oil. Toss with vinaigrette as directed.

IF FOLLOWING A LOW-FIBER DIET AND AVOIDING DIFFICULT-TO-DIGEST FOODS...

Trim the ends off the green beans and pull off stringy veins, then boil until soft (or use canned beans).

Vegan choice

Higher-calorie choice

Lower-fiber choice

Lactose-free choice

MAKES 4 SERVINGS

IBD Tips

- Orange juice is rich in potassium, but the amount in this recipe is relatively small.

- Zest is the outer skin of a citrus fruit such as an orange or lemon. The oils it contains add a strong flavor to foods. However, the white membrane under the zest is usually bitter, so don't scrape too deep with your grater or peeler.

- Choose canola oil or olive oil for their favorable fatty acid profiles. Canola oil is a plant source of omega-3 fat, and olive oil is a high source of monounsaturated fat.

Nutrients Per Serving	
Calories	201
Fat	18 g
Fiber	2 g
Protein	1 g
Carbohydrate	8 g

MAKES 4 SERVINGS

IBD Tips

- Carrots are high in beta carotene, an antioxidant.
- Carrots are a source of potassium; while orange juice is rich in potassium, the amount used in this recipe is small.
- If you use margarine, this recipe is a lactose-free choice.

Honey-Glazed Carrots

1 lb	carrots, cut into 1-inch (2.5 cm) pieces	500 g
1 tbsp	liquid honey or brown sugar	15 mL
1 tbsp	orange juice	15 mL
2 tsp	butter or margarine	10 mL
1/2 tsp	ground ginger	2 mL
1/2 tsp	grated orange zest (optional)	2 mL

1. In a medium saucepan over high heat, boil carrots until tender-crisp; drain. Add honey, orange juice, butter, ginger and, if using, orange zest. Quickly stir for 2 to 3 minutes or until glaze forms.

> **IF FOLLOWING A LOW-FIBER DIET AND AVOIDING DIFFICULT-TO-DIGEST FOODS...**
> Cook the carrots until soft.

Nutrients Per Serving	
Calories	77
Fat	2 g
Fiber	2 g
Protein	1 g
Carbohydrate	16 g

Ginger Carrots

Here's a delicious way to enjoy carrots that provides an excellent source of vitamin A.

4 cups	chopped carrots	1 L
½ cup	vegetable or chicken stock	125 mL
2 tsp	minced gingerroot	10 mL
1 tsp	minced garlic	5 mL
1 tsp	packed brown sugar	5 mL
¼ tsp	freshly squeezed lemon juice	1 mL

1. In a large saucepan, combine carrots, stock, ginger, garlic, brown sugar and lemon juice. Bring to a boil, then reduce heat, cover and simmer for about 20 minutes or until carrots are tender-crisp and liquid is absorbed.

IF FOLLOWING A LOW-FIBER DIET AND AVOIDING DIFFICULT-TO-DIGEST FOODS...

Cook the carrots until soft so they can be easily chewed well.

Vegan choice

Lower-calorie choice

Lower-fat choice

Lower-fiber choice

Lactose-free choice

Source of sodium

MAKES 6 SERVINGS

IBD Tips

- Commercial vegetable stock and chicken stock provide sodium (unless labeled "no-salt-added").

- Minced gingerroot is available at most grocery stores. Ginger aids digestion and, for some, may improve appetite and reduce nausea. If mincing your own gingerroot, use the side of a spoon to scrape off the skin first. Gingerroot keeps well in the freezer for up to 3 months and can be grated from frozen.

- Carrots are high in beta carotene, an antioxidant, and moderately high in potassium.

Nutrients Per Serving	
Calories	41
Fat	0 g
Fiber	3 g
Protein	1 g
Carbohydrate	10 g

MAKES 3 TO 4 SERVINGS

Tip

- If some of the skin adheres to the flesh after the peppers have cooled, use your fingers to peel it off.

IBD Tips

- This recipe is appropriate for a low-fiber diet because the skins of the peppers are removed. Be sure to finely grind the black pepper.

- Red bell peppers have more beta carotene and vitamin C than yellow or green bell peppers.

Roasted Bell Peppers

These multipurpose peppers are always great to have on hand, as they can be used in a number of recipes. Use a variety of colored peppers, such as yellow, red, orange and green, to add vibrancy to pasta sauces and salads or to use in one of the variations below.

- *Preheat oven to 350°F (180°C)*
- *13- by 9-inch (33 by 23 cm) baking dish, greased*

3	bell peppers, seeds and ribs removed, quartered	3
2 tbsp	garlic-infused oil	30 mL
1 tbsp	garlic powder	15 mL
	Salt and freshly ground black pepper	

1. Place peppers in prepared baking dish. Brush both sides of each pepper piece with garlic oil and sprinkle with garlic powder and salt and pepper to taste. Bake for 45 to 50 minutes or until very soft and wrinkled.

2. Transfer to a bowl, cover with a plate and let cool to room temperature. The skins will naturally separate from the flesh of the pepper (see tip, at left). Store in an airtight container and refrigerate for up to 4 days.

Variations

Balsamic Marinated Peppers: Cut peeled roasted peppers into quarters. Add ½ cup (125 mL) balsamic vinegar and toss to coat. Cover and refrigerate for 8 hours or for up to 1 week.

Garlic Marinated Peppers: Toss peeled roasted peppers with 2 cloves garlic, thinly sliced, and ¼ cup (60 mL) extra-virgin olive oil. Marinate for several hours or overnight, then remove the garlic. Add sea salt and freshly ground black pepper to taste and serve immediately.

Nutrients Per Serving	
Calories	90
Fat	7 g
Fiber	2 g
Protein	1 g
Carbohydrate	7 g

Stewed Okra

A staple of Southern cooking, okra is the magical ingredient that can be used to thicken gumbo or, when breaded and deep fried, served as a crunchy snack. This okra recipe concentrates on the sweet-tart taste of okra itself.

2	tomatoes	2
1 lb	okra	500 g
2 tbsp	butter (optional)	30 mL
1 tbsp	olive oil	15 mL
½ tsp	hot pepper flakes	2 mL
4	cloves garlic, thinly sliced	4
½ tsp	freshly ground black pepper	2 mL
1 cup	water	250 mL
1 tbsp	freshly squeezed lime juice	15 mL
½ tsp	salt	2 mL
	Few sprigs fresh coriander, chopped	

1. Blanch tomatoes in boiling water for 30 seconds. Over a bowl, peel, core and deseed them. Chop tomatoes into chunks and set aside. Strain any accumulated tomato juices from bowl; add the juices to the tomatoes.

2. With a sharp knife, trim ¼ inch (0.5 cm) from the okra stems. Cut a vertical slit, 1 inch (2.5 cm) long, through the bellies of the okras, taking care not to slice them in half.

3. In a large frying pan, heat butter, if using, and oil over high heat until sizzling. Add hot pepper flakes and stir-fry for 30 seconds. Add okras and fry, actively tossing and turning for about 5 minutes, until they are scorched on both sides. Add garlic and black pepper; toss-fry for just under 1 minute until the garlic is frying (but before it burns).

4. Immediately add reserved tomato and tomato juice. Stir-fry for 1 minute until the tomato is beginning to fry. Add water and stir until it begins to boil around the okras. Reduce heat to simmer and cook for 20 minutes, gently folding and stirring every few minutes. (The okras will become increasingly tender and the sauce will thicken.)

5. Sprinkle okra with lime juice and salt. Gently fold and stir for under a minute and remove from heat. Transfer to a serving dish and garnish with chopped coriander. The okra can be served immediately but will improve if allowed to rest for about 30 minutes.

Vegan choice

Lower-calorie choice

Lactose-free choice

Source of soluble fiber

Source of potassium

MAKES 4 SERVINGS

IBD Tips

- Okra is not typically found in low-fiber diets, but can be included if eaten in small amounts and cooked until the seeds are very soft. You can also use canned okra.

- Okra has thickening properties and is often used in soups and stews. It is a source of soluble fiber.

- Okra and tomatoes provide potassium.

IF FOLLOWING A LOW-FIBER DIET...

Finely grind the black pepper, use ground hot pepper, and finely chop the coriander (do not include stems). If you experience soreness in the anal area from frequent loose stools, you may want to omit the hot pepper flakes.

Nutrients Per Serving

Calories	88
Fat	4 g
Fiber	4 g
Protein	3 g
Carbohydrate	12 g

Vegetarian choice

Lower-calorie choice

Lower-fat choice

Higher-protein choice

Source of sodium

MAKES 8 SERVINGS

Tip

- If there is not enough soup for the amount of vegetables, add a little water.

IBD Tips

- This recipe is appropriate for a low-fiber diet, as long as the cauliflower is cooked until soft. Cauliflower and broccoli are gas-producing, so start with small portions.

- Cauliflower is a member of the anticarcinogenic cabbage family and can be found in white, orange and purple varieties.

- Boost calories by choosing full-fat soup and mozzarella.

Nutrients Per Serving	
Calories	70
Fat	1 g
Fiber	3 g
Protein	7 g
Carbohydrate	8 g

Cauliflower au Gratin

A simple way of preparing cauliflower that can be put together in a flash.

- *Preheat oven to 350°F (180°C)*
- *9-inch (23 cm) casserole dish with cover, lightly greased*

1	large cauliflower, cut into florets	1
1	green onion, finely chopped	1
1	can (10 oz/284 mL) condensed reduced-fat cream of broccoli soup, undiluted	1
1 cup	shredded skim-milk mozzarella cheese	250 mL

1. Bring 6 cups (1.5 L) water to a boil. Drop cauliflower into boiling water and cook for 2 minutes; drain well.

2. Place cauliflower in prepared casserole dish and sprinkle with green onion. Stir in soup. Sprinkle with cheese.

3. Cover and bake in preheated oven for 20 minutes or until cauliflower is tender and cheese is melted. Uncover and broil until cheese is browned.

IF YOU ARE WELL...

If there is no medical reason for you to avoid fiber or difficult-to-digest foods, you can substitute broccoli for the cauliflower.

Cheesy Broccoli and Potato Casserole

- *Preheat oven to 350°F (180°C)*
- *8-cup (2 L) baking dish, lightly greased*

6	potatoes, cubed	6
¼ cup	2% milk	60 mL
1 tsp	butter or margarine	5 mL
½ tsp	freshly ground white pepper	2 mL
½ tsp	dried parsley	2 mL
2 cups	broccoli florets	500 mL
1	small onion, sliced	1
1 cup	shredded old Cheddar cheese	250 mL

1. In a large saucepan, cook potatoes in boiling water until tender; drain well. Mash potatoes with milk, butter and seasonings.

2. Meanwhile, steam broccoli and onion until barely tender, or microwave on High for 5 to 8 minutes.

3. Spread potato mixture in lightly greased 8-cup (2 L) baking dish; top with broccoli, onion and cheese. Bake, covered, in preheated oven for 10 minutes; remove cover and bake for 5 minutes longer or until cheese is melted. Or microwave, covered, on High for about 8 minutes.

IF FOLLOWING A LOW-FIBER DIET AND AVOIDING DIFFICULT-TO-DIGEST FOODS...

Peel the potatoes, finely chop the onion and steam until soft, and omit the broccoli or substitute a cooked or canned lower-fiber vegetable such as cauliflower florets or asparagus tips.

Vegetarian choice

Higher-calorie choice

Higher-protein choice

Source of potassium

MAKES 6 SERVINGS

Tip

- This creamy, fiber-rich casserole can be served with plainer meats such as grilled chicken. Made with cheese and milk, it is a great way to add calcium to your diet. If you are lactose-intolerant, use lactose-reduced milk or a fortified soy beverage.

IBD Tips

- Potatoes are rich in potassium; broccoli also supplies some.

- Don't skip this recipe just because it's made with broccoli! If you are well and there is no medical reason for you to avoid fiber or difficult-to-digest foods, include broccoli in your diet. Broccoli is a source of beta carotene, vitamins C and E, folate, calcium and potassium.

Nutrients Per Serving	
Calories	223
Fat	7 g
Fiber	4 g
Protein	9 g
Carbohydrate	32 g

MAKES 6 TO 8 SERVINGS

Tips

- Substitute sweet potato for squash.

- For a gingerbread taste, try adding 1 tbsp (15 mL) molasses and reducing maple syrup to 3 tbsp (45 mL).

- Egg whites can now be purchased in containers at grocery stores.

- Prepare recipe to end of step 1 up to 2 days in advance.

- Can be baked early in the day and reheated.

IBD Tips

- Butternut squash is rich in beta carotene and potassium. The cream-colored skin is easy to remove.

- To boost calories, use full-fat sour cream.

- If you use margarine, this recipe is a lactose-free choice.

Nutrients Per Serving	
Calories	99
Fat	3 g
Fiber	0 g
Protein	3 g
Carbohydrate	17 g

Butternut Squash with Maple Syrup

- *Preheat oven to 350°F (180°C)*
- *8-inch (20 cm) square baking dish, sprayed with vegetable spray*

1 lb	diced peeled butternut squash	500 g
1/3 cup	dried bread crumbs	75 mL
1/4 cup	light sour cream	60 mL
1/4 cup	maple syrup	60 mL
2 tsp	margarine or butter	10 mL
2 tsp	grated orange zest	10 mL
3/4 tsp	ground cinnamon	4 mL
1/4 tsp	ground ginger	1 mL
3	eggs, separated	3
1/2 cup	canned corn kernels, drained	125 mL
Pinch	salt	Pinch

1. In a pot of boiling water, cook squash for 8 minutes or until tender; drain. Put in a food processor along with bread crumbs, sour cream, maple syrup, margarine, orange zest, cinnamon, ginger and 2 egg yolks. (Discard third egg yolk.) Process until smooth. Transfer to a large bowl; cool. Add corn.

2. In a bowl, with an electric mixer, beat 3 egg whites with salt until stiff peaks form. Stir one-quarter of egg whites into squash mixture. Gently fold remaining egg whites into squash mixture. Pour into prepared pan. Bake 25 minutes or until set.

IF FOLLOWING A LOW-FIBER DIET AND AVOIDING DIFFICULT-TO-DIGEST FOODS...

Use white bread crumbs, and omit the corn kernels.

Crispy Sweet Potato Cakes

Sweet potatoes, which are loaded with beta carotene, are delicious when made into a crispy cake.

1 lb	sweet potato, peeled and grated	500 g
1 tbsp	finely chopped fresh basil	15 mL
1 tbsp	chopped fresh Italian parsley	15 mL
1 tbsp	orange juice	15 mL
½ tsp	salt	2 mL
¼ tsp	freshly ground black pepper	1 mL
3 tbsp	all-purpose flour, divided	45 mL
	Vegetable oil for frying	
	Salt (optional)	

1. In a bowl, combine sweet potato, basil, parsley, orange juice, salt and pepper. Set aside for 15 minutes to draw out juices. Sprinkle 1 tbsp (15 mL) flour over top and stir well. Divide mixture into 12 equal portions.

2. Lightly dust work surface with 1 tbsp (15 mL) of the remaining flour. Place portions of sweet potato mixture on the work surface. Using hands, roll each into a ball. Sprinkle with remaining flour, evenly covering the outside of each ball.

3. Into a large skillet, pour oil to a depth of ¼ inch (0.5 cm). Heat over high heat for 30 seconds or until hot but not smoking. Working in batches as necessary, place balls in skillet, about 2 inches (5 cm) apart. Using a metal spatula, press each flat into a patty shape. Reduce heat to medium-high and cook, turning and checking bottoms to ensure even cooking, for 2 to 3 minutes per side or until well browned and crispy. Transfer to a paper towel–lined plate and keep warm. Repeat with remaining cakes, adding and heating oil as necessary between batches.

4. Sprinkle with salt, if using, before serving. Serve immediately or let cool, cover and refrigerate for up to 3 days. Reheat in 375°F (190°C) oven for 10 minutes.

Variations

Make these cakes using equal amounts of sweet potato and another vegetable. Mix 8 oz (250 g) white potatoes, carrots, parsnips or turnips, peeled and grated, with 8 oz (250 g) sweet potato.

If you like the taste of orange, add ½ tsp (2 mL) grated orange zest to the mixture.

Vegan choice

Lower-calorie choice

Lower-fat choice

Lactose-free choice

Source of potassium

MAKES 4 TO 6 SERVINGS

Tip

- One large or 2 small sweet potatoes weigh about 1 lb (500 g).

IBD Tip

- Sweet potatoes are rich in potassium and beta carotene. Orange juice is also rich in potassium, but the amount used in this recipe is small.

IF FOLLOWING A LOW-FIBER DIET...

Finely chop the basil and parsley (do not include stems), finely grind the black pepper, and adjust cooking time to make sure the grated sweet potatoes are soft. To further reduce fiber, try a mixture of grated sweet potatoes and regular potatoes.

Nutrients Per Serving	
Calories	97
Fat	Trace
Fiber	3 g
Protein	2 g
Carbohydrate	22 g

Sweet Potato Fries

When you sub in sweet potatoes for the potatoes and bake them instead of frying, fries actually become good for you as well as delicious!

MAKES 4 SERVINGS

IBD Tips

- This recipe is suitable for vegetarians who eat dairy, and is easily converted to vegan if the cheese is omitted.

- To boost calories in this recipe, add more oil. Boost the sodium by adding a liberal amount of salt.

- Sweet potatoes are a high source of potassium and the antioxidant beta carotene.

- If you are sensitive to the milk sugar lactose, you may still be able to tolerate aged hard cheeses such as Parmesan and Romano, as they have relatively small amounts of lactose.

- *Preheat oven to 350°F (180°C)*
- *Rimmed baking sheet, lined with parchment paper*

1 lb	sweet potatoes, peeled and cut into ¼-inch (0.5 cm) thick slices	500 g
2 tsp	grapeseed oil	10 mL
2 tbsp	grated Romano cheese	30 mL
	Salt and freshly ground black pepper	

1. In a large bowl, toss sweet potatoes, oil and cheese until sweet potatoes are well coated. Spread out in a single layer on prepared baking sheet.

2. Bake in preheated oven for 20 to 30 minutes, turning halfway through, until crispy and golden. Season to taste with salt and pepper.

> **IF FOLLOWING A LOW-FIBER DIET AND AVOIDING DIFFICULT-TO-DIGEST FOODS...**
>
> Be sure to finely grind the black pepper. This recipe already calls for the sweet potatoes to be peeled.

Nutrients Per Serving	
Calories	120
Fat	3 g
Fiber	3 g
Protein	3 g
Carbohydrate	20 g

Baked French Wedge Potatoes

These "french fries" beat those cooked in lots of oil. Children and adults can't stop eating them. Try different spices.

- *Preheat oven to 375°F (190°C)*
- *Baking sheet, sprayed with nonstick vegetable spray*

4	potatoes, unpeeled	4
2 tbsp	margarine, melted	30 mL
1/2 tsp	chili powder	2 mL
1/2 tsp	dried basil	2 mL
1 tsp	crushed garlic	5 mL
1 1/2 tsp	chopped fresh parsley	7 mL
1 tbsp	freshly grated Parmesan cheese	15 mL

1. Scrub potatoes; cut each into 8 wedges. Place on baking sheet.

2. In small bowl, combine margarine, chili powder, basil, garlic and parsley; brush half over potatoes. Sprinkle with half of the Parmesan; bake for 30 minutes. Turn wedges over; brush with remaining mixture and sprinkle with remaining cheese. Bake for 30 minutes longer.

IF FOLLOWING A LOW-FIBER DIET AND AVOIDING DIFFICULT-TO-DIGEST FOODS...

Peel the potatoes, and finely chop the parsley (do not include stems).

MAKES 6 SERVINGS

Tip

- Potatoes should be firm, heavy and smooth. Keep in a cool place for 2 to 3 weeks where there is ventilation to keep them dry.

IBD Tips

- Don't be afraid to experiment with herbs and spices. Chili powder adds great flavor and should be avoided only if necessary during times of illness or when you are experiencing anal soreness from frequent loose stools.

- If you are sensitive to lactose, you may still be able to tolerate Parmesan, as it has a relatively small amount of lactose.

- Potatoes pack the potassium in this recipe.

Nutrients Per Serving	
Calories	127
Fat	4 g
Fiber	2 g
Protein	2 g
Carbohydrate	21 g

MAKES 8 SERVINGS

Tips

- For a change, try using Swiss instead of Cheddar cheese.

- Want to bake potatoes in a hurry? Use your microwave! A medium potato (6 to 8 oz/175 to 250 g) takes only 3 to 4 minutes to cook on High. Pierce with a fork before cooking. Let stand for 2 minutes to soften before serving. Alternatively, you can start baked potatoes in the microwave and crisp them up in a toaster oven or on the barbecue.

IBD Tips

- Potatoes are rich in potassium.

- Canned soup and cheese are sources of sodium.

- If you're trying to gain weight, select full-fat canned soup, milk and cheese. Otherwise, choose lower-fat versions.

Nutrients Per Serving	
Calories	149
Fat	5 g
Fiber	1 g
Protein	5 g
Carbohydrate	22 g

Easy Scalloped Potatoes

- *Preheat oven to 325°F (160°C)*
- *13- by 9-inch (33 by 23 cm) baking dish, greased*

1	can (10 oz/284 mL) condensed cream of celery soup	1
1¼ cups	milk (1 full soup can)	300 mL
½ cup	sliced onion	125 mL
3 cups	potatoes, cut into ¼-inch (5 mm) thick slices	750 mL
½ cup	shredded Cheddar cheese	125 mL
	Freshly ground black pepper	
	Paprika	

1. In a large bowl, stir together soup, milk, onion and potatoes. Pour into prepared baking dish; sprinkle with cheese. Season with pepper and paprika to taste. Bake in preheated oven for 65 to 75 minutes or until potatoes are tender.

> **IF FOLLOWING A LOW-FIBER DIET AND AVOIDING DIFFICULT-TO-DIGEST FOODS...**
> Finely chop the onion, peel the potatoes, and finely grind the black pepper.

Garlic Mashed Potatoes

The texture of mashed potatoes is really a matter of taste. Some like them smooth, others prefer the odd lump or two. Whichever you prefer, these flavorful potatoes are a great accompaniment to many dishes.

4	large potatoes, peeled and cut in half	4
3 tbsp	soy margarine	45 mL
4	cloves garlic, minced (about 4 tsp/20 mL)	4
1 cup	vanilla-flavor or plain soy milk	250 mL
	Salt and freshly ground black pepper	

1. In a large pot, combine potatoes with cold water to cover, then bring to a boil over high heat. Reduce heat to low and simmer for 25 to 30 minutes or until potatoes are easily pierced with a fork. Drain and return to pot.

2. Meanwhile, in a small saucepan, melt margarine over low heat until bubbling. Add garlic and cook, stirring, for 30 to 60 seconds or until fragrant but not browned. Add soy milk. Increase heat to medium and bring to a boil. Remove from heat and let steep while mashing potatoes.

3. Using a potato masher, mash potatoes. (If you prefer a smoother texture, put the potatoes through a ricer.) Add soy milk mixture, stirring constantly until desired consistency is achieved. Season with salt and pepper to taste. Mix well.

Variation

Add 2 tbsp (30 mL) finely chopped fresh chives or garlic chives along with the soy milk. Serve with vegan sour cream alternative on the side.

> **IF FOLLOWING A LOW-FIBER DIET AND AVOIDING DIFFICULT-TO-DIGEST FOODS...**
>
> Finely grind the black pepper (larger pieces can increase the risk of a food-related obstruction).

Vegan choice

Higher-calorie choice

Lactose-free choice

Source of potassium

MAKES 4 TO 5 SERVINGS

IBD Tips

- If you consume dairy products, substitute regular margarine for soy margarine, cow's milk for soy milk and, in the variation, regular sour cream for vegan sour cream alternative. The recipe will no longer be lactose-free.

- Soy milk provides high-quality protein, has no cholesterol, and contains primarily unsaturated fat. Soy also supplies isoflavones, which are phytonutrients. Most varieties are fortified with calcium and vitamin D, but be sure to shake the carton, as calcium settles at the bottom.

Nutrients Per Serving	
Calories	263
Fat	8 g
Fiber	3 g
Protein	5 g
Carbohydrate	44 g

MAKES 4 TO 6 SERVINGS

Tip

- Depending on the type of stove you have and the kind of pot you are using, the cooking times may vary. Check rice after 30 minutes to see how much of the liquid has been absorbed. If there is liquid left, replace the lid and cook longer, lifting the lid as little as possible.

IBD Tips

- Coconut milk is surprisingly high in saturated fat, and thus calories, but reduced-fat versions are available.

- Most varieties of soy milk are fortified with calcium. Research suggests that calcium carbonate is absorbed as well as the calcium in cow's milk. However, other forms, such as tricalcium phosphate, are not, so you need to drink more to get the same amount of calcium as you'd get from cow's milk.

Nutrients Per Serving	
Calories	187
Fat	16 g
Fiber	Trace
Protein	3 g
Carbohydrate	11 g

Coconut Rice

1	can (14 oz/398 mL) coconut milk	1
½ cup	vanilla-flavor soy milk	125 mL
1 cup	basmati or jasmine rice	250 mL
¼ tsp	salt, or to taste	1 mL
2 tbsp	unsweetened shredded coconut	30 mL

1. In a pot, bring coconut milk and soy milk just to a boil over medium-high heat. Watch carefully, because once the liquid reaches the boiling point, it will boil over.

2. Stir in rice and salt. Reduce heat to low, cover and cook for 30 to 40 minutes or until liquid is absorbed and rice is tender.

3. Fluff with a fork and stir in coconut. Serve immediately.

IF FOLLOWING A LOW-FIBER DIET AND AVOIDING DIFFICULT-TO-DIGEST FOODS...

Omit the shredded coconut.

The Facts About Rice

Next to wheat, rice is the largest food crop in the world. There are over 40,000 varieties of rice. The food industry classifies rices according to whether they are short-, medium- or long-grain. In addition, specialty rices such as jasmine, basmati and Arborio are distinguished by such characteristics as aroma. Wild rice is not technically a rice at all; rather, it is a long-grain marsh grass.

Brown rice is more nutritious and flavorful than white rice, but it also has more fiber, which can make it difficult for some people with IBD to digest. If you are following a low-fiber diet, use white rice. Soft cooked white rice is one of the foods known to help thicken loose stool. If you are well and there is no medical reason for you to avoid fiber or difficult-to-digest foods, include brown rice and wild rice in your diet. Be sure to adjust cooking times if you substitute them for their more refined counterparts in recipes.

Looking for added flavor and color? Cook rice in vegetable or tomato juice! If using commercially prepared juice, you will also be adding potassium and sodium.

Levantine Rice

A perfect rice for entertaining, this slightly sweet yet savory pilaf can be enjoyed warm or at room temperature, and robustly accompanies just about anything you wish to serve with it.

¼ cup	olive oil	60 mL
¼ tsp	salt	1 mL
¼ tsp	freshly ground black pepper	1 mL
½ tsp	ground cinnamon	2 mL
2	onions, finely diced	2
1 cup	short-grain rice (preferably Arborio or Vialone Nano)	250 mL
½ tsp	granulated sugar	2 mL
2 tbsp	raisins	30 mL
1¾ cups	boiling water	425 mL
⅓ cup	toasted pine nuts	75 mL
	Few sprigs fresh parsley, chopped	

1. In a heavy-bottomed pot with a tight-fitting lid, heat oil over high heat for 30 seconds. Add salt, pepper and cinnamon and stir-fry for just under 1 minute, until cinnamon darkens. Add onions and stir-fry for 2 minutes until softened.

2. Add rice and stir-fry actively for 3 minutes, until all of it has been exposed to the oil and is heated through. Add sugar and raisins and stir to mix.

3. Immediately add boiling water (use ¼ cup/60 mL less water if you like rice al dente), and pull pot off heat as it sizzles and splutters for 30 seconds. Mix well and reduce heat to low. Cover pot tightly. Let simmer undisturbed for 20 minutes, then remove from heat; do not uncover, but let it rest for 10 minutes to temper. (For up to 30 or 40 minutes, it will stay warm and improve.)

4. When ready to serve, fluff the rice, folding from the bottom up to redistribute the onions that have risen to the top, and transfer to a serving dish. Garnish liberally with pine nuts and parsley.

IF FOLLOWING A LOW-FIBER DIET AND AVOIDING DIFFICULT-TO-DIGEST FOODS...

Omit the raisins and pine nuts, finely grind the black pepper, and finely chop the parsley (do not include stems).

Vegan choice

Lactose-free choice

MAKES 4 TO 6 SERVINGS

IBD Tips

- Olive oil is a high source of monounsaturated fat.
- Vialone Nano is an Italian white rice with short, plump grains. It has a high starch content and is often used in risottos, as it has a creamy consistency when cooked.

Nutrients Per Serving	
Calories	199
Fat	14 g
Fiber	3 g
Protein	4 g
Carbohydrate	17 g

MAKES 6 SERVINGS

IBD Tips

- Cottage cheese, Cheddar and added salt provide sodium.

- If you're trying to gain weight, choose full-fat sour cream, cottage cheese and Cheddar. Otherwise, select reduced-fat or fat-free dairy products.

- There are many varieties of mushrooms, including button, portobello, oyster and shiitake; all add great flavor to recipes. Store them in a paper bag in the fridge and wash just before using.

California Casserole

Here's a recipe that will satisfy even the pickiest vegetarians in your family. For added flavor, substitute vegetable broth for the water.

- *Preheat oven to 350°F (180°C)*
- *6-cup (1.5 L) baking dish, lightly greased*

2 cups	water	500 mL
¾ cup	long-grain white rice	175 mL
1 cup	light sour cream	250 mL
1 cup	shredded medium Cheddar cheese	250 mL
½ cup	lower-fat cottage cheese	125 mL
½ cup	chopped onion	125 mL
¼ cup	chopped mushrooms	60 mL
¼ cup	chopped green bell pepper	60 mL
½ tsp	salt	2 mL
¼ tsp	freshly ground black pepper	1 mL

1. In a large saucepan, bring water to a boil; add rice. Cover and cook on low for about 20 minutes or until rice is tender and water is absorbed. Let stand for 5 minutes.

2. Combine hot rice, sour cream, Cheddar and cottage cheese, onion, mushrooms, green pepper and seasonings. Pour into a lightly greased 6-cup (1.5 L) baking dish. Bake, uncovered, in preheated oven for about 25 minutes.

> **IF FOLLOWING A LOW-FIBER DIET AND AVOIDING DIFFICULT-TO-DIGEST FOODS...**
>
> Finely chop the onion, use canned mushrooms and finely chop or purée them, peel the green pepper, and finely grind the black pepper.

Nutrients Per Serving	
Calories	220
Fat	9 g
Fiber	1 g
Protein	10 g
Carbohydrate	23 g

Rice Cakes with Tomato Purée

- *Preheat oven to 425°F (220°C)*
- *Baking sheet, sprayed with vegetable spray*

Rice Cakes

4 cups	Basic Vegetable Stock (see recipe, page 171)	1 L
½ cup	wild rice	125 mL
½ cup	white rice	125 mL
1 tsp	minced garlic	5 mL
½ cup	shredded part-skim mozzarella cheese (about 2 oz/50 g)	125 mL
¼ cup	shredded Swiss cheese (about ½ oz/15 g)	60 mL
¼ cup	chopped green onions	60 mL
2 tbsp	freshly grated Parmesan cheese	30 mL
1 tsp	dried basil	5 mL
1	egg	1
2	egg whites	2

Sauce

½ cup	prepared tomato pasta sauce	125 mL
2 tbsp	2% milk	30 mL
¼ tsp	dried basil	1 mL

1. *Prepare the rice cakes:* In a saucepan, bring stock to a boil; stir in wild rice and white rice; cover, reduce heat to medium-low and cook 35 minutes or until rice is tender. Let rice cool slightly. Drain any excess liquid. Rinse with cold water.

2. In a bowl, stir together cooled rice, garlic, mozzarella, Swiss, green onions, Parmesan, basil, whole egg and egg whites until well mixed. Using a ¼-cup (60 mL) measure, form mixture into 10 patties.

3. Place on prepared baking sheet. Bake approximately 10 minutes per side until browned.

4. *Meanwhile, prepare the sauce:* In a small saucepan, heat tomato sauce, milk and basil. Serve with rice cakes.

IF FOLLOWING A LOW-FIBER DIET AND AVOIDING DIFFICULT-TO-DIGEST FOODS...

Omit the wild rice and use 1 cup (250 mL) white rice, finely chop the green onions, and choose a plain pasta sauce. If you decide to make your own tomato sauce, be sure to peel and seed the tomatoes (see page 169).

Vegetarian choice

Lower-fiber choice

Higher-protein choice

MAKES 10 CAKES (1 per serving)

Tips

- These cakes can also be sautéed in a nonstick skillet sprayed with vegetable spray.
- Prepare cakes up to 1 day in advance; keep refrigerated until ready to bake.

IBD Tips

- This recipe is surprisingly low in sodium per serving, considering it contains prepared pasta sauce, cheese and vegetable stock.
- To boost calories, choose full-fat cheeses and milk or cream.
- Although tomato pasta sauce is rich in potassium, the amount used with each rice cake is small.

Nutrients Per Serving	
Calories	114
Fat	3 g
Fiber	1 g
Protein	6 g
Carbohydrate	16 g

Simple Risotto

MAKES 6 SERVINGS

Tip

- While adding the chicken broth, be careful to stir gently so rice kernels do not break up and become mushy. As a timeline guide, when you add the first quantity of chicken broth, set a timer for 22 minutes.

IBD Tips

- Commercial chicken broth contains more sodium than homemade.

- If you are sensitive to lactose, you may still be able to tolerate Parmesan, as it has a relatively small amount of lactose.

- The alcohol content of wine evaporates with cooking.

There are many variations on risotto, a creamy Italian rice dish made with short-grain Arborio rice. Risotto can be served as a one-dish main course with the addition of seafood, meat or vegetables, or as a sophisticated side dish.

4 cups	chicken broth	1 L
¼ cup	finely chopped onion	60 mL
1 tbsp	olive oil	15 mL
1 cup	Arborio rice or other Italian short-grain rice	250 mL
¼ cup	dry white wine	60 mL
3 tbsp	freshly grated Parmesan cheese	45 mL
	Freshly ground black pepper	

1. In a large covered saucepan, bring chicken broth to a boil.

2. Meanwhile, in a large saucepan over medium heat, cook onion in oil for about 5 minutes or until tender but not browned, stirring frequently. Stir in rice; cook until all grains are coated, about 1 minute. Add wine and cook until almost evaporated. Add ½ cup (125 mL) of the hot chicken broth.

3. Cook, stirring gently with a wooden spoon, until almost all liquid has been absorbed. Continue adding chicken broth in ½-cup (125 mL) amounts until all broth has been used, stirring constantly. This technique will require about 22 minutes total cooking time. The rice will be creamy, moist and tender but firm. Remove from heat; stir in Parmesan cheese. Add freshly ground pepper to taste.

> **IF FOLLOWING A LOW-FIBER DIET AND AVOIDING DIFFICULT-TO-DIGEST FOODS...**
>
> Finely grind the black pepper (larger pieces can increase the risk of a food-related obstruction).

Nutrients Per Serving	
Calories	131
Fat	4 g
Fiber	1 g
Protein	6 g
Carbohydrate	18 g

Spinach Risotto

- *Preheat oven to 400°F (200°C)*
- *Ovenproof saucepan with heatproof handle (see tip, at right)*

2 tbsp	butter	30 mL
1 cup	diced onion	250 mL
1 cup	Arborio rice	250 mL
1 tbsp	minced garlic	15 mL
1	package (10 oz/300 g) frozen spinach, partially thawed (see tip, at right)	1
3 cups	vegetable stock	750 mL
3 tbsp	prepared sun-dried tomato pesto	45 mL
	Freshly grated Parmesan cheese	

1. In an ovenproof saucepan, melt butter over medium heat. Add onion and cook until softened, about 3 minutes. Add rice and garlic; cook, stirring, until the grains of rice are coated with butter, about 1 minute. Add spinach and cook, breaking up with a spoon, until thoroughly integrated into the rice, about 2 minutes. Stir in stock and pesto. Bring to a boil.

2. Transfer saucepan to preheated oven and bake, stirring partway through, until rice has absorbed the liquid, about 30 minutes. Remove from oven and sprinkle Parmesan over top. Serve immediately.

IF FOLLOWING A LOW-FIBER DIET AND AVOIDING DIFFICULT-TO-DIGEST FOODS...

Finely dice the onion and use about 1 cup (250 mL) spinach purée, strained if possible, instead of the spinach.

Vegetarian choice

Higher-calorie choice

Source of potassium

MAKES 4 SERVINGS

Tips

- If you don't have a saucepan with an ovenproof handle, transfer the mixture to a deep 6-cup (1.5 L) baking dish after completing Step 1.

- To partially thaw the spinach for this recipe, place the package in a microwave and heat on High for 3 minutes. It can easily be separated using a fork but will still have some ice crystals. Do not drain before adding to rice.

IBD Tips

- Spinach is not typically found in a low-fiber diet, but puréeing it reduces the obstruction risk.

- Spinach is packed with nutrients and is worth including in your diet if you are well. If it's been awhile since you've eaten it, start with a small amount of cooked chopped spinach. Cooked spinach provides potassium.

Nutrients Per Serving	
Calories	222
Fat	8 g
Fiber	7 g
Protein	7 g
Carbohydrate	34 g

MAKES 8 SERVINGS

IBD Tips

- Risotto is known to help thicken loose stool
- Olive oil is a rich source of monounsaturated fat.
- Arborio rice is a round white rice popular in Italian dishes. It is known for its ability to absorb large quantities of liquid without becoming mushy.
- If you are sensitive to lactose, you may still be able to tolerate Parmesan, as it has a relatively small amount of lactose.
- Boost sodium by using commercial chicken broth.

Nutrients Per Serving	
Calories	138
Fat	3 g
Fiber	1 g
Protein	4 g
Carbohydrate	23 g

Baked Springtime Risotto

Here's another great oven-baked rice dish that cooks unsupervised while you spend time with your family preparing the rest of the meal.

- *Preheat oven to 350°F (180°C)*
- *12-cup (3 L) casserole dish with cover*
- *Baking sheet*

1 tbsp	olive oil	15 mL
1	small onion, diced	1
1	clove garlic, minced	1
1 cup	Arborio rice	250 mL
3 cups	hot chicken broth, divided	750 mL
½ tsp	salt (or to taste)	2 mL
10	thin spears asparagus, cut into short pieces	10
1	red bell pepper, cut into thin strips	1
¼ cup	freshly grated Parmesan cheese	60 mL
¼ cup	minced fresh parsley	60 mL
	Freshly ground black pepper	

1. In a medium saucepan, heat oil over medium heat. Sauté onion and garlic for 5 minutes or until softened. Add rice and cook, stirring, for about 1 minute or until evenly coated. Add 2 cups (500 mL) of the broth and salt; bring to a simmer. Transfer to casserole dish, cover and place on baking sheet.

2. Bake in preheated oven for 15 minutes. Remove from oven and stir in the remaining broth, asparagus and red pepper. Cover and bake for 15 minutes or until rice is al dente (tender to the bite) and most of the liquid is absorbed.

3. Ladle into serving bowls and sprinkle each serving with cheese, parsley and pepper to taste.

Variation

The first time you add broth, replace ½ cup (125 mL) of the chicken broth with an equal amount of dry white wine.

IF FOLLOWING A LOW-FIBER DIET AND AVOIDING DIFFICULT-TO-DIGEST FOODS...

Finely dice the onion, use canned asparagus tips, peel the red pepper, finely mince the parsley (do not include stems), and finely grind the black pepper.

Curried Squash Risotto with Apricots and Dates

Vegan choice

Higher-calorie choice

Lower-fat choice

Lactose-free choice

Source of potassium

True risotto requires that you add hot liquid in small amounts, stirring constantly until absorbed. Use this technique (if you have time) for a creamier texture. (Keep in mind that you'll also need to add a larger quantity of stock.)

1 tsp	vegetable oil	5 mL
2 tsp	minced garlic	10 mL
¾ cup	chopped onions	175 mL
1½ tsp	curry powder	7 mL
¾ cup	wild rice	175 mL
¾ cup	white rice	175 mL
3½ cups	Basic Vegetable Stock (see recipe, page 171)	875 mL
1 cup	diced butternut squash	250 mL
⅓ cup	chopped dried apricots	75 mL
⅓ cup	chopped dates	75 mL

1. In a nonstick saucepan sprayed with vegetable spray, heat oil over medium heat. Add garlic, onions and curry powder; cook 4 minutes or until softened. Add wild rice and white rice; cook, stirring, 2 minutes.

2. Add the stock; bring to a boil. Reduce heat to low, cover and cook 20 minutes. Stir in squash. Increase heat to medium; cover and cook another 10 minutes or until liquid is absorbed and rice and squash are tender.

3. Stir in apricots and dates. Let stand, covered, 10 minutes before serving.

IF FOLLOWING A LOW-FIBER DIET AND AVOIDING DIFFICULT-TO-DIGEST FOODS...

Finely chop the onions, omit the wild rice and use 1½ cups (375 mL) white rice, use soft ripe fresh apricots with skins removed instead of the dried apricots, and omit the dates.

MAKES 4 TO 6 SERVINGS

Tips

- Try replacing squash with diced sweet potatoes.
- Prepare up to 1 day in advance. Reheat gently.

IBD Tips

- Don't be afraid to use herbs and spices. Curry powder adds great flavor and should be avoided only if necessary during times of illness or when you're experiencing anal soreness from frequent loose stools.

- Butternut squash has a high beta carotene content. Precut butternut squash, often available fresh or frozen, is a great help when your energy is down.

- Olive oil and canola oil are heart-healthy choices.

- Butternut squash, dried apricots and dates are all rich in potassium.

Nutrients Per Serving	
Calories	223
Fat	1 g
Fiber	3 g
Protein	6 g
Carbohydrate	49 g

MAKES 4 TO 6 SERVINGS

Tips

- If the handle of your skillet is not ovenproof, wrap it in aluminum foil.
- For best results, stir the risotto partway through cooking. This prevents the grains on top from drying out.

IBD Tips

- Sausage may contain hidden sources of lactose; read the ingredient list.
- If you don't like spicy Italian sausage, substitute turkey kielbasa; it is milder and lower in fat.
- Sausage, added salt and commercial chicken stock provide sodium.

Nutrients Per Serving	
Calories	357
Fat	20 g
Fiber	1 g
Protein	6 g
Carbohydrate	25 g

Sausage and Red Pepper Risotto

Although this recipe has a fairly long cooking time, it is actually convenient as it eliminates the constant stirring usually associated with cooking risotto.

- *Preheat oven to 350°F (180°C)*
- *Ovenproof saucepan with heatproof handle (see tip, at left)*

1 tbsp	vegetable oil	15 mL
1 lb	Italian sausage, removed from casings	500 g
1 cup	diced onion	250 mL
1 tbsp	minced garlic	15 mL
1/2 tsp	salt	2 mL
	Freshly ground black pepper	
1 1/2 cups	Arborio rice	375 mL
3 cups	chicken stock	750 mL
1/2 cup	white wine or water	125 mL
2	roasted red bell peppers, chopped	2

1. In an ovenproof saucepan, heat oil over medium heat. Add sausage and cook, breaking up with a wooden spoon, until lightly browned and no longer pink inside, about 5 minutes. Using a slotted spoon, transfer to a bowl and keep warm. Drain off all but 1 tbsp (15 mL) fat.

2. Add onion to pan and cook, stirring, until softened, about 3 minutes. Add garlic, salt and black pepper to taste. Cook, stirring, for 1 minute. Add rice and cook, stirring, until all the grains are coated with oil.

3. Add stock and wine. Bring to a boil. Stir in roasted red peppers and reserved sausage meat. Bake in preheated oven, stirring partway through cooking, until rice has absorbed liquid, about 30 minutes.

> **IF FOLLOWING A LOW-FIBER DIET AND AVOIDING DIFFICULT-TO-DIGEST FOODS...**
>
> Remove any casing from the sausage, finely dice the onion, finely grind the black pepper, and peel the roasted red peppers.

Barley Risotto with Grilled Peppers

- *Preheat broiler*
- *Baking sheet*

1	red bell pepper	1
1	yellow bell pepper	1
3½ to 4 cups	vegetable or chicken stock	875 mL to 1 L
1 cup	pearl barley	250 mL
1 cup	chopped onions	250 mL
2 tsp	minced garlic	10 mL
3 tbsp	freshly grated low-fat Parmesan cheese	45 mL
¼ tsp	freshly ground black pepper	1 mL

1. Place red pepper and yellow pepper on baking sheet. Cook under preheated broiler, turning occasionally, for 20 minutes or until charred on all sides; remove from oven. When cool enough to handle, peel, stem and core peppers. Cut into chunks; set aside.

2. In a saucepan over medium-high heat, combine 2 cups (500 mL) stock with barley. Bring to a boil; reduce heat to low. Cook, stirring occasionally, for 30 minutes or until tender but firm. Set aside.

3. In a large nonstick frying pan sprayed with vegetable spray, cook onions and garlic over medium-high heat for 4 minutes or until softened. Add 1½ cups (375 mL) remaining stock; bring to a boil. Add cooked barley and roasted peppers; bring to a boil, stirring often. Reduce heat to medium-low; cook, stirring often, for 10 minutes or until barley is creamy. Add extra stock as needed. Add Parmesan cheese and pepper. Serve immediately.

IF FOLLOWING A LOW-FIBER DIET AND AVOIDING DIFFICULT-TO-DIGEST FOODS...

Finely chop the onions, and finely grind the black pepper. Consume only a small portion to limit the amount of fiber provided by the barley.

Vegetarian choice

Higher-calorie choice

Lower-fat choice

Higher-protein choice

Source of soluble fiber

MAKES 4 SERVINGS

Tip

- To ensure that you always have some roasted peppers on hand, prepare them in large batches. When cool enough to handle, remove the skin and seeds, slice the peppers, and freeze them in airtight containers. When needed, they defrost quickly.

IBD Tips

- This recipe provides sodium and a good dose of fiber. When targeting soluble fiber in your diet, it is wise to introduce small amounts and gradually increase to avoid the potential side effects of gas and bloating.

- If you're trying to gain weight, select full-fat Parmesan cheese.

Nutrients Per Serving	
Calories	253
Fat	4 g
Fiber	10 g
Protein	10 g
Carbohydrate	47 g

Barley with Sautéed Vegetables and Feta Cheese

MAKES 5 TO 6 SERVINGS

Tip

- Make early in day and refrigerate; reheat on low to serve. Also delicious at room temperature.

IBD Tips

- Barley is a great substitute for rice as a side dish and is an excellent source of soluble fiber. Be sure to cook it until it is soft rather than chewy if you are concerned about digestion or obstruction.

- Choose canola oil or olive oil for their favorable fatty acid profiles. Canola oil is a plant source of omega-3 fat, and olive oil is a high source of monounsaturated fat.

- Feta cheese is a source of sodium.

- Tomatoes are rich in potassium.

Although barley is rarely used this way, this dish proves how wonderful it is with tomatoes and feta cheese.

1 tbsp	vegetable oil	15 mL
2 tsp	crushed garlic	10 mL
¾ cup	chopped green bell pepper	175 mL
¾ cup	chopped mushrooms	175 mL
¾ cup	pot barley	175 mL
1½ cups	crushed canned tomatoes	375 mL
3 cups	chicken stock	750 mL
1½ tsp	dried basil (or 2 tbsp/30 mL chopped fresh)	7 mL
½ tsp	dried oregano	2 mL
3 oz	feta cheese, crumbled	90 g

1. In large nonstick saucepan, heat oil; sauté garlic, green pepper and mushrooms until softened, approximately 5 minutes. Add barley and sauté for 2 minutes, stirring constantly.

2. Add tomatoes, stock, basil and oregano; cover and simmer for approximately 30 minutes or until barley is tender. Pour into serving dish and sprinkle with cheese.

> **IF FOLLOWING A LOW-FIBER DIET AND AVOIDING DIFFICULT-TO-DIGEST FOODS...**
>
> Peel and finely chop the green pepper, use canned mushrooms and finely chop or purée them, and peel and seed an equivalent amount of fresh tomatoes (see page 169), then crush them yourself.

Nutrients Per Serving	
Calories	185
Fat	6 g
Fiber	4 g
Protein	8 g
Carbohydrate	25 g

Desserts

Desserts can be included in a healthy diet and are a tasty way to end a meal. They are usually associated with high-calorie and high-fat foods, and while these can be helpful when you are trying to gain weight, most people should aim to eat occasional small portions. Instead, select lower-calorie, lower-fat choices that are packed with vitamins and minerals — fruit, for example. Desserts are a great way to add fruit to your diet. Fruit salads or fruit kabobs with a dipping sauce of vanilla pudding or yogurt are fresh and tasty, and can work for those on a low-fiber diet. Let seasonal fruit guide your choices. Other options that will satisfy your sweet tooth without expanding your waistline include frozen yogurt, applesauce, biscotti, low-fat pudding and angel food cake.

And now for some really good news: many ingredients traditionally used in desserts, including bananas, oats, oat bran, tapioca pudding, applesauce, soft cooked white rice, smooth peanut butter, cheese, marshmallows and gelatin, are known to help thicken loose stool. So you can have your cake and eat it too!

Enjoy Chocolate in Moderation

Many individuals with IBD ask if they can still eat chocolate, and the answer is yes! Chocolate is a plant food made from the bean of a South American tree, and like other plant foods it contains phytochemicals such as antioxidants. Unfortunately, the more processed it is, the less phytochemicals it contains. Darker chocolate contains the most flavonoids, so be sure to look for dark chocolate with a high cocoa content.

The key is to enjoy small amounts in moderation, as even dark chocolate is high in fat. Commercial chocolate is processed and includes ingredients such as cocoa butter (fat), cocoa powder, sugar and milk. (White chocolate is not really chocolate at all; it is just cocoa fat, sugar and flavorings.) Remember, too, that chocolate contains some caffeine; for sensitive individuals, this may be enough to stimulate cramping or more frequent bowel movements.

If you are following a low-fiber diet, choose chocolate without dried or candied fruits, coconut or nuts. Chocolate that contains caramel, wafers, biscuits, smooth peanut butter or marshmallow is fine.

> Many dessert foods make great snacks at any time of the day.

> Frozen desserts made from soy taste great! There is a wide array of products available, including dessert bars, sandwiches and frozen cones.

Butter vs. Margarine

Butter and margarine are both fats. Butter is flavorful in baked goods, but it is high in saturated fat, which your liver uses to make cholesterol. Therefore, it should be used occasionally and in small amounts. Margarine is higher in monounsaturated and polyunsaturated fats and lower in saturated fat. Select non-hydrogenated margarine, as it is lower in trans fats and is considered a healthier heart choice.

Be Wary of "Portion Distortion"

In North America, the food industry pushes value marketing, which encourages consumers to purchase larger portions for just a little more money. The goal is to make you feel like you are getting more for your money while industry profits increase. It leads us to eat bigger portions of less healthy food and contributes to weight gain. To combat this, order smaller sizes, share with a friend, choose single rather than double serving sizes and eat slowly. Stop eating when you are comfortably full, rather than feeling like you have to finish what's on your plate. Enjoy the leftovers — even dessert leftovers — another day. Be sure to include snacks between meals if you are likely to get very hungry and overeat at mealtime.

KEEP YOUR BAKED GOODS TENDER

You will create a tougher batter by stirring too much (overmixing). Start by combining all the dry ingredients in your recipe, then add the liquids, mixing only until they are evenly blended.

Cinnamon Baked Pears

- *Preheat oven to 350°F (180°C)*
- *Baking dish*

4	pears	4
½ cup	blueberries	125 mL
½ cup	water	125 mL
2 tbsp	packed brown sugar	30 mL
1 tbsp	freshly squeezed lemon juice	15 mL
¼ tsp	ground cinnamon	1 mL

Yogurt Sauce

½ cup	lower-fat plain yogurt	125 mL
1 tbsp	packed brown sugar	15 mL
½ tsp	ground cinnamon	2 mL
½ tsp	vanilla	2 mL

1. Peel pears and cut in half lengthwise; scoop out core. Place cut side down in shallow baking dish. Sprinkle blueberries around pears.

2. Combine water, brown sugar, lemon juice and cinnamon; pour over pears. Bake, covered, in preheated oven for about 45 minutes or until pears are tender, basting occasionally with pan juices.

3. *Prepare the yogurt sauce:* In a small bowl, combine yogurt, brown sugar, cinnamon and vanilla. Serve pears with pan juices; spoon a dollop of yogurt sauce over cooked pear halves.

IF FOLLOWING A LOW-FIBER DIET AND AVOIDING DIFFICULT-TO-DIGEST FOODS...

Omit the blueberries.

MAKES 4 SERVINGS

Tip

- Most pears are shipped before they are fully ripe in order to avoid damage. If your pears are overly firm, store them in a cool place to ripen before using in this recipe.

IBD Tips

- Some fruits, such as pears, contain higher amounts of fructose, which may contribute to diarrhea if large amounts are eaten. This recipe uses 4 pears divided into 4 servings, so it shouldn't be a problem.

- Poached fruit is one way to eat a lower-fat dessert while also getting vitamins and minerals. Sometimes a light, fresh taste is just what you want!

- Boost calories in this recipe by preparing the sauce with full-fat yogurt.

Nutrients Per Serving	
Calories	167
Fat	1 g
Fiber	3 g
Protein	2 g
Carbohydrate	40 g

MAKES 8 SERVINGS

Tip

• You can make these tarts up to 2 days before you plan to serve them. Cover each ramekin with plastic wrap and refrigerate. Remove from refrigerator 30 minutes before serving.

IBD Tips

• This recipe is suitable for vegetarians who eat dairy and eggs.

• Almonds are a good source of calcium and, together with condensed milk, boost calories and protein in this recipe.

• Pumpkin provides the bulk of the potassium in this recipe, but almonds and condensed milk contribute as well.

• Ginger aids digestion and, for some, may improve appetite and reduce nausea.

Pumpkin Pie Tarts with Ground Almond Crust

These tarts give you all the flavor of pumpkin pie without the heavy pastry crust.

• *Preheat oven to 400°F (200°C)*
• *Eight ¹/₂-cup (125 mL) heatproof ramekins, greased*
• *2 baking sheets*

¹/₂ cup	ground almonds	125 mL
2	eggs, beaten	2
1¹/₄ cups	canned pumpkin purée (not pie filling)	300 mL
¹/₂ cup	sweetened condensed milk	125 mL
1 tsp	ground cinnamon	5 mL
¹/₂ tsp	ground ginger	2 mL
¹/₄ tsp	ground cloves	1 mL
¹/₄ tsp	ground nutmeg	1 mL

1. Place 4 ramekins on each baking sheet. Divide ground almonds among prepared ramekins.

2. In a medium bowl, whisk together eggs, pumpkin, milk, cinnamon, ginger, cloves and nutmeg until well blended. Divide evenly among ramekins.

3. Bake in preheated oven for 10 minutes. Reduce oven temperature to 350°F (180°C) and bake for 12 to 15 minutes or until mostly set (the middle of the tarts should still jiggle slightly). Let cool completely in ramekins on a wire rack.

Variation

Use ground pecans instead of almonds.

IF FOLLOWING A LOW-FIBER DIET AND AVOIDING DIFFICULT-TO-DIGEST FOODS...

Make sure the almonds are finely ground.

Pumpkin

Bright orange vegetables like pumpkin are an excellent way to increase antioxidants, such as beta carotene, and boost potassium. Canned pumpkin purée is convenient and can be kept in your pantry for whenever you wish to make a pumpkin recipe.

Nutrients Per Serving	
Calories	121
Fat	6 g
Fiber	1 g
Protein	5 g
Carbohydrate	14 g

Buttermilk Oat-Banana Cake

- *Preheat oven to 350°F (180°C)*
- *8-inch (20 cm) square baking pan, lightly greased and floured*

1 cup	buttermilk	250 mL
2/3 cup	rolled oats	150 mL
1/3 cup	oat bran or wheat bran	75 mL
1/4 cup	butter or margarine	60 mL
1 cup	granulated sugar	250 mL
1	egg	1
1 tsp	vanilla	5 mL
2	ripe bananas, mashed	2
1 1/2 cups	all-purpose flour	375 mL
1 tsp	baking soda	5 mL
1 tsp	baking powder	5 mL

Glaze

1/2 cup	granulated sugar	125 mL
1/2 cup	buttermilk	125 mL
1/4 cup	butter or margarine	60 mL
1/2 tsp	baking soda	2 mL

1. In a small bowl, pour buttermilk over rolled oats and oat bran. Let stand for 10 minutes.

2. In a medium bowl, cream butter and sugar. Beat in egg and vanilla. Combine bananas and buttermilk mixture with creamed ingredients. Sift together flour, baking soda and baking powder. Stir dry ingredients into banana mixture; blend well.

3. Pour batter into prepared pan. Bake in preheated oven for 45 minutes or until tester inserted in center comes out clean. Let stand for 5 minutes.

4. *Prepare the glaze:* In a small saucepan over medium heat, combine ingredients; bring just to a boil. (Watch closely; mixture will foam.)

5. Poke holes with tester (a metal skewer or a wooden toothpick) all over cake surface; pour glaze over cake while still warm. Cool cake before cutting.

IF FOLLOWING A LOW-FIBER DIET AND AVOIDING DIFFICULT-TO-DIGEST FOODS...

Avoid the wheat bran.

MAKES 12 SERVINGS

Tip

- This recipe is a great way to use over-ripe bananas. If you can't use bananas that are becoming ripe, pop them into a resealable plastic bag and freeze them. They will turn black, but once they are thawed and the skins are removed, they will be perfect for this recipe.

IBD Tips

- This recipe packs three foods known to help thicken loose stool: oats, oat bran and bananas!

- Buttermilk is made commercially by adding bacterial culture to milk. To make your own, add 2 tsp (10 mL) vinegar or lemon juice to 1 cup (250 mL) milk.

- Bananas provide the potassium in this recipe.

Nutrients Per Serving	
Calories	277
Fat	9 g
Fiber	1 g
Protein	4 g
Carbohydrate	46 g

Vegetarian choice

Higher-calorie choice

Lower-fat choice

Lower-fiber choice

Chocolate Marble Vanilla Cheesecake

- *Preheat oven to 350°F (180°C)*
- *9-inch (23 cm) springform pan sprayed with vegetable spray*

MAKES 20 SERVINGS

Tips

- This recipe can be cut in half, but use only 2 tbsp (30 mL) flour. Bake for 35 minutes, or until slightly loose at the center.

- For a mocha flavor, dissolve 2 tsp (10 mL) instant coffee in same amount of water and add to batter.

- When using margarine, choose a soft (non-hydrogenated) version to limit consumption of trans fats.

- Prepare up to 2 days ahead. Freeze for up to 6 weeks.

IBD Tips

- This recipe is appropriate for a low-fiber diet.

- Cheese and cheesecake are known to help thicken stool.

- To boost calories in this recipe, select full-fat ricotta, cottage cheese and sour cream.

Crust

2 cups	chocolate wafer crumbs	500 mL
3 tbsp	water	45 mL
1½ tbsp	margarine or butter, melted	20 mL

Filling

2 cups	ricotta cheese	500 mL
2 cups	2% cottage cheese	500 mL
1¾ cups	granulated sugar	425 mL
2	large eggs	2
⅓ cup	all-purpose flour	75 mL
⅔ cup	light sour cream	150 mL
2 tsp	vanilla	10 mL
2 oz	semi-sweet chocolate	50 g
2 tbsp	water	30 mL

1. *Prepare the crust:* In bowl, combine crumbs, water and margarine; mix well. Press onto sides and bottom of springform pan; refrigerate.

2. *Prepare the filling:* In food processor, combine ricotta and cottage cheeses, sugar and eggs; process until completely smooth. Add flour, sour cream and vanilla; process until well combined. Pour into pan. Melt chocolate with water and stir until smooth. Spoon onto cake in several places and swirl through lightly with a knife. Bake for 65 minutes or until set around edge but still slightly loose in center. Let cool; refrigerate until well chilled.

Chocolate

The health benefits of chocolate are related to the flavonol content (phytochemicals from the cocoa bean). The processing of cocoa affects the amount of flavonols, and it's difficult to know the flavonol content of a particular chocolate, even if it's labeled "dark chocolate" or "70% cacao." Chocolate boosts calories but also provides high amounts of saturated fat. In larger amounts, it can contribute to loose frequent stool.

Nutrients Per Serving

Calories	215
Fat	5 g
Fiber	1 g
Protein	7 g
Carbohydrate	31 g

The Original Dad's Cookie

- *Preheat oven to 300°F (150°C)*
- *Baking sheet, ungreased*

1 cup	all-purpose flour	250 mL
¾ cup	oat bran	175 mL
1 cup	quick-cooking oats	250 mL
1 tsp	baking powder	5 mL
1 tsp	baking soda	5 mL
1½ tsp	ground cinnamon	7 mL
1 tsp	ground nutmeg	5 mL
1 tsp	ground allspice	5 mL
1 cup	butter or margarine, softened	250 mL
¼ cup	lightly packed brown sugar	60 mL
¾ cup	granulated sugar	175 mL
2 tbsp	molasses	30 mL
1	egg	1
1 tsp	vanilla	5 mL

1. In a medium bowl, mix together flour, oat bran, oats, baking powder, baking soda, cinnamon, nutmeg and allspice.

2. In a large bowl, beat butter or margarine and sugars until smooth. Beat in molasses, egg and vanilla until well blended. Add flour mixture and mix well.

3. Shape dough into 1-inch (2.5 cm) balls and place about 2 inches (5 cm) apart on baking sheet. Using the tines of a fork dipped in flour, flatten. Bake in preheated oven for 15 minutes or until golden brown. Let cool on baking sheet for 2 to 3 minutes, then transfer to wire racks to cool completely.

Vegetarian choice

Lower-calorie choice

Lower-fiber choice

Source of potassium

MAKES ABOUT 5 DOZEN COOKIES (1 per serving)

IBD Tips

- This recipe is appropriate for a low-fiber diet.

- Oats and oat bran provide soluble fiber and help thicken loose stool. Because of this desirable effect, many low-fiber diets include oats and oat products despite their increased fiber content.

- Margarine and butter are both fats, but non-hydrogenated margarine is considered a healthier heart choice.

- If you select blackstrap molasses, it will provide additional calcium and iron. Molasses provides the potassium in this recipe.

- These cookies are perfect for a midday snack! Pack a couple in your knapsack or briefcase before leaving home.

- If you use margarine, this recipe is lactose-free.

Nutrients Per Serving	
Calories	64
Fat	3 g
Fiber	1 g
Protein	1 g
Carbohydrate	8 g

MAKES 2 DOZEN COOKIES (1 PER SERVING)

Tip

- Stone-ground flours give a grainier texture to cookies than refined flours. Look for them at health food or natural foods stores or well-stocked supermarkets.

IBD Tips

- This recipe is suitable for vegetarians who eat dairy and eggs.

- Brown sugar is granulated sugar with added molasses. Molasses does contribute some nutrients, but not enough to make a health difference in the amounts people typically consume.

- Chocolate chips may contain milk; however, the amount is usually small, a consideration only for severe cases of lactose intolerance.

- Chocolate provides the potassium in this recipe.

Nutrients Per Serving	
Calories	129
Fat	6 g
Fiber	2 g
Protein	2 g
Carbohydrate	18 g

Ancient Grains Chocolate Chip Cookies

This recipe uses two wonderful stone-ground ancient grains. Kamut and spelt are varieties of wheat and are not gluten-free, so if you live with celiac disease or non-celiac gluten sensitivity, they are not suitable for you.

- *Preheat oven to 350°F (180°C)*
- *Baking sheets, greased or lined with parchment paper*

½ cup	lightly packed brown sugar	125 mL
⅓ cup	non-hydrogenated margarine	75 mL
¼ cup	ground flaxseeds	60 mL
¼ cup	granulated sugar	60 mL
1	egg	1
1 tsp	vanilla extract	5 mL
¾ cup	stone-ground Kamut flour	175 mL
¾ cup	stone-ground spelt flour	175 mL
½ tsp	baking soda	2 mL
¼ tsp	salt	1 mL
1 cup	semisweet chocolate chips	250 mL

1. In a large bowl, using an electric mixer on high speed, cream brown sugar, margarine, flaxseeds and granulated sugar for 1 minute. Beat in egg and vanilla until blended. Add Kamut flour, spelt flour, baking soda and salt; mix until well blended. Stir in chocolate chips.

2. Drop by tablespoonfuls (15 mL) about 2 inches (5 cm) apart on prepared baking sheets. Bake in preheated oven for 12 to 15 minutes or until bottoms are lightly browned. Let cool on pans on a wire rack for 5 minutes, then transfer to rack to cool completely.

> **IF FOLLOWING A LOW-FIBER DIET AND AVOIDING DIFFICULT-TO-DIGEST FOODS...**
> Select finely ground versions of Kamut and spelt and make sure the flaxseeds are finely ground. Many individuals with IBD report that they can tolerate ground flaxseeds.

Peanut Butter Flaxseed Cookies

Although these cookies appear rich, they contain wholesome ingredients and beat traditional coffee-shop fare by a long shot!

- *Preheat oven to 350°F (180°C)*
- *Baking sheets, lightly greased or lined with parchment paper*

1¼ cups	all-purpose flour	300 mL
½ cup	ground flaxseed	125 mL
1 tsp	baking soda	5 mL
Pinch	salt	Pinch
½ cup	granulated sugar	125 mL
½ cup	packed brown sugar	125 mL
½ cup	butter, softened	125 mL
1	egg	1
1 tsp	vanilla	5 mL
½ cup	creamy peanut butter	125 mL

1. In a small bowl, combine flour, flaxseed, baking soda and salt.

2. In a large bowl, cream granulated sugar, brown sugar and butter. Beat in egg and vanilla. Beat in peanut butter until smooth. Fold in flour mixture.

3. Shape dough into balls, using about 1 tbsp (15 mL) dough per cookie, and place 2 inches (5 cm) apart on prepared baking sheets. Using a fork, flatten cookies in a crisscross pattern.

4. Bake in preheated oven for 8 to 10 minutes or until lightly browned. Let cool on baking sheets on a wire rack for 5 minutes, then remove to rack to cool completely.

MAKES 28 COOKIES (1 per serving)

IBD Tips

- These cookies are appropriate for a low-fiber diet.

- Peanut butter is known to help thicken stool. When choosing peanut butter, select one made from peanuts alone. You can always add salt yourself if you prefer the taste. Other brands of peanut butter, especially those that don't require refrigeration after opening, have been processed with sugar and trans fats and are less heart healthy.

- Per serving, these cookies are very low in lactose and are not likely to cause symptoms for many people with lactose intolerance.

- Ground flaxseed is a plant source of omega-3 fat, which has anti-inflammatory properties. Many individuals with IBD report that they can tolerate ground flaxseed.

Nutrients Per Serving	
Calories	118
Fat	7 g
Fiber	1 g
Protein	2 g
Carbohydrate	13 g

Vegetarian choice

Lower-calorie choice

Lower-fiber choice

Lactose-free choice

**MAKES ABOUT
1 DOZEN COOKIES
(1 per serving)**

Tip

- This recipe makes a smaller batch of cookies than usual, but it can be doubled, if desired.

IBD Tips

- Oats and oat bran provide soluble fiber and help thicken loose stool. Because of this desirable effect, many low-fiber diets include oats and oat products despite their increased fiber content.

- Rolled oats are the flat flakes obtained by steaming and rolling the hulled grains. Old-fashioned rolled oats take longer to cook than the finely cut quick-cooking oats.

Nutrients Per Serving	
Calories	72
Fat	3 g
Fiber	1 g
Protein	1 g
Carbohydrate	10 g

Oat Bran Raisin Cookies

- *Preheat oven to 350°F (180°C)*
- *Baking sheet, greased*

²⁄₃ cup	uncooked oat bran cereal	150 mL
¼ cup	old-fashioned rolled oats	60 mL
3 tbsp	all-purpose flour	45 mL
½ tsp	baking powder	2 mL
3 tbsp	margarine, softened	45 mL
¼ cup	firmly packed brown sugar	60 mL
1	egg white, lightly beaten	1
2 tsp	water	10 mL
¼ tsp	vanilla	1 mL
2 tbsp	raisins	30 mL

1. In a small bowl, mix together oat bran, rolled oats, flour and baking powder.

2. In a large bowl, beat together margarine and brown sugar until smooth and creamy. Stir in egg white, water and vanilla, mixing until thoroughly incorporated. Add flour mixture and mix well. Fold in raisins.

3. Drop by level tablespoonfuls (15 mL), about 2 inches (5 cm) apart, onto prepared baking sheet. Using a fork or the bottom of a glass, flatten slightly. Bake in preheated oven for 12 to 15 minutes or until bottoms are slightly browned. Cool on sheet for 3 minutes, then transfer to wire racks to cool completely.

IF FOLLOWING A LOW-FIBER DIET AND AVOIDING DIFFICULT-TO-DIGEST FOODS...

Omit the raisins.

Passover Almond Cookies

- Preheat oven to 300°F (150°C)
- Baking sheet, lightly greased

3	eggs	3
½ cup	granulated sugar	125 mL
1 tbsp	matzo meal	15 mL
2 tbsp	brandy	30 mL
2¼ cups	finely ground almonds or hazelnuts	550 mL
	Halved blanched almonds	

1. In a medium bowl, whisk eggs until light and fluffy. Add sugar and matzo meal and mix well. Stir in brandy. Fold in nuts until well combined.

2. Shape dough into 1-inch (2.5 cm) balls. Place about 2 inches (5 cm) apart on prepared baking sheet and gently press half a nut in the center of each. Bake in preheated oven for 20 minutes or until lightly browned. Immediately transfer to wire racks to cool.

IF FOLLOWING A LOW-FIBER DIET AND AVOIDING DIFFICULT-TO-DIGEST FOODS...

Omit the halved blanched almonds (the finely ground nuts are okay), and use matzo meal made with white flour.

Vegetarian choice

Lower-calorie choice

Lower-fiber choice

Lactose-free choice

Source of potassium

MAKES ABOUT 2½ DOZEN COOKIES (1 per serving)

IBD Tips

- Matzo is an unleavened bread made from wheat flour, water and sometimes salt. Matzo meal is made by grinding matzo into fine crumbs after baking. Unleavened bread products can help thicken loose stool.

- Nuts are high in unsaturated fat, which makes them a healthy high-calorie addition to a recipe.

- The brandy in this recipe is unlikely to cause problems for individuals with IBD, as the alcohol content evaporates with cooking.

- Nuts are a rich source of potassium.

Nutrients Per Serving	
Calories	66
Fat	4 g
Fiber	1 g
Protein	2 g
Carbohydrate	5 g

**MAKES
30 COOKIES
(1 PER SERVING)**

Tip

- Store the cooled cookies in an airtight container in the refrigerator for up to 5 days.

IBD Tips

- This recipe is gluten-free.
- To make this recipe lactose-free, substitute non-hydrogenated margarine or vegetable oil for the butter. This also reduces saturated fat and is a more heart-healthy choice.
- Don't be afraid to use spice to add flavor and appeal. Ground ginger, cinnamon and cloves are appropriate for a low-fiber diet.
- Molasses provides the potassium in this recipe. If you select blackstrap molasses, it will provide additional calcium and iron.

Nutrients Per Serving	
Calories	75
Fat	3 g
Fiber	1 g
Protein	1 g
Carbohydrate	12 g

Ginger Quinoa Crinkles

Turbinado sugar (sometimes called raw sugar) adds a sophisticated sparkle and crunch to these spicy favorites. The nutty-sweet flavor of quinoa flour boosts the deep flavor of the molasses and spices.

- *2 large baking sheets, lined with parchment paper*

1⅓ cups	quinoa flour	325 mL
2½ tsp	ground ginger	12 mL
2 tsp	baking soda	10 mL
1 tsp	ground cinnamon	5 mL
¼ tsp	ground cloves	1 mL
¼ tsp	fine sea salt	1 mL
⅔ cup	natural cane sugar or packed dark brown sugar	150 mL
⅓ cup	unsalted butter, softened	75 mL
1	egg	1
¼ cup	dark (cooking) molasses	60 mL
¾ cup	cooked quinoa, cooled	175 mL
3 tbsp	turbinado sugar	45 mL

1. In a small bowl, whisk together quinoa flour, ginger, baking soda, cinnamon, cloves and salt.

2. In a large bowl, using an electric mixer on medium speed, beat cane sugar and butter until light and fluffy. Beat in egg and molasses until blended. Using a wooden spoon, stir in quinoa. Stir in flour mixture until just blended. Cover and refrigerate for 1 hour.

3. Preheat oven to 350°F (180°C).

4. Roll dough into thirty 1-inch (2.5 cm) balls. Place turbinado sugar in a shallow dish and roll balls in sugar to coat. Place balls 2 inches (5 cm) apart on prepared baking sheets.

5. Bake, one sheet at a time, for 9 to 12 minutes or until puffed and set at the edges. Let cool on pan on a wire rack for 3 minutes, then transfer to the rack to cool.

> **IF FOLLOWING A LOW-FIBER DIET AND AVOIDING DIFFICULT-TO-DIGEST FOODS...**
>
> Omit the cooked quinoa and substitute additional quinoa flour or quinoa flakes. Depending on how quinoa is cooked, it can have a crunchy texture.

Peanut Butter Marshmallow Treats

- *Preheat oven to 325°F (160°C)*
- *13- by 9-inch (33 by 23 cm) cake pan, greased*

Base

1½ cups	packed brown sugar	375 mL
½ cup	butter, softened	125 mL
½ cup	peanut butter (smooth or crunchy)	125 mL
2	eggs	2
1 tsp	vanilla	5 mL
1½ cups	quick-cooking rolled oats	375 mL
1 cup	all-purpose flour	250 mL

Topping

3 cups	miniature marshmallows	750 mL

Frosting

¼ cup	smooth peanut butter	60 mL
¼ cup	butter or margarine, softened	60 mL
2 tbsp	milk	30 mL
1 tsp	vanilla	5 mL
1⅓ cups	confectioner's (icing) sugar, sifted	325 mL

1. *Prepare the base:* In a large bowl, beat brown sugar, butter and peanut butter until smooth. Beat in eggs, then vanilla, until blended. Blend in oats and flour. Press evenly into prepared pan. Bake in preheated oven for 25 to 30 minutes or until lightly browned around the edges.

2. *Prepare the topping:* Sprinkle marshmallows evenly over base. Bake 1 to 2 minutes longer or until marshmallows puff up slightly. Place pan on a wire rack to cool completely.

3. *Prepare the frosting:* In a small bowl, beat peanut butter, butter, milk and vanilla until smooth and creamy. Gradually add confectioner's sugar, beating until mixture is smooth and spreadable. Spread evenly over marshmallow layer, then cut into bars.

IF AVOIDING DIFFICULT-TO-DIGEST FOODS...

Use only smooth peanut butter.

Lower-fiber choice

MAKES 36 BARS (1 per serving)

IBD Tips

- This recipe packs three foods known to help thicken loose stool: smooth peanut butter, oats and marshmallows.

- Oats are one of the best sources of a soluble fiber called beta glucan. Despite the increased fiber content, many low-fiber diets include oats and oat products because they have the desirable effect of thickening, or "gelling," loose stool.

- Drizzle these bars with chocolate for added delight!

- Non-hydrogenated margarine is lower in trans fats and is considered a healthier heart choice.

Nutrients Per Serving	
Calories	159
Fat	7 g
Fiber	1 g
Protein	3 g
Carbohydrate	23 g

**MAKES 30 BARS
(1 per serving)**

Tip

- For the best texture, these bars are best eaten within 3 days. Store them in a cookie tin or another airtight container at room temperature.

IBD Tips

- This recipe is appropriate for a low-fiber diet.

- Soy margarine is used in place of butter or regular margarine as it does not contain whey, a dairy product. If you are not vegan, you can use butter and regular granulated sugar in this recipe.

- Zest is the outer skin, or peel, of a citrus fruit such as an orange or lemon. This is where the flavorful oils are found, but make sure you don't grate too deep, as the white membrane under the zest is bitter.

Nutrients Per Serving	
Calories	116
Fat	6 g
Fiber	Trace
Protein	1 g
Carbohydrate	15 g

Lemon Shortbread Bars

- *Preheat oven to 325°F (160°C)*
- *13- by 9-inch (33 by 23 cm) baking pan, ungreased*

2½ cups	all-purpose flour	625 mL
1 cup	granulated natural cane sugar	250 mL
1 cup	cold soy margarine	250 mL
2 tsp	finely grated lemon zest	10 mL
3 tbsp	freshly squeezed lemon juice	30 mL
1 to 2 tsp	water (optional)	5 to 10 mL
2 tbsp	confectioner's (icing) sugar, sifted	15 mL

1. In a large bowl, combine flour with sugar. Using two knives, a pastry blender or your fingers, cut in margarine until mixture resembles coarse crumbs. Add lemon zest and juice. Stir with a fork until dough comes together. If dough doesn't hold together, gradually add just enough water to make a dry dough.

2. Shape dough into a ball and press evenly into pan. Bake in preheated oven for 40 to 45 minutes or until a tester inserted in the center comes out clean. Remove from oven and immediately dust evenly with confectioner's sugar. Let cool in pan on a rack for 15 minutes. Cut into 2-inch by 1-inch (5 cm by 2.5 cm) bars.

Lemon Mousse

Lower-fat evaporated milk replaces whipping cream in this melt-in-your-mouth lemon mousse.

¼ cup	2% evaporated milk	60 mL
1 tsp	unflavored gelatin	5 mL
1½ tsp	grated lemon zest	7 mL
⅓ cup	freshly squeezed lemon juice	75 mL
	Yellow food coloring (optional)	
½ cup	granulated sugar	125 mL
⅓ cup	water	75 mL
2	egg whites	2
	Fresh berries	
	Mint leaves (optional)	

1. Pour evaporated milk into a small bowl; chill in freezer along with beaters.

2. In a small saucepan, sprinkle gelatin over lemon zest and juice; heat over low heat until dissolved. Add a few drops of food coloring, if desired. Cool.

3. In another small saucepan, cook sugar and water over high heat until candy thermometer reaches 234° to 240°F (112° to 116°C) or soft ball stage (syrup dropped into cold water forms soft ball).

4. In a bowl and using electric mixer, beat egg whites until soft peaks form; gradually pour in syrup, beating constantly. Beat until cool and very stiff. Fold in gelatin mixture.

5. Beat evaporated milk until soft peaks form; fold into egg white mixture. Pour into 5 dessert glasses. Refrigerate for 3 to 4 hours or until set. Serve topped with fresh berries, and mint leaves, if desired.

IF FOLLOWING A LOW-FIBER DIET AND AVOIDING DIFFICULT-TO-DIGEST FOODS...
Omit the fresh berries.

Lower-fat choice

Lower-fiber choice

MAKES 5 SERVINGS

Tip

- This delicious mousse uses an Italian meringue, which adds a hot sugar syrup to beaten egg whites. It is a little more work than regular meringue, but it's worth it.

IBD Tips

- Gelatin is known to help thicken loose stool.
- Boost calories in this recipe by using homogenized milk or cream.

Nutrients Per Serving	
Calories	101
Fat	Trace
Fiber	Trace
Protein	3 g
Carbohydrate	23 g

MAKES 6 TO 8 SERVINGS

IBD Tips

- Bananas are known to thicken loose stool. They also provide potassium in this recipe.

- This pudding makes a great high-calorie dessert or snack if you are trying to gain weight. The bananas provide a light taste that balances the richness of the cream.

Banana Cream Pudding

- 8-cup (2 L) glass bowl (as you would use for trifle)

⅔ cup	firmly packed brown sugar	150 mL
⅓ cup	all-purpose flour	75 mL
2 cups	milk	500 mL
2	egg yolks, beaten	2
2 tbsp	butter or margarine	30 mL
1 tsp	vanilla	5 mL
1 cup	whipping (35%) cream, whipped	250 mL
6	ripe but firm bananas, sliced	6
⅓ cup	chopped nuts (optional)	75 mL

1. In a medium saucepan, over medium heat, mix together brown sugar and flour. Stir in milk and, stirring constantly, cook until bubbly and thickened. Continue cooking for 1 minute longer, then remove from heat.

2. Take a cupful (250 mL) of the hot mixture and stir into the beaten egg yolks; return this mixture to the saucepan. Bring to a boil and boil gently for 3 minutes, stirring constantly. Remove from heat. Add the butter and vanilla and stir until blended and smooth. Set aside to cool, stirring occasionally. When at room temperature, fold in the whipped cream.

3. Spoon about one-third of the pudding into the glass bowl. Spread half of the sliced bananas over top. Repeat the layers and top with the remaining pudding. Sprinkle the chopped nuts over top, if desired, or add a few extra slices of banana for decoration, or both. Cover tightly with plastic wrap and chill in refrigerator for at least 1 hour or until ready to serve.

> **IF FOLLOWING A LOW-FIBER DIET AND AVOIDING DIFFICULT-TO-DIGEST FOODS...**
> Omit the chopped nuts.

Nutrients Per Serving	
Calories	329
Fat	15 g
Fiber	2 g
Protein	5 g
Carbohydrate	46 g

Raspberry Tapioca Pudding

1	package (10 oz/300 g) frozen sweetened raspberries, thawed	1
1	lemon peel strip (1 inch/2.5 cm)	1
1 cup	red grape juice	250 mL
1/3 cup	granulated sugar	75 mL
1/4 cup	quick-cooking tapioca	60 mL
1/2 cup	whipping (35%) cream	125 mL
2 tbsp	confectioner's (icing) sugar, sifted	30 mL

1. Pour raspberries into a strainer and reserve the juice, but throw away the seeds. Add enough water to the juice to make it 2 cups (500 mL). Pour into a large saucepan. Add lemon peel, grape juice and sugar. Bring to a boil over medium heat, then reduce heat to low and simmer, uncovered, for 10 minutes.

2. Remove the lemon peel and add the tapioca. Cook, stirring constantly, for 10 minutes. Spoon into 6 individual serving dishes, cover each tightly with plastic wrap and chill in refrigerator for 4 to 5 hours, or until set.

3. In a small mixer bowl, on high speed, beat whipping cream and confectioner's sugar until soft peaks form. Spoon over puddings.

Vegetarian choice

Higher-calorie choice

Lower-fiber choice

MAKES 6 SERVINGS

IBD Tips

- This recipe is appropriate for a low-fiber diet, as the raspberry seeds are removed and only the juice is used. The recipe also calls for grape juice, but the amount per serving is minimal and therefore unlikely to cause intolerance symptoms even for sensitive individuals.

- Tapioca is known to help thicken loose stool. Tapioca comes from the starch of the manioc root (also known as cassava or yucca), a tuber vegetable grown in tropical and subtropical climates. Used to thicken many dishes, it is a bland food that absorbs the flavor of the ingredients it is added to, in this case raspberry and grape juice.

- The whipping cream makes this dessert a high-calorie choice for when you are trying to gain weight.

Nutrients Per Serving	
Calories	217
Fat	7 g
Fiber	2 g
Protein	1 g
Carbohydrate	39 g

MAKES 4 SERVINGS

Tips

- Milk, cream and sour cream are scalded when bubbles form around the edge of the pan.

- Top each dish with a dollop of whipped cream or sprinkle some granulated sugar and cinnamon on top.

IBD Tips

- This recipe is appropriate for a low-fiber diet.

- White rice is known to help thicken stool.

- Add a pinch of ground cinnamon or nutmeg for a more traditional flavor.

- To boost calories in this recipe, try higher-fat dairy products. While boosting fat in the diet is not a long-term healthy strategy, it is okay to help you achieve short-term weight gain goals, especially after times of illness.

Nutrients Per Serving	
Calories	219
Fat	8 g
Fiber	Trace
Protein	7 g
Carbohydrate	31 g

Hint of Orange Creamy Rice Pudding

- *Double boiler*

½	orange	½
2 cups	milk, scalded	500 mL
¼ cup	long-grain rice	60 mL
¼ cup	granulated sugar	60 mL
¼ tsp	salt	1 mL
1	egg yolk, lightly beaten	1
½ cup	light (5%) cream	125 mL
¼ tsp	vanilla	1 mL

1. Pare the orange half so that the peel is in one long continuous spiral.

2. In the top of a double boiler, over gently boiling water, combine orange peel, milk, rice, sugar and salt. Cook for about 15 minutes, stirring occasionally, until rice is tender. Remove the orange peel.

3. In a small bowl, whisk egg yolk and cream. Stir in a small amount of the hot mixture, then pour into hot mixture and blend thoroughly. Cover and continue cooking for 45 to 50 minutes, stirring several times, until mixture thickens. Remove from heat and stir in vanilla.

4. Spoon into 4 individual dessert dishes or glasses. Serve warm or chilled.

Maple Barley Pudding

Barley isn't a traditional dessert ingredient, but here, sweetened with maple syrup, it makes a delicious pudding. Leftovers make a delicious breakfast!

- Preheat oven to 350°F (180°C)
- 8-inch (20 cm) square glass baking dish, greased

2	eggs, beaten	2
1 tsp	ground cinnamon	5 mL
1 tsp	ground cardamom	5 mL
Pinch	salt	Pinch
1½ cups	2% milk	375 mL
½ cup	pure maple syrup	125 mL
1 tsp	vanilla extract	5 mL
2 cups	cooked pearl barley (see box, below), cooled	500 mL
½ cup	dried cherries	125 mL

1. In a large bowl, whisk together eggs, cinnamon, cardamom, salt, milk, maple syrup and vanilla. Stir in barley and cherries. Pour into prepared baking dish.
2. Bake in preheated oven for 55 minutes or until set. Serve warm or cold.

Variations

Use soy milk instead of milk for a lactose-free version.

When you are well and there is no medical reason to reduce fiber and avoid difficult-to-digest foods, try replacing the cherries with your favorite dried fruit, such as raisins, cranberries or blueberries.

IF FOLLOWING A LOW-FIBER DIET AND AVOIDING DIFFICULT-TO-DIGEST FOODS...

Omit the dried cherries. Low-fiber diets often include barley, despite its fiber content, because it provides soluble fiber, which has the desirable effect of thickening, or "gelling," loose stool.

How to Cook Pearl Barley

To make 2 cups (500 mL) cooked pearl barley, combine ⅔ cup (150 mL) barley and 2 cups (500 mL) water in a medium saucepan with a tight-fitting lid. Bring to a boil over high heat. Reduce heat to low, cover and simmer for 35 minutes or until liquid is absorbed. Fluff with a fork.

Vegetarian choice

Higher-calorie choice

Lower-fat choice

Source of soluble fiber

Source of potassium

MAKES 8 SERVINGS

IBD Tips

- This recipe is suitable for vegetarians who eat dairy and eggs.
- To decrease calories in this recipe, select lower-fat milk; to increase them, choose whole milk.
- Barley is a rich source of soluble fiber and also supplies potassium.
- Dried fruit, such as cherries, provides potassium and antioxidants.
- Cardamom is an aromatic spice, which may heighten your interest in eating and boost your flavor experience.

Nutrients Per Serving	
Calories	171
Fat	2 g
Fiber	3 g
Protein	4 g
Carbohydrate	34 g

Contributing Authors

Byron Ayanoglu
125 Best Vegetarian Recipes
Recipes from this book appear on pages 187, 249, 251, 267, 287 and 297.

Esther Brody
500 Best Cookies, Bars & Squares
Recipes from this book appear on pages 313, 316, 317 and 319.

Esther Brody
250 Best Cobblers, Custards, Cupcakes, Bread Puddings & More
Recipes from this book appear on pages 322, 323 and 324.

Johanna Burkhard
500 Best Comfort Food Recipes
A recipe from this book appears on page 219.

Johanna Burkhard and Barbara Allan
The Diabetes Prevention & Management Cookbook
A recipe from this book appears on page 230.

Andrew Chase and Nicole Young
The Blender Bible
Recipes from this book appear on pages 172 and 174.

Maxine Effenson Chuck and Beth Gurney
125 Best Vegan Recipes
Recipes from this book appear on pages 148, 149, 154, 255, 256, 258, 260, 261, 262, 263, 268, 283, 286, 291, 295, 296 and 320.

Tiffany Collins
200 Best Panini Recipes
A recipe from this book appears on page 210.

Tiffany Collins
300 Best Casserole Recipes
Recipes from this book appear on pages 116 and 203.

Pat Crocker
The Smoothies Bible
Recipes from this book appear on pages 161, 162, 163, 164 and 166.

Dietitians of Canada
Dietitians of Canada Cook!
Recipes from this book appear on pages 151, 186, 250, 254, 310, 314 and 325.

Dietitians of Canada
Dietitians of Canada Cook Great Food
Recipes from this book appear on pages 120, 125, 126, 127, 128, 132, 145, 153, 157, 173, 178, 182, 192, 194, 196, 197, 205, 208, 212, 214, 215, 217, 221, 225, 241, 253, 269, 272, 274, 275, 279, 280, 284, 289, 294, 298, 300, 309, 311 and 321.

Dietitians of Canada
Dietitians of Canada Simply Great Food
Recipes from this book appear on pages 117, 118, 122, 123, 129, 130, 133, 135, 140, 146, 150, 155, 156, 158, 159, 165, 175, 189, 202, 222, 227, 229, 252, 259, 264, 285, 288, 302 and 315.

Judith Finlayson
The Convenience Cook
Recipes from this book appear on pages 176, 188, 191, 204, 207, 209, 216, 220, 228, 234, 235, 242, 243, 248, 257, 270, 301 and 304.

Judith Finlayson
The Vegetarian Slow Cooker
A recipe from this book appears on page 177.

George Geary and Judith Finlayson
650 Best Food Processor Recipes
A recipe from this book appears on page 198.

Lynn Roblin, Nutrition Editor
500 Best Healthy Recipes
Recipes from this book appear on pages 147, 152, 171, 179, 180, 190, 195, 206, 213, 218, 226, 244, 271, 273, 276, 277, 278, 290, 293, 299, 303, 305, 306 and 312.

Susan Sampson
200 Best Canned Fish & Seafood Recipes
Recipes from this book appear on pages 193, 231, 232, 236, 237 and 238.

Camilla V. Saulsbury
150 Best Gluten-Free Muffin Recipes
Recipes from this book appear on pages 136 and 139.

Camilla V. Saulsbury
500 Best Quinoa Recipes
Recipes from this book appear on pages 119, 121, 134, 138, 160 and 318.

Carla Snyder and Meredith Deeds
300 Sensational Soups
A recipe from this book appears on page 181.

Donna Washburn and Heather Butt
Complete Gluten-Free Cookbook
Recipes from this book appear on pages 124, 211 and 292.

Index

Library and Archives Canada Cataloguing in Publication

Steinhart, Allan Hillary, 1959-, author
Crohn's & colitis diet guide / Dr. A. Hillary Steinhart, MD, MSc, FRCP(C), Division Head, Gastroenterology, Mount Sinai Hospital & Julie Cepo, BSc, BASc, RD. — Second edition.

Includes index.
ISBN 978-0-7788-0478-9 (pbk.)

1. Crohn's disease—Diet therapy. 2. Colitis—Diet therapy. 3. Crohn's disease—Diet therapy—Recipes. 4. Colitis—Diet therapy—Recipes. 5. Inflammatory bowel diseases. 6. Cookbooks. I. Cepo, Julie, author II. Title. III. Title: Crohn's and colitis diet guide.

RC862.E52S735 2014   616.3'440654   C2013-908435-5